Social determinants approaches to public health:

from concept to practice

Editors

Erik Blas, Johannes Sommerfeld and Anand Sivasankara Kurup

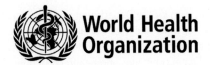

World Health Organization

For further information, please contact:

Department of Ethics, Equity, Trade, and Human Rights Health (ETH)
World Health Organization
20, Avenue Appia, CH-1211 Geneva 27, SWITZERLAND

http://www.who.int/social_determinants
e-mail: pphc@who.int

About this book

The thirteen case studies contained in this publication were commissioned by the research node of the Knowledge Network on Priority Public Health Conditions (PPHC-KN), a WHO-based interdepartmental working group associated with the WHO Commission on Social Determinants of Health. The publication is a joint product of the Department of Ethics, Equity, Trade and Human Rights (ETH), Special Programme for Research and Training in Tropical Diseases (TDR), Special Programme of Research, Development and Research Training in Human Reproduction (HRP), and Alliance for Health Policy and Systems Research (AHPSR). The case studies describe a wealth of experiences with implementing public health programmes that intend to address social determinants and to have a great impact on health equity. They also document the real-life challenges in implementing such programmes, including those in scaling up, managing policy changes, managing intersectoral processes, adjusting design and ensuring sustainability.

This publication complements the previous publication by the Department of Ethics, Equity, Trade and Human Rights entitled *Equity, social determinants and public health programmes*, which analysed social determinants and health equity issues in 13 public health programmes, and identified possible entry points for interventions to address those social determinants and inequities at the levels of socioeconomic context, exposure, vulnerability, health outcomes and health consequences.

Acknowledgements

The book is a joint initiative of the WHO Department of Ethics, Equity, Trade and Human Rights (ETH), Special Programme of Research, Development and Research Training in Human Reproduction (HRP), Special Programme for Research and Training in Tropical Diseases (TDR), and the Alliance for Health Policy and Systems Research (AHPSR).

The authors of the various chapters of the book are listed below:

Carlos Acosta-Saal, Ajmal Agha, Irene Agurto, Halida Hanum Akhter, Laura C. Altobelli, Erik Blas, Chris Bonell, Joanna Busza, Jia Cheng, Uche Ezeoke, Abigail Hatcher, James Hargreaves, Patrick Harris, Sara Javanparast, Heidi Bart Johnston, Kausar S Khan, Julia Kim, Kathi Avery Kinew, Jaap Koot, Amanda Meawasige, Romanus Mtung'e, Jane Miller, Linda Morison, Joel Negin, Elizabeth Oliveras, Obinna Onwujekwe, Benjamin Onwughalu, Godfrey Phetla, John Porter, Paul Pronyk, Lorena Rodriguez, Anna Schurmann, Evie Sopacua, Stephanie Sinclair, Johannes Sommerfeld, Siswanto Siswanto, Anand Sivasankara Kurup, Tony Lower, Jan Ritchie, Vicki Strange, Graham Tabi, Yeşim Tozan, Daniel Umeh, Benjamin Uzochukwu, James Ogola Wariero, Charlotte Watts, Su Xu, Isabel Zacarías, Shaokang Zhan and Chanjuan Zhuang.

The study design and implementation team consisted of Erik Blas, Johannes Sommerfeld, Sara Bennett, Shawn Malarcher and Anand Sivasankara Kurup. Bo Eriksson, Jens Aagaard-Hansen and Norman Hearst reviewed and provided inputs to the publication at different stages. Valuable inputs in terms of contributions, peer reviews and suggestions on various chapters were also received from a number of WHO staff at headquarters, regional offices and country offices, as well as other partners and collaborators. The editors would like to acknowledge specifically the contributions of Marco Ackerman, Anjana Bhushan, Davison Munodawafa, Benjamin Nganda, Sarah Simpson, Susan Watts, Erio Ziglio and Ramesh Shademani. The editorial team consisted of Erik Blas, Johannes Sommerfeld and Anand Sivasankara Kurup.

The text was copyedited by Bandana Malhotra and publication design and layout was done by Netra Shyam.

Foreword

The health of a population is measured by the level of health and how this health is distributed within the population. The WHO publication from early 2010, entitled *Equity, social determinants and public health programmes* analysed from the perspective of thirteen priority public health conditions their social determinants and explored possible entry points for addressing the avoidable and unfair inequities at the levels of socioeconomic context, exposure, vulnerability, health-care outcome and social consequences. However, the analysis needs to go beyond concepts to explore how the social determinants of health and equity can be addressed in the real world. This publication takes the discussion on social determinants of health and health equity to a practical level of how programmes have actually addressed the challenges faced during implementation.

Social determinants approaches to public health: from concept to practice is a joint publication of the Department of Ethics, Equity, Trade and Human Rights (ETH), Special Programme for Research and Training in Tropical Diseases (TDR), Special Programme of Research, Development and Research Training in Human Reproduction (HRP), and Alliance for Health Policy and Systems Research (AHPSR). The case studies presented in this volume cover public health programme implementation in widely varied settings, ranging from menstrual regulation in Bangladesh and suicide prevention in Canada to malaria control in Tanzania and prevention of chronic noncommunicable diseases in Vanuatu.

The book does not provide a one-size-fits-all blueprint for success; rather, it analyses from different perspectives and within different contexts programmatic approaches that led to success or to failure. The final chapter synthesizes these experiences and draws the combined lessons learned. These lessons include: the need for understanding equity as a key value in public health programming and for working not only across sectors but also across health conditions. This requires a combination of visionary technical and political leadership, an appreciation that long-term sustainability depends on integration and institutionalization, and that there are no quick fixes to public health challenges. Programmes must get out of their comfort zones and, in addition to applying traditional biomedical and programmatic tools, they have to learn to address the economic, social, cultural and political realities in which public health conditions and inequities exist.

A common lesson learned from all the analysed cases is to not wait to identify what went right or wrong until after the programme has elapsed or failed. Research is a necessary component of any implementation to routinely explore, gauge, and adjust strategies and approaches in a timely manner. We believe that this publication will inspire programme managers, policy-makers and researchers to work hand-in-hand to launch new and better public health programmes and to further strengthen existing ones.

Erik Blas   Johannes Sommerfeld   Anand Sivasankara Kurup

Acronyms and abbreviations

AHPSR	Alliance for Health Policy and Systems Research
AJK	Azad Kashmir
AKU	Aga Khan University
ALGON	Association of Local Governments of Nigeria
AMC	Assembly of Manitoba Chiefs
ANIS I	Anthropometric Nutritional Indicators Survey
ARI	acute respiratory infections
ASIST	applied suicide intervention skills training
AusAID	Australian Agency for International Development
BAPSA	Bangladesh Association for the Prevention of Septic Abortion
BCC	behaviour change communication
BWHC	Bangladesh Women's Health Coalition
CEPS	cultural, economic, political and social
CHEW	community health extension worker
CIE	communication, information and education
CLAS*	Local Health Administration Communities
CLTS	community-led total sanitation
CNCDs	chronic non-communicable diseases
CO	community organizer
CSDH	Commission on Social Determinants of Health
DFID	Department for International Development (UK)
DGFP	Directorate General of Family Planning
DHS	Demographic and Health Survey
DIRESA*	Regional Health Directorate
DPT3	diphtheria, pertussis and tetanus third dose
DSNC	District School Nutrition Committee
ERC	Research Ethics Review Committee
ERC	Expert Review Committee
FANA	federally administered northern areas
FATA	federally administered tribal areas
FGD	focus group discussion
FMOH	Federal Ministry of Health
FNIHB	First Nations and Inuit Health Branch

FW	field worker
FWV	family welfare visitor
GAVI	Global Alliance for Vaccines and Immunizations
HMIS	Health Management Information System
HNPSP	Health and Nutrition Population Sector Programme
HPSP	Health and Population Sector Programme
HRP	Special Programme of Research, Development and Research Training in Human Reproduction
IBRD	International Bank for Reconstruction and Development
ICC	Interagency Coordinating Committee
ICDDR,B	International Centre for Diarrhoeal Disease Research, Bangladesh
ICPD	International Conference on Population and Development
IDB	Inter-American Development Bank
IDRC	International Development Research Centre
IMAGE	Intervention with Microfinance for AIDS and Gender Equity
IMCI	Integrated Management of Childhood Illnesses
INAC	Indian and Northern Affairs
IPD	immunization plus days
IPV	intimate-partner violence
IRKs	insecticide retreatment kits
ITN	insecticide-treated nets
KINET	Kilombero Net Project
KYI	Keewatin Youth Initiative
LGA	local government area
LLIN	long-lasting insecticidal net
MCH	Maternal and Child Health
MDG	Millennium Development Goal
MEF	Ministry of Economy and Finance
MFI	microfinance initiative
MFN	Manitoba First Nations
MOE	Ministry of Education
MOH	Ministry of Health
MOHFW	Ministry of Health and Family Welfare
MOHSW	Ministry of Health and Social Welfare
MoWD	Ministry of Women and Development
MR	Menstrual Regulation
MRTSP	Menstrual Regulation Training and Services Programme

MSF	Medecins sans Frontieres
MVP	Millennium Villages Project
MVU	mobile video unit
NAB	National Accountability Bureau
NATNETS	National Insecticide Treated Nets programme
NAYSPS	National Aboriginal Youth Suicide Prevention Strategy
NCD	noncommunicable disease
NGO	nongovernmental organization
NIPORT	National Institute of Population Research and Training
NIU	National Implementation Unit
NMCP	National Malaria Control Programme
NPC	National Population Commission
NPHCDA	National Primary Health Care Development Agency
NPI	National Programme on Immunization
NWFP	North West Frontier Province
ORT	oral rehydration therapy
PAC*	Shared Administration Programme
PACFARM*	Shared Administration Programme for Pharmaceuticals
PAHP	Pacific Action for Health Project
PATH	Planning Alternative Tomorrows with Hope
PBM	Pakistan Baitul Maal
PHC	primary health care
PMI	President's Malaria Initiative
PPHC	Priority Public Health Conditions
PSBPT*	Basic Health for All Programme
PSI	Population Services International
PSL*	Local Health Plan
PSRL	Programmatic Social Reform Loan
RADAR	Rural AIDS & Development Action Research Programme
REC	Reaching Every Child
RED	Reach Every District
REW	Reach Every Ward
RHSTEP	Reproductive Health Services Training and Education Programme
SDH	social determinants of health
SEF	Small Enterprise Foundation
SEG*	Free School Insurance
SES	socioeconomic strata

SFL	Sisters-for-Life
SIA	supplemental immunization activity
Sida	Swedish International Development Cooperation Agency
SIS*	Integrated Health Insurance
SMI*	Maternal–Child Insurance
SMOH	State Ministries of Health
SNP	School Nutrition Project
STC	School Tawana Committee
TDR	Special Programme for Research and Training in Tropical Diseases
TFI	Task Force on Immunization
TNVS	Tanzanian National Voucher Scheme
TOT	training of trainers
UNDP	United Nations Development Programme
UNICEF	United Nations Children's Fund
USAID	United States Agency for International Development
VCT	voluntary counselling and testing
W/U	weighed/under-fives
WFP	World Food Programme
WHO	World Health Organization
WSP-EAP	Water and Sanitation Programme East Asia and Pacific
YAC	Youth Advisory Council
YSPI	Youth Suicide Prevention Initiative

---

* Spanish acronym

Contents

Introduction and methods of work

1

Erik Blas,[1] Anand Sivasankara Kurup,[1,*] and Johannes Sommerfeld[1,2]

[1] World Health Organization (WHO)
[2] Special Programme for Research and Training in Tropical Diseases (TDR)
* Corresponding author: sivasankarakurupa@who.int

1.1 Background

Achieving greater equity in health is a goal in itself, and achieving the various specific global health and development targets without ensuring equitable distribution across and within populations is of limited value (Blas and and Sivasankara Kurup, 2010). Although many public health programmes have achieved considerable success in reducing mortality and morbidity, they often fail to capitalize on interventions that address the social context and conditions in which people live, i.e. interventions that have a potential to contribute to greater health equity. Moreover, national-level statistics often mask unfair disparities within and between population groups in terms of health outcomes resulting from unequal access, extreme vulnerabilities and exposure to various risk factors. It has also been acknowledged that many key public health targets, including the health-related Millennium Development Goals (MDGs), are not easily attainable even if there is a massive scale-up of available technologies (Maher et al., 2007; Lönnroth et al., 2010). Often, even simple and effective tools, such as vaccines against childhood diseases, are unable to reach those most in need due to several social and structural factors (United Nations, 2010). This calls for a broader approach that addresses the social determinants to reduce inequities in programme performance and health outcomes through intersectoral action, community participation and empowerment of populations that are most vulnerable to health threats (Hasan et al., 2005).

Health equity has increasingly been on the agenda of the World Health Organization (WHO) in recent years. As part of a comprehensive effort to promote greater equity in global health, in a spirit of social justice, the Commission on Social Determinants of Health (CSDH) was convened by WHO to gather and review evidence on what needs to be done to reduce health inequities and provide guidance for Member States and WHO itself on how to reduce those avoidable, unfair and remediable differences in health outcomes between population groups both within and among countries (Lee, 2004). The CSDH submitted its report in 2008 with overarching recommendations to close the equity gap in a generation by improving daily living conditions, tackling inequitable distribution of power, money and resources, measuring and understanding the problem, and assessing the impact of action (CSDH, 2008). Apart from this, the *World health report* in 2008 placed health equity as the central value underpinning the renewal of primary health care (PHC) and called for priority public health programmes

to align with the associated principles and approaches (WHO, 2008). In May 2009, the World Health Assembly called upon the international community and urged WHO Member States to tackle health inequities within and across countries through political commitment to the main principles of "closing the gap in a generation". It emphasized the need to generate new, or make use of existing, methods and evidence, tailored to national contexts in order to address the social determinants and social gradients of health and health inequities. The Assembly requested the WHO Director-General to promote addressing of the social determinants of health to reduce health inequities as an objective of all areas of the Organization's work, especially priority public health programmes, and research on effective policies and interventions (World Health Assembly of the World Health Organization, 2009).

Effectively addressing inequities in health involves not only new sets of interventions, but modifications to the way that public health programmes are organized and operate, as well as redefinition of what constitutes a public health intervention (Blas and Sivasankara Kurup, 2010). The Priority Public Health Conditions Knowledge Network (PPHC-KN) (WHO, 2007), one of nine Knowledge Networks supporting the CSDH, was established as an interdepartmental working group involving 16 public health programmes of WHO. The PPHC-KN has helped to widen the discussion on what constitutes public health interventions by identifying inequities in the social determinants of health, and promoting appropriate interventions to address those inequities through public health programmes (Blas and Sivasankara Kurup, 2010).

To analyse issues related to social determinants and equity within public health programmes, the PPHC-KN developed and applied a five-level framework, informed by discussion papers prepared for the WHO Regional Office for Europe (Dahlgren and Whitehead, 2006; Diderichsen et al., 2001; and the comprehensive conceptual framework of the CSDH [Solar and Irwin, 2007]). The framework has five levels of analysis: socioeconomic context and position, differential exposure, differential vulnerability, differential health outcomes and differential consequences (Blas and Sivasankara Kurup, 2010). For each level, the analysis established and documented the social determinants at play and their contribution to inequity, for example, pathways, magnitude and social gradients in outcomes; promising entry points for intervention; potential adverse effects of eventual change; possible sources of resistance

Figure 1: Priority public health conditions analytical framework

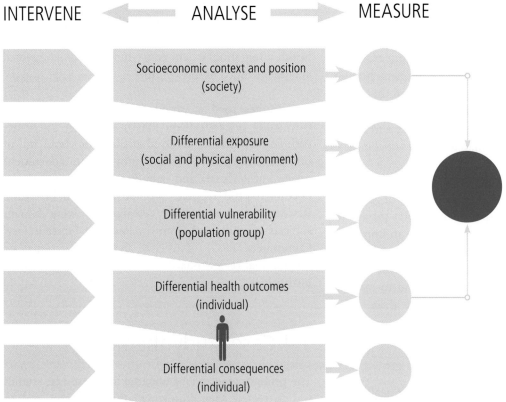

Source: Blas and Sivasankara Kurup, 2010, p. 7

to change; and what has been tried and what were the lessons learned.

As part of the WHO-led PPHC-KN, a research node was created and charged with substantiating, through empirical case study research, how specific public health programmes have addressed issues related to the social determinants of health and equity. This effort involved 13 institutions and more than 40 researchers. The current volume is a compilation and synthesis of these 13 case studies. The case studies examine the implementation challenges of addressing the social determinants of health, especially in low- and middle-income settings.

1.2 Rationale

To have meaning in public health, ideas and concepts need to be translated into concrete action, and interventions need to be implemented at the scale of populations. The transition from the drawing board, the experiment, or the pilot project into the real-life situation has challenged many a public health programme. This is particularly true when programmes address social determinants of health conditions and how health is distributed in a population. Programmes will inevitably have to deal with fundamental structures of societies, including who controls power and resources. One can appear to do *all the right things and still not get the right results*. It may be tempting to do a two-by-two matrix.

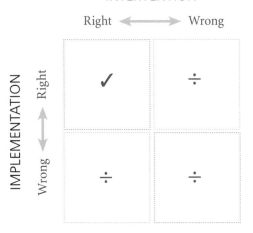

The matrix indicates that if we have the right interventions and implement them in the right way, we get the right results. While this is hard to dispute, when it comes to the real world, there may be no such thing as 100% right or wrong; instead, there may be a range of nuances and grey zones. There is a lot of learning to be done from examples where both the interventions and the implementation were right. However, these cases are rare, and there may be much more learning from cases where interventions and their implementation were almost right and where the results were almost there than from cases of complete perfection or failure.

A critical phase in most programmes is that of going to scale – moving from the experiment or pilot project to the full-scale intervention required to have an impact at the population level. Another critical phase is when the programme is to be sustained, for example, to be funded and institutionalized for the long term and to operate without the day-to-day involvement of those who conceived the project and worked in it. This transition process may also offer many insights and opportunities for learning.

Most research on the social determinants of health and equity has focused on possible causal relationships. The set of case studies presented here focused on programmatic issues concerning the organization of public health programmes and the process of implementation. In particular, the case studies document the challenges faced and how they were dealt with in practical local situations.

1.3 Process and methods

In order to commission case studies on a wide range of public health programmes and a representative set of countries, a call for letters of interest was issued jointly by the WHO Department of Ethics, Equity, Trade and Human Rights in collaboration with the Special Programme of Research, Development and Research Training in Human Reproduction (HRP), the Special Programme for Research and Training in Tropical Diseases (TDR), and the Alliance for Health Policy and Systems Research (AHPSR). The call attracted 70 letters of interest from all WHO Regions. All letters of interest were peer reviewed and scored on a set of pre-established selection criteria. Evaluation of the proposals included criteria such as the quality of the proposal, feasibility and potential to contribute new knowledge on implementing

programmes addressing the social determinants of health and health inequities. Mean scores were computed and the 14 highest-ranking projects were then selected to examine the implementation challenges faced by them in addressing the social determinants of health in public health programmes. Thirteen studies were completed and are included in this volume.

The studies used a variety of standard methods in case study research (Yin, 2003), including interviews with key informants involved at the policy level and in implementing the respective programmes, document review of official and unofficial statistics, project documents and reports, and the published literature. Review and clearance for research involving human subjects was obtained from the Research Ethics Review Committee (ERC) of WHO, and from national or institutional review boards of the participating research institutions.

1.4 Case study themes

The primary objective of undertaking these case studies was to review their implementation processes and to draw lessons that can be learned by others embarking on the difficult path to correct inequities in health by addressing the social determinants. The objective was thus not to evaluate the performance and outcomes of these programmes, but to understand how they addressed the challenges to implementation. Therefore, the case studies focused on the following five types of processes of implementation, and the learning and challenges thereof – going to scale, managing policy change, managing intersectoral processes, adjusting design and ensuring sustainability.

Going to scale

Many successful programmes are often conceived by visionaries, and carried forward by dedicated personnel, who understand the ideas, purposes and ideologies behind the programmes. However, while moving from small-scale pilot programmes to large interventions covering and benefiting a whole population, these programmes often face considerable challenges. The case studies documented the learning from such projects on the processes of moving from a small to a large scale, the challenges encountered on the way, how they overcame the challenges, and what were the barriers and facilitators.

Managing policy change

It is important to understand the challenges associated with policy formulation and change, particularly in relation to policies benefiting the poor and vulnerable, the influence of the political environment, the role of individuals as policy champions, and managing opposing professional views. The case studies documented how these processes were managed – from the initial evidence of the need for change to completion of the policy formulation process, e.g. in relation to shifting resources or power from one group to another. Several of the case studies also assessed the influence of the political environment, and the roles and effect on the process of individuals as policy champions.

Managing intersectoral processes

In order to create a comprehensive response to public health challenges, including addressing the social determinants of health and health inequities, managing intersectoral processes is a key challenge. It requires specific skills and methods that public health professionals often lack and, in the process, they often fail. Learning from managing the stewardship challenges in working with other sectors can guide new programmes.

Adjusting design

Any programme that aims to address inequity should adapt not only to the changing needs and priorities of the population that it proposes to address, but also to the programmatic challenges and opportunities experienced during implementation. Integral elements of managing programmes include designing and redesigning them according to experiences gained and making adjustments to the original design during implementation. The issues, reasons and sequence of various elements of such adjustments to the programme, and their effects on the design, were also documented through the case studies.

Ensuring sustainability

Considerations regarding financial and institutional sustainability have to be built into the programmes from the start. Different concepts of sustainability, the lessons learned and issues in securing ongoing financial support for the programme, as well as promoting institutional sustainability, are discussed in the case studies.

1.5 Summary

The individual case studies are presented in Chapters 2 to 14 of the volume, and a synthesis on the lessons learned is presented in Chapter 15.

Chapter 2. Bangladesh
Bangladesh's menstrual regulation programme

Collaborative work between donors, the government and NGOs increased the country's capacity to address an important element of equity in health, namely, increased access to safe abortion, and for women to be part of a decision that affects their health and lives. The case study documented the learning from a three-pronged approach involving the government, NGO and donor. This approach has been skillfully and successfully pursued in the menstrual regulation programme in Bangladesh for more than three decades.

Chapter 3. Canada
Manitoba First Nations suicide prevention programme

When the socially excluded try to do something about their situation, they are faced with a double burden: the exclusion itself, and being excluded from dealing with the exclusion. The Canada case study documents the learning from the Manitoba First Nations suicide prevention programme. It describes the effects of leadership, which have been nurtured and developed over time, both within disadvantaged population groups and through formation of strategic alliances with outsiders who are willing to lend some of their leadership capacity to the programme.

Chapter 4. Chile
Food and vegetable promotion and the 5-a-day programme

It is imperative to foster intersectoral action in order to ensure equity. Structural interventions need to be in place to address equity, with improved coordination between the ministries of Health, Education and Agriculture to increase consumption of healthy food and vegetables among the most vulnerable populations. The Chile experience of intersectoral collaboration and public–private partnerships for fruit and vegetable consumption to prevent noncommunicable diseases is an indicator that intragovernment leadership and commitment is necessary for multisectoral policy development, implementation and monitoring, and effective scaling up.

Chapter 5. China
Dedicated delivery centre for migrants in Minhang District, Shanghai

Lessons learned from the China case study suggest that a values-based project requires particular considerations to go to scale. Policy change requires innovative thinking, questioning of conventional wisdom, and diligently taking on both higher authorities and health professionals. In the practical implementation, priority-setting, technical approaches, values and staff, and institutional development had to be considered and addressed simultaneously. The case demonstrates that inequity in pregnancy outcomes between migrants and residents is avoidable, and that at least some among the public, authorities and within the health-care profession find them unfair.

Chapter 6. Indonesia
Reviving health posts as an entry point for community development: *Gerbangmas* movement in Lumajang district, Indonesia

The *Gerbangmas* movement in Lumajang district, Indonesia is an innovation within a decentralized health system. The policy change of the *Gerbangmas* initiative was an incremental process that took approximately five years. The *Gerbangmas* movement has encouraged multiple sectors to set programmes for community empowerment and to bring these together through a common indicator framework controlled by the community. The study suggests that for conducting community empowerment to address the social determinants of health, it is of importance to use a non-sectoral mechanism that can accommodate multisectoral interests.

Chapter 7. Iran
Child malnutrition: engaging health and other sectors

Intersectoral collaboration becomes difficult when resources are limited. Highest-level government commitment is a must when going to scale. Establishing effective intersectoral action needs more than building organizational capacity through upgrading staff knowledge and skills; it also requires health objectives to be translated into the interests of and institutionalized within government sectors as well as community organizations. Having a visionary and energetic champion, if not a must, will greatly facilitate the process.

Chapter 8. Kenya
The Millennium Villages Project to improve health and eliminate extreme poverty in rural African communities

This case study reviews early experience with a multisectoral development project, the Millennium Villages Project (MVP), in rural African communities. The MVP tests the key recommendations of the UN Millennium Project and demonstrates in practice at the village level how to achieve the Millennium Development Goals (MDGs). It demonstrates that integrated interventions that simultaneously target the availability, acceptability and accessibility dimensions are feasible and can lead to high-impact programmes at the village level but there are important contextual constraints as well.

Chapter 9. Nigeria
Immunization programme in Anambra State

Despite continued attempts, routine immunization coverage in some areas of Nigeria has remained very low. Local ownership of the programme is the key to sustainability of the programme; involvement at the political level is necessary but not sufficient. Local-level administrative integration is indispensable. This study explores the roles of stakeholders in the development and implementation of the Reaching Every Ward (REW) policy for delivering immunization services in Nigeria, and the factors influencing their roles in keeping and not keeping the focus of the REW.

Chapter 10. Pakistan
Multipartner national project to reduce malnutrition among rural girls in Pakistan – Tawana

Malnutrition figures for children below the age of 5 years have been stagnant in Pakistan over the past several years. The Tawana project, initiated by the Federal Ministry of Women and Development, following a pilot project undertaken by the Aga Khan University, was a national project launched in 29 districts. It focused on empowering local women by giving them the opportunity to plan and manage a feeding programme, and demonstrates how malnutrition could be reduced. Enrolment and retention of girls in government primary schools increased through a concerted approach. However, the project also demonstrated that showing results and impact is not sufficient to maintain political and administrative support.

Chapter 11. Peru
Local Health Administration Committees (CLAS)

Local Health Administration Communities (CLAS) in Peru are non-profit civil associations that enter into agreements with the government and receive public funds to administer PHC services, applying private sector law for contracting and purchasing. It is an example of a strategy that effectively addresses the social determinants of health. These refer to social, cultural and economic barriers at the local level which keep people from effectively utilizing health-care services. This case study describes the political and professional opportunities as well as threats that such programmes face in the long run.

Chapter 12. South Africa
Intervention with Microfinance for AIDS and Gender Equity (IMAGE)

The Intervention with Microfinance for AIDS and Gender Equity (IMAGE) was an attempt to design, implement and evaluate a cross-sectoral intervention that aimed to improve health outcomes by targeting their social determinants in rural South Africa. The intervention combined an established microfinance programme with gender and HIV/AIDS training, and activities to support community mobilization. The case study highlights key lessons from the experiences of developing an intersectoral collaboration, expanding the scale of intervention delivery following a trial, and exploring models for long-term sustainable delivery.

Chapter 13. Tanzania
Insecticide-treated nets in Tanzania

This case study analyses the national programme for insecticide-treated nets (ITNs) in Tanzania during the period 1995–2008, focusing on implementation issues in relation to the social determinants of health and how to benefit the poorest, most exposed and most vulnerable groups in society. The case study describes the importance of monitoring and research in such programmes as well as the influence of shifting donor interests and approaches.

Chapter 14. Vanuatu
Pacific Action for Health Project: addressing the social determinants of alcohol use and abuse with adolescents

Young people in the Republic of Vanuatu are increasingly being faced with rapid urbanization, lack of education, consumption of unhealthy foods, limited job opportunities, and the widespread availability and accessibility of inexpensive cigarettes and alcohol. This case study covers an integrated health promotion and community development programme, the Pacific Action for Health Project (PAHP), set up to address the social determinants for noncommunicable diseases in the capital of Vanuatu, Port Vila.

Chapter 15. From concept to practice – synthesis of findings

The synthesis process involved analysing the five key aspects of the programmes that have been covered by the case studies: going to scale, managing policy change, managing intersectoral processes, adjusting design and ensuring sustainability. It looked closely at the common lessons learned under each of these five aspects of the programme. Among the key messages emerging from the synthesis are: the importance of evidence and baseline; that in the long haul, the battle for equity takes place in the public space through intelligent use of the evidence and partners; and finally, that scale-up should consider three phases – providing proof of principle; testing the scalability of the programme with particular focus on the drivers of expansion and how to transfer the values torch; and roll-out with systematic monitoring, repeated evaluation and timely adjustments to the programme.

References

1. Blas E and Sivasankara Kurup A (2010). *Equity, social determinants and public health programmes*. Geneva, World Health Organization.

2. CSDH (2008). *Closing the gap in a generation: health equity through action on the social determinants of health*. Final report of the Commission on Social Determinants of Health. Geneva, World Health Organization.

3. Dahlgren G, Whitehead M (2006). *Levelling up: a discussion paper on European strategies for tackling social inequities in health (part 2).* Copenhagen, WHO Regional Office for Europe.

4. Diderichsen F, Evans T, Whitehead M (2001). The social basis of disparities in health. In: Evans T et al., eds. *Challenging inequities in health.* New York, Oxford University Press:12–23.

5. Hasan A, Patel S, Satterthwait D (2005). How to meet the Millennium Development Goals (MDGs) in urban areas. *Environment and Urbanization,* 17:3–19.

6. Lee JW (2004). *Address to the 57th World Health Assembly,* 17 May 2004. Geneva, World Health Organization. (http://www.who.int/dg/lee/speeches/2004/wha57/en/index.html, accessed on 06 November 2010).

7. Lönnroth K et al. (2010). Tuberculosis: the role of risk factors and social determinants. In: Blas E and Sivasankara Kurup A, eds. *Equity, social determinants and public health programmes.* Geneva, World Health Organization:219–241.

8. Maher D et al. (2007). Planning to improve global health: the next decade of tuberculosis control. *Bulletin of the World Health Organization,* 85:341–347.

9. Solar O, Irwin A (2007). *A conceptual framework for action on the social determinants of health.* Discussion paper for the Commission on Social Determinants of Health. Geneva, World Health Organization.

10. United Nations (2010). *The Millennium Development Goals report.* New York, United Nations.

11. Yin RK (2003). *Case study research – design and methods.* Thousand Oaks, California, Sage Publications Inc.

12. WHO (2008). *The world health report 2008. Primary health care: now more than ever.* Geneva, World Health Organization.

13. World Health Assembly of the World Health Organization. *Resolution WHA62.14. Reducing health inequities through action on the social determinants of health.* Geneva, World Health Organization, 2009:21–25. (http://apps.who.int/gb/ebwha/pdf_files/WHA62-REC1/WHA62_REC1-en-P2.pdf, accessed 20 October 2009).

14. WHO (2007). *Priority Public Health Conditions Knowledge Network scoping paper.* (http://www.who.int/social_determinants/resources/pphc_scoping_paper.pdf, accessed on 10 October 2010).

Scaled up and marginalized

A review of Bangladesh's menstrual regulation programme and its impact[1]

2

Heidi Bart Johnston,[2,*] Anna Schurmann,[3] Elizabeth Oliveras,[4] and Halida Hanum Akhter[5]

[1] This work was made possible through funding provided by the World Health Organization (WHO) and the UK Department for International Development (DFID) to ICDDR,B.

[2] Independent Consultant, previously at ICDDR,B, Dhaka, Bangladesh

[3] Carolina Population Center, University of North Carolina Chapel Hill, USA

[4] Pathfinder International, Watertown, MA, USA. Previously at ICDDR,B, Dhaka, Bangladesh

[5] Retired. Previously at Family Planning Association of Bangladesh

* Corresponding author: heidibartjohnston@gmail.com

Abstract

Every year, globally, an estimated 66 500 women die attempting to terminate a pregnancy. To the extent that women's lives and futures are influenced by childbirth, access to contraception and safe abortion services is fundamental to gender equity. Yet many countries legally restrict access to safe abortion. In these countries, women with a socioeconomic advantage are more able to circumvent restrictive abortion laws and access safe abortion services; poor and less educated women are more likely to use unsafe methods and suffer serious morbidity and death. This is particularly egregious as deaths from unsafe abortion are entirely preventable, given access to modern contraception and safe abortion services. Bangladesh's Menstrual Regulation (MR) Programme is an example of a programme with the potential to reduce morbidity and mortality related to unsafe abortion in the context of a restrictive abortion law. We describe how Bangladesh's MR Programme evolved from an urban-based relief effort in 1972 to a nationwide primary care-level programme; review intersectoral processes that have and continue to influence policy development and programme implementation; assess the impact of the programme; explore contextual factors that have influenced the potential of the programme over time; and comment on issues of programme sustainability and replicability in settings beyond Bangladesh. Available evidence suggests that the MR Programme has contributed to a reduction in maternal mortality; however, mortality from unsafe abortion continues to disproportionately impact the socioeconomically disadvantaged.

2.1 Background

Access to contraception and safe abortion services is critical to gender equity, particularly in contexts in which women bear the primary responsibility for child care, and forgo educational and career opportunities if unplanned or mistimed pregnancy and childbirth takes place. By legally restricting safe methods of fertility control, women's lives, careers and futures can be fundamentally altered by pregnancy and childbirth. In these environments, women who try to take control of their future by terminating a mistimed pregnancy, particularly those with few socioeconomic resources, risk their lives and health.

Deaths from unsafe abortion – one of the five leading causes of maternal mortality – vividly illustrate inequity in access to health care. Internationally, 98% of the estimated 66 500 abortion-related deaths that occur each year take place in developing countries (World Health Organization, 2007a). Socioeconomic disparities in mortality and morbidity related to unsafe abortion continue at all levels, from regional to national to community. In rural Bangladesh, an analysis showed that women from the poorest-asset quintile were more than twice as likely to die from complications of abortion compared with women from the wealthiest-asset quintile; those with no formal education were more than 11 times more likely to die of unsafe abortion than those with 8 or more years of formal education (Chowdhury et al., 2007). Guaranteeing equitable access to contraceptive and safe abortion services would prevent the vast majority of these deaths, and provide women and couples with the means of determining the timing and spacing of their children.

To address the high rates of mortality and morbidity from unsafe abortion, governments at the International Conference on Population and Development (ICPD) five-year anniversary Special Session of the United Nations General Assembly in June 1999 strengthened the 1994 ICPD Program of Action Language on abortion, agreeing that where abortion is legal it should be safe and accessible. In 2003, the World Health Organization (WHO) published a guidance of best practices to support this 1999 agreement (WHO, 2003). The recommendations include interventions such as providing abortion services at primary-care facilities and, to enable this, fostering mid-level clinician provision of abortion, and replacing dilatation and curettage with safer and simpler vacuum aspiration or medical abortion technology for uterine evacuation. The guidance further recommends contraceptive counselling and services before abortion clients leave a health-care facility to decrease the likelihood of a subsequent unintended pregnancy.

Most of these recommendations have been in place in Bangladesh for over 30 years. In Bangladesh, where abortion is illegal except to save a woman's life, mid-level clinicians in the MR Programme have been using vacuum aspiration for uterine evacuation at the primary-care level since 1977. The government has mandated that MR services be available at all of the more than 4500 Union Health and Family Welfare Centres, as well as secondary- and tertiary-care facilities to make MR services accessible throughout the country (Akhter, 2001). Since 1975, fertility has dropped from 6.9 to 2.7 births per woman (NIPORT et al., 2007) and, while the number of MR and abortions has increased, deaths from unsafe abortion have decreased (Oliveras et al., 2008).

In this chapter, we describe how the MR Programme evolved from an urban-based relief effort in 1972 to a nationwide primary-care level programme. We review the intersectoral processes that influenced and continue to influence policy development and programme implementation; assess the impact of the programme; explore the social, economic, political and cultural factors that have influenced the potential of the programme over time; and comment on programme sustainability and replicability in settings beyond Bangladesh.

2.2 Methods

Our study questions were:

1. How did Bangladesh's MR Programme develop, and what key factors influenced its evolution over time?

2. Is the strategy of MR service delivery in a restrictive abortion law environment sustainable if implemented by a strong public sector–NGO–donor partnership? If so, what are the forces that sustain the programme? If not, what necessary forces are missing?

3. Has the MR Programme had a positive and equitable impact on reducing mortality and morbidity from abortion complications? What are the social, economic, political and cultural barriers and facilitators to programme success?

4. What lessons, if any, can be transferred from the MR Programme experience to other countries with high maternal mortality from unsafe abortion and restrictive abortion laws?

We employed a case study design to facilitate in-depth exploration of the forces that have shaped and continue

to shape the MR Programme. We conducted an extensive review of the published and peer-reviewed literature, and grey literature related to the MR Programme. We collected the grey literature via a systematic search for documents relating to the MR Programme, including official government publications, agendas and minutes of relevant meetings, formal studies and evaluations of the MR Programme, and conducted fact-checking with different levels of MR Programme stakeholders, including programme managers, service providers and researchers.

2.3 Findings

Evolution of the MR programme in three phases

In Bangladesh, the British Penal Code of 1860, Section 312, criminalizes abortion except to save the life of the woman, and penalizes providers of abortion with fines and imprisonment (Ministry of Law, Justice and Parliamentary Affairs, 1977). Yet MR, or evacuation of the uterus of a woman at risk of being pregnant to "ensure a state of non-pregnancy", is sanctioned by the government, and provided by public sector clinicians at primary, secondary and tertiary levels of the health-care system (Population Control and Family Planning Division, 1979).

The evolution of Bangladesh's MR Programme can be divided into three phases: conceptualization (1971–1981); distancing of MR activities from the State (1982–1998); and marginalization of MR (1998–till date).

Phase 1: Conceptualization (1971–1981)

The MR Programme was conceptualized in the early years of Bangladesh's Independence as part of a solution to unsustainable population growth. Three leading forces drove the early stages of the MR Programme: the temporary waiving of the strict abortion law immediately post Independence; concern regarding population growth; and the development of new uterine evacuation technology. In this section, we describe the context in which the Programme was initiated and implemented, identifying drivers of change and barriers to success.

The liberation war

In 1971, Bangladesh fought a nine-month war of

liberation with Pakistan. Pakistani forces raped 200 000–400 000 Bangladeshi women, prompting international media coverage that highlighted for the first time the use of rape as a weapon of war (Drummond, 1971; Brownmiller, 1975; Mookherjee, 2008), and national and international support for the rape victims.

In 1972, the restrictive abortion law was waived for "heroines of war" who had been raped and were pregnant. International feminist and aid organizations arranged for medical teams from India, Australia and the UK to perform medical terminations of pregnancy at district hospitals in Bangladesh (Akhter, 1988; Ross, 2002). While working with the international medical teams, the Bangladeshi doctors received not only technical training but also exposure to the concept of abortion as a woman's right (Ross, 2002). This temporary sanctioning of abortion eased public opinion toward uterine evacuation procedures and solidified a cadre of professional elite prepared to defend a woman's right to control her fertility (Potts and Diggory, 1977; Amin, 1996; Piet-Pelon, 1998; Khan, 2000).

The population control agenda

At Independence, Bangladesh was one of the most densely populated countries in the world; it had a population of 70 million and a fertility rate of almost seven children per woman. In the 1970s, concern with rapid population growth dominated the international development agenda (Donaldson and Tsui, 1990). Bangladesh was heavily reliant on donor support to recover from the cyclone of 1970, the liberation war of 1971 and the famine of 1974, and was under pressure to curb population growth. This pressure intensified after the famine gave rise to fears of a Malthusian crisis (Lee et al., 1995).

The Bangladeshi Government embraced the population control agenda and allocated 6% of the development budget and 5% of the revenue budget to family planning between 1974–75 and 1986–87 (Islam and Tahir, 2002; Lee et al., 1995). In 1978, the Government of Bangladesh declared population control the country's main priority. Resource allocation for the first four five-year health and population programmes privileged vertical family planning service delivery above all other health priorities. Within the Ministry of Health and Population Control, abortion was seen as an important complement to family planning in terms of the population control agenda. In the early 1970s, the modern contraception prevalence rate was 4.7% (Ministry of Health and Population Control, 1978).

Development of service infrastructure for safe pregnancy terminations

During the 1970s, an infrastructure for safe, voluntary pregnancy termination was established. In 1974, the government encouraged the introduction of a pilot uterine evacuation programme in a few family planning clinics. This was funded by the United States Agency for International Development (USAID) through the nongovernmental organization (NGO) The Pathfinder Fund, as part of a national postpartum programme that included provision of contraception and family planning services (Piet-Pelon, 1998).

The Pathfinder Fund played a lead role in the campaign to train paramedics – called family welfare visitors (FWVs) – in uterine evacuation care. FWVs have a minimum of 10 years of basic education, followed by 18 months of reproductive health training. Some have an additional three months of training in uterine evacuation. While the medical community resisted the authorization of paramedics to provide uterine evacuation services, arguments to employ FWVs to make the simple procedure accessible to women in rural and less affluent areas prevailed (Ross, 2002).

Vacuum aspiration using the Karman cannula revolutionized pregnancy termination service delivery, allowing uterine evacuation without the need for anaesthetics or an operating theatre (Karman, 1972; Ekwempu, 1990). Vacuum aspiration is safer than dilatation and curettage, recovery is fast (WHO, 2003), it can be performed safely by mid-level providers at outpatient facilities (Bhatia et al., 1980; Warriner et al., 2006), and the equipment is portable and does not require electricity.

In 1978, the Ministry of Health and Population Control in collaboration with The Pathfinder Fund initiated a uterine evacuation training and services programme in seven government medical colleges and two district hospitals for government doctors, FWVs and a few private doctors (Akhter, 1988). American medical consultants came to Bangladesh to train providers in the use of manual vacuum aspiration, and doctors were also sent to Singapore for training (Piet-Pelon, 1998; Ross, 2002).

Policy development

The combination of multiple factors described earlier contributed to a policy environment conducive to a liberalization of the abortion law.

In 1973, the first five-year plan highlighted the importance of abortion as an important means of controlling fertility despite social censure, putting it firmly on the country's policy agenda. The 1976 National Population Policy Outline (Government of the People's Republic of Bangladesh, 1976) proposed the legalization of medical termination of pregnancy as it was practised at the time. Though the Population Policy Outline recommended liberalization of the abortion law up to 12 weeks of pregnancy, this recommendation was not acted upon.

Legalization of abortion was considered further in 1977 when the Population Control and Family Planning Division commissioned the Bangladesh Institute of Law and International Affairs to report on the laws pertaining to population growth, and recommend new legislation as necessary. The report suggested legalizing abortion for the first 12 weeks of pregnancy by licensed paramedics or medical doctors under safe medical conditions on the basis of humanitarian, eugenic, socioeconomic, or contraceptive failure – according to the best judgement of the clinician. However, in 1977, General Zia assumed the presidency, augmenting his political support by appealing to religious conservatives (Lee et al., 1995). As with the National Population Policy Outline, the recommendations of the Institute of Law were not enacted, on the basis that uterine evacuation was already available, and a concern that explicit legislation might arouse religious opposition (Ross, 2002).

Responding to domestic and international interests, the government gradually introduced a uterine evacuation training and service delivery programme. In 1979, the Population Control and Family Planning Division of the Ministry of Health and Population Control circulated a memorandum with a legal interpretation by the Bangladesh Institute of Law and International Affairs to authorize MR services to be included in the national family planning programme (Ali et al., 1978; Ross, 2002). Technically competent and politically savvy champions in the Ministry of Health and Population Control provided strong support for the MR Programme, ordering medical doctors and paramedics to offer MR services in all government hospitals, and at primary care-level health and family planning complexes throughout the country.

Phase 2: Distancing of MR activities from the State (1982–1997)

Since inception, the MR Programme in Bangladesh has been vulnerable to donors' changing priorities. Three important international policy changes during this second phase impacted the MR Programme: an increased emphasis on funding NGOs rather than the State; the US Government's restrictive Mexico City Policy, and the reproductive health and rights approach to population promulgated by the 1994 ICPD.

Tensions in donor priorities: the United States' Mexico City Policy and the International Conference on Population and Development Programme of Action

In the 1980s, fertility decline had begun in Bangladesh and donors moved away from their strong emphasis on fertility control. Population dynamics came to be regarded in a more nuanced way, as the effects of population pressures on poverty and health proved difficult to quantify (Lakshminaranayan, 2007). In 1994, the ICPD called for, and Bangladesh signed onto, expanding women's life choices, achieving gender equity, and paying greater attention to sexual and reproductive health and rights (Germain, 1998). This more comprehensive approach superseded vertical programmes with their narrow focus on fertility control (Lakshminaranayan, 2007).

Until 1983, USAID supported the MR Programme through the NGO The Pathfinder Fund. Increased religious conservatism in the United States led to the imposition of the Reagan administration's Mexico City Policy in 1984. This policy bars US financial and technical family planning assistance to foreign NGOs which, with their own funds, provide safe abortion services, referrals to abortion services or any kind of advocacy around abortion issues (Blane and Friedman, 1990; Crane and Dusenberry, 2004). The Pathfinder Fund relinquished all MR-related activities. The model MR clinics and training programme became a "special project" of the Ministry of Health, called the Menstrual Regulation Training and Services Programme (MRTSP, which later became the RHSTEP[1]). The programme was run by a steering committee of doctors and government bureaucrats chaired by the secretary of health (Ross, 2002). Financing of the MR Programme was taken over by the Population Crisis Committee, the Ford Foundation, and the Swedish International Development Cooperation Agency (Sida). By 1998, the other donors had pulled out of Bangladesh and Sida was the sole donor supporting the MR Programme.

---

[1] In 2003, MRTSP changed its name to Reproductive Health Services Training Education Project, or RHSTEP. To minimize confusion in this paper, we will refer to the organization as RHSTEP.

Devolution from the State to NGOs

From the 1980s, NGOs in Bangladesh became increasingly responsible for the essential functions of the MR Programme. A confluence of factors contributed to the transition of the MR Programme from a purely public sector programme to a public–NGO sector partnership. First, a key MR Programme champion within the Ministry of Health and Population Control left the Ministry to take a position at an international organization (Ross, 2002). The weight of programme leadership was then in the NGO sector. A conflict between the government and The Pathfinder Fund over the training of paramedics in MR services delivery possibly contributed to the transition, as did strong conservative religious and even specific anti-abortion sentiment from important international political and economic partners. The transition was not unique, as the 1980s saw a trend in international development programming of increasing investments in NGO rather than public sector programmes (White, 1999; Schurmann and Mahmud, 2009).

Three different NGOs were established to manage the MR Programme, all with complementary roles. In 1982, The Pathfinder Fund assisted in the establishment of the Bangladesh Association for the Prevention of Septic Abortion (BAPSA) to research and monitor the MR Programme, and contribute to programme logistics (Dixon-Mueller, 1988; Ross, 2002). The Bangladesh Women's Health Coalition (BWHC) was also formed at this time to provide MR training, service delivery and advocacy. In 1991, RHSTEP became a nationally registered NGO when the Ministry of Health eliminated all special projects. Donors funded these NGOs directly, and provided no financial or technical MR Programme support to the government. While the aim of the Ford Foundation and Sida was to have the Ministry of Health and Family Welfare (MOHFW) eventually take over responsibility for the MR Programme, under this structure, government involvement with the essential training, service delivery and logistical aspects of the programme diminished (Ross, 2002; Paulin and Ahsan, 2003).

The MR Programme was and continues to be administratively based in the Directorate General of Family Planning (DGFP) within the MOHFW. The DGFP works closely with the three NGOs – RHSTEP, BAPSA and BWHC – in implementing the programme. The MOHFW provides considerable support to the NGOs in the form of clinic space and equipment for MR training and services (Akhter, 2001). RHSTEP remains the primary MR training organization in the country with training facilities located in 18 medical college and district hospitals (RHSTEP, 2006); BAPSA remains responsible for coordinating the logistics of the MR Programme including liaising between MR trainees and training institutions, monitoring the distribution of MR equipment, and publishing the quarterly newsletter *Health and Rights*[2] (BAPSA, 2006; Hossain, 2008). BWHC continues to provide MR services and paramedic FWV training in MR and other reproductive health services (Ahmed and Afroze, 2006).

As well as the three implementing NGOs, several committees are in place to advise and supervise the MR Programme. The Coordination Committee of MR Activities in Bangladesh was established in 1987 with the membership of four MR organizations. The Technical Advisory Committee for MR Activities was established in 1990 with the Director General of the DGFP as chairperson, and the Line Director of Maternal and Child Health as secretary. While well designed in principle, in practice these committees rarely meet and have little impact on programme coordination.

In 1997, a National Reproductive Health Strategy was developed, prioritizing four services in the area of reproductive health: safe motherhood, family planning, MR and post-abortion care, and the management of reproductive tract infections and sexually transmitted infections. This was followed by the Maternal Health Strategy in 2001, which gave less emphasis to MR. Both these documents were designed to inform the Health and Population Sector Programme (HPSP). Since 1997, MR is mentioned less frequently and less explicitly in policy documents.

Phase 3: The marginalization of MR (1998–till date)

During the current phase, characterized by the implementation of health sector reform, the official

---

[2] Formerly *The MR Newsletter*, *Health and Rights* is distributed to 13 000 readers each quarter, and has four main aims: (1) provide clinicians with essential information on sexual and reproductive health and rights; (2) sensitize public opinion on the consequences of septic abortion, (3) provide clinicians with updated technical knowledge and guidance in order to facilitate improvement in the quality of services, and (4) highlight the MR training needs among the potential providers of MR (BAPSA, 2005).

language in the 2000 National Population Policy shifted from the legalization language of 1976 to language emphasizing the need to reduce unsafe abortion. A continued conservative climate internationally, driven in part by the re-instituted US Mexico City Policy, contributed to the limited dynamism of the MR Programme. NGOs receiving USAID funds and providing MR services lost funding; monitoring and evaluation of the programme came to a near standstill. Feminist and women's organizations in Bangladesh have not embraced the MR agenda (Ross, 2002). Despite these hurdles, at present there is a nascent sense of optimism for the provision of MR services in Bangladesh.

Health sector reform

The health sector reform process of the HPSP (1998–2003) presents another chapter in the evolution of reproductive health policy in Bangladesh. The goals of the policy – in line with the ICPD agenda – were primarily to reduce maternal and infant mortality and morbidity by reducing fertility to replacement level by the year 2005 and by improving nutritional status (Germain, 1997; Bates et al., 2003). The reform process was coordinated by the World Bank and included a consortium of other donors and the Government of Bangladesh. Donor investment was over US$ 350 million between 1999 and 2003. The most significant change of the HPSP was the merging of the Health and Family Planning Directorates of the MOHFW, which allowed for sectorwide provision of family planning and primary health-care services (however, this merging never effectively occurred). The integrated programme replaced the 125 vertical projects previously managed under the MOHFW (Chowdhury et al., 2003).

With the implementation of the HPSP in 1998, Sida and other donors began contributing non-earmarked funds directly to the MOHFW. Allocation of funds was to be guided by the five-year sectorwide programme, with the shared assumption that the MOHFW would continue to issue contracts with the three MR NGOs as outlined in the HPSP Programme Implementation Plan. One expected benefit was enhanced government ownership, and thus enhanced sustainability of the programme (Ross, 2002). However, the mechanism for funding the MR NGOs was unclear. After a lengthy competitive bidding process during which the MR NGOs received no funding, in June 2002, the MOHFW signed a contract with one of the MR NGOs for the last year of the five-year HPSP. This funding gap brought the MR NGOs to a near-collapse, and the quality of service provision was compromised

(Chowdhury et al., 2003; Johnston, 2004). In 2003, the MOHFW formally requested Sida to renew direct support to the MR NGOs. Sida responded positively and agreed to fund the MR NGOs for one more year (Paulin and Ahsan, 2003).

Sida revised its funding strategy to reimburse NGOs for the number of services performed. Tellingly, and in line with this implicit emphasis on service delivery, BAPSA, the MR research and monitoring organization, shifted its agenda to service delivery with some monitoring and logistics functions.

The 2001 reimposition of the US Government's Mexico City Policy had a more widespread effect on MR service delivery compared with the original 1984 imposition because, over time in Bangladesh, numerous health-care service delivery NGOs had grown to play a role in MR service delivery. These NGOs tended to interpret the policy cautiously, ending MR service provision and minimizing collaborations with MR NGOs in areas such as training, workshops and referrals, leading to the isolation of the MR NGOs from the wider reproductive health professionals' community.

While USAID actively opposed MR service delivery under the Mexico City Policy, most other donors have been more neutral in their attitude toward MR. Donor neutrality has had the negative effect of allowing less controversial priorities, such as Safe Motherhood, to consume the MOHFW's finite resources and attention, leaving MR services relatively neglected. One example of this neglect is that no new FWVs have been recruited since 1994. As the last generation of FWVs nears retirement, no new cadre of paramedic providers is being trained in MR services. Such a provider gap will cripple the programme.

The HPSP was followed by the Health and Nutrition Population Sector Programme (HNPSP: 2003–2010), which formally re-established family planning and primary health programmes as separate programmes. With delays in the implementation of the new plan, Sida agreed to continue to provide funding to the three MR NGOs from 2003 to 2010.

There is a sense of optimism for MR service delivery due to the growth of internationally affiliated Bangladeshi-run NGOs (Marie Stopes Clinical Society and Family Planning Association of Bangladesh) making a commitment to scale up safe MR services. Additionally, international donors including Sida and the Royal Netherlands Embassy have demonstrated their commitment to a sustainable MR Programme (Paulin and Ahsan, 2003; Johnson et al., 2006). The Asian Development Bank is also supporting MR as a core service in its widespread public–private partnership Urban Primary Health Care Project. However, the private sector remains largely unregulated, and untrained providers offer what may seem to the client to be convenient and relatively inexpensive services. This is considered in the following discussion on programme impact.

Impact of the MR Programme

The challenges of collecting data on abortion, a marginalized and stigmatized topic in Bangladesh, limit our ability to assess the impact of the MR Programme on reducing abortion-related mortality and morbidity or the equitability of impact. However, we can identify general trends. For example, abortion data from the International Centre for Diarrhoeal Disease Research, Bangladesh (ICDDR,B) demographic surveillance sites in the predominately rural areas of Matlab, Abhoynagar and Mirsarai suggest that marital abortion ratios (the number of reported abortions divided by the number of reported births in a given time period) and total marital abortion rates (the number of abortions a married woman would have over her lifetime if current age-specific abortion rates prevailed) have on the whole increased over the time. In the rural riverine area of Matlab, with a population of around 200 000, ICDDR,B administers an intensive family planning programme in half of the surveillance site, the other half benefits from the government programme and is considered more representative of national trends. In the Matlab surveillance area under the government family planning programme, the marital abortion ratio has increased more than fivefold from the early 1980s, when it was close to 20 abortions per 1000 live births, to over 100 abortions per 1000 live births in 2004 (Oliveras et al., 2008).

Abortion-related deaths have decreased dramatically from 17.7 to 2.4 per 100 000 women of reproductive age annually from 1976 to 2005 in the ICDDR,B programme area, and from 16.8

to 2.2 per 100 000 in the government programme area of ICDDR,B's Matlab Demographic Surveillance (Figure 1). The decrease in mortality is in part attributable to increase in the use of contraception in both areas, from 46% in 1984 to 71% in 2005 in the ICDDR,B programme area, and from 16% in 1984 to 47% in 2005 in the government programme area (*see* Rahman et al., 2001). That the differences in rates of abortion-related mortality are minimal between the two areas while the differences in rates of contraceptive prevalence are substantial suggests that factors in addition to contraceptive use are at work in reducing abortion-related mortality.

Verbal autopsy data from the Matlab ICDDR,B programme area show a decrease in abortion-related mortality as a percentage of maternal mortality, from 24% of maternal mortality in the decade 1976–1985 to 11% of maternal mortality in the period 1996–2005. The shift has been less dramatic in the comparison area, from 17% of maternal mortality to 15% of maternal mortality in the same time periods (data not shown) (Chowdhury et al., 2007; Oliveras et al., 2008). The Matlab government area estimate of 15% of maternal mortality caused by unsafe abortion is considered the best estimate of abortion-related mortality as a percentage of maternal mortality for Bangladesh.

These data show that along with the scale up of the MR Programme, there has been an increase in reported MR and a decrease in deaths from unsafe abortion. While

Figure 1. Abortion-related deaths per 100 000 women of reproductive age, Matlab 1976–2005

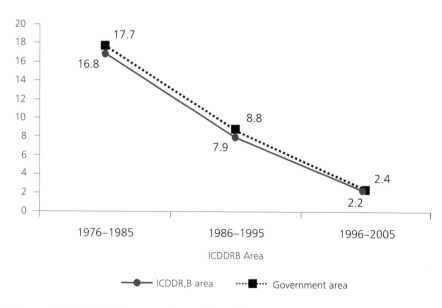

Data sources: ICDDR,B's Matlab maternal mortality verbal autopsy 1976–2005 dataset and ICDDR,B Matlab health and demographic surveillance system dataset

this does not imply causality, it is consistent with MR Programme success in reducing mortality related to unsafe abortion (Oliveras et al., 2008).

The volume of services provided also speaks of the impact of this programme. The MOHFW reports 124 045 MR procedures performed at government and MR NGO facilities in 2006. About half of these were performed at government clinics, and half at the MR NGO facilities. MR NGOs reported providing over 60 000 MR services in 2004–05 and 2005–06, with the bulk of these procedures performed at RHSTEP clinics located in government facilities. These data are widely believed to substantially underestimate the number of MR procedures provided in the public and NGO sectors and do not include MRs performed in the for-profit private sector (Begum et al., 1987; Amin et al., 1989; Chowdhury et al., 2003).

While few studies have been conducted, the available data suggest that vulnerable populations remain at relatively high risk of death from unsafe abortion. Complementing quantitative data from Matlab, which highlight the relationships between socioeconomic status and unsafe abortion, qualitative data suggest that materially impoverished women prefer informal sector services as providers in the public sector are rude to poor women (Johnston, 1999).

In a study conducted in 1997 in rural Bangladesh, women reported that the readily available, informally trained, unauthorized private sector providers in their communities better met their priorities of confidential services, good behaviour to the client, and low cost – at least initially. The study showed that among the 108 attempted pregnancy terminations that were reported, 27 women (25%) accessed care from the trained government provider. Thirty-one women (29%) attempted to self-induce abortion; 29 women (27%) used village homeopath techniques to abort; 13 women (12%) used techniques from the informally trained village pharmacist; and 8 (7%) went to the *kabiraj* or traditional healer for an abortion. Sixty-two per cent of first attempts at abortion failed, leaving women to attempt abortion a second and, for some, a third time (Johnston, 1999). The leading medical college hospital in the capital city, Dhaka, reports that the majority of patients in their obstetrics and gynaecology ward are women presenting with complications of unsafe abortion (Rashid M, Professor and Head, Department of Obstetrics and Gynecology, Dhaka Medical College and Hospital, Dhaka, Bangladesh, personal communication, 28 March 2009).

Despite the successes of the MR Programme, many socially and economically disadvantaged women still do not access government services and, for a number of reasons considered below, turn to the informal sector for pregnancy termination. That an estimated 15% of 21 000 pregnancy-related deaths (Oliveras et al., 2008; WHO, 2007b), or 3150 lives in Bangladesh are lost annually to unsafe abortion, and that these deaths are concentrated among the poor and uneducated, demonstrates a need to rethink the strategies of this innovative and life-saving programme to make it better meet the needs of all women, regardless of socioeconomic status.

Socioeconomic context: barriers to equitable access

For the programme to meet the needs of women regardless of socioeconomic status, the strategies of the MR Programme must reach beyond the health system and address the social, cultural, political and economic determinants of health. In this section, we briefly describe the societal barriers that can prevent women from accessing safe MR care.

Poor quality of care can turn clients away from public sector facilities. Qualitative studies indicate that clinicians provide an uneven quality of services depending on the characteristics of the client. Examples of poor quality service include clinicians not eliciting patient histories, not listening to patients, allowing patients to plead for services and charging for services that are meant to be free (Schuler and Hossain, 1998). Clinicians sometimes unfairly refuse to provide MR – especially in circumstances in which the client is unmarried or the pregnancy is the result of rape (Begum et al., 1987).

Despite MR services ostensibly being provided free of charge in government clinics, few women pay nothing. In one study, only 11% of women reported receiving services free of charge (Akhter, 1988). Reported expenditures varied greatly – 19% paid less than 100 taka (US$ 1.47), 18% paid 500–1000 taka (US$ 7.35–14.70) and 19% paid over 1000 taka. Other evidence suggests that MR services can be refused in the free clinic and instead provided after hours at a charge, sometimes using the public facilities (Piet-Pelon, 1998; Caldwell et al., 1999).

Unofficial fees often coexist with "free services" in Bangladesh. Illegal fees inordinately affect the poor, who are less likely to question the provider or understand the health-care system. The lowest income category has been found to pay 143% of the charges of the highest income category for public sector care (Killingsworth et al., 1999).

The high level of variation in fees reflects inequity in access to services. Reasons for variation in patient fees for MR include: marital status, with unmarried women paying more; duration of gestation, with women with longer gestation periods paying more; and the different types of pain management provided. In addition to such fees are the cost of patient travel, opportunity costs and lost income for the client and accompanying caregivers, drugs, and clinic or hospital admission fees. Fees for the treatment of abortion complications follow a similar pattern.

In Bangladesh, client–patron relationships shape power hierarchies. As such, clients are beneficiaries of patron "favours" rather than citizens with rights (Blair, 2005). Patron–client relationships impact the health sector as clients rely on personal relationships to get better quality or lower cost services, through waiving of unofficial fees, for example. Schuler et al. (2002) found a perception that without such a relationship, service quality for the poor would be lower and the price higher, and that "only the wealthy can get good health care". The wealthy are less often approached for unofficial fees, and are better positioned to demand quality services due to their higher level of institutional literacy, and peer-like relationships with medical professionals.

Level of education is an important determinant of health-seeking behaviour for women in Bangladesh (Chakraborty et al., 2003; Ahmed et al., 2005). Education, or literacy, determines access to information and comfort with and ability to negotiate the formal health-care system. The likelihood of seeking abortion or MR, especially with a licensed provider, increases with women's education. MR and induced abortions are more common among educated women, but educated women suffer less in terms of abortion-related mortality, suggesting access to better care (Ahmed et al., 2005; Chowdhury et al., 2007).

Bangladesh achieved gender parity in primary and lower secondary school enrolments in the 1990s. However, schoolgirls and schoolboys are rarely taught about reproductive health or family planning. Furthermore, initiation of discussion about sex, family planning or reproduction is almost always the responsibility of men; talking about sex, even to husbands, is considered shameful (Khan, 2002).

Knowledge of MR has increased over the duration of the programme, with just over 22% of women interviewed in a contraceptive prevalence survey in 1979 reporting that they had heard of MR, compared with over 80% in all Demographic and Health Surveys (DHS) since 1999. Knowledge of MR is higher in urban areas (87% vs 79%), and increases with educational attainment and socioeconomic status. Knowledge is lower among adolescents, with 74% of girls under 20 years knowing of MR. Despite this growing awareness, confusion about MR remains a barrier, especially in terms of accessing the service within 10 weeks of the last menstrual period and finding a safe provider (Singh et al., 1997).

Purdah is a custom that generally secludes women from society at the onset of menarche. *Purdah*-related restrictions on Bangladeshi women's mobility are a significant barrier to accessing health care, especially if women are seeking care for a stigmatized procedure such as MR. Women would normally not seek care on their own but would be accompanied by a male relative, which imposes additional opportunity costs. As informal sector providers such as *kabiraj* live in rural areas in closer proximity to most women than a clinic, *purdah* is likely to be a strong motivator to women accessing care in the informal sector.

In Bangladesh, efforts to allow women reproductive freedom are feared to promote promiscuity (Khan, 2002). Thus, abortion can be considered controversial and a threat to the social order (Maloney et al., 1981; Ross, 2002). Hence, there is little policy dialogue or debate concerning abortion. A community-based study conducted in rural Bangladesh found that factors such as shame, blame, embarrassment, pregnancy outside marriage and religious disapproval cause women to be silent about MR and abortion (Bhuiya et al., 2001).

A few existing public opinion studies show that educated and wealthier participants were more likely to have supportive attitudes toward legalizing abortion (Chaudhury, 1980), and some professions also had relatively supportive attitudes – for example, 75% of government officials expressed their support, compared with 32% of the medical faculty (Chaudhury, 1975). Although one study found that people consider MR an essential service under certain circumstances such as poverty, a large family, pregnancy in elderly women, and pre- or extramarital pregnancy (Chowdhury et al., 2003), MR clients are inclined to think that societal attitudes are more negative. A qualitative study from 2002 showed that most clients thought the community had a negative opinion of MR (Islam et al., 2004); such perceptions are likely to affect the way in which women consider and use services.

We were not able to identify any studies on religious attitudes towards abortion, but religious conservatism is often cited as a barrier to programme improvements. According to *Hanafi* jurists, the school of legal interpretation followed by most Bangladeshis, abortion is permitted until the end of the fourth month of pregnancy (Amin, 1996); however, the popular perception is that abortion is a religious sin. While Islamic-based political parties such as the *Jamat-I-Islam* have fluctuating levels of political influence, they generally have little influence among the policy elite. Their impact is more strongly felt at the local level (Ross, 2002).

2.4 Discussion

This analysis of the evolution of the MR Programme through 30 years of implementation may offer lessons for its future sustainability, and for the design of programmes aiming to reduce mortality and morbidity related to unsafe abortion in other contexts. We show that mortality from unsafe abortion has declined but persists, particularly among the poor and less educated, and highlight the social, economic, political and cultural barriers to safe MR services. In this section, we consider issues of going to scale, managing policy change, managing intersectoral processes, adjusting design and ensuring sustainability. Finally, we consider the generalizability of the strategies of the Bangladesh MR Programme to other settings.

Going to scale

The development of Bangladesh's MR Programme was based on the local cultural context, the human and technical resources available, and the priorities of national and international technocrats and bureaucrats. The programme was built around the recognized need that to promote equitable access, family planning and MR services needed to be available at the primary-care level. The promise that the new manual vacuum aspiration technology could be used by paramedics to perform uterine evacuation services at the primary-care level contributed to the design stage of the MR Programme, and was characterized by a spirit of innovation. Despite this innovation around a potentially controversial service, the nationwide scaling up of the MR Programme was managed without a visible backlash.

Like many developing countries, Bangladesh has inadequate numbers of physicians to deliver health-care services to its predominantly rural population. In the 1970s, the family planning programme relied heavily on paramedics. The NGO Gonoshyasta Kendra (People's Health Centre) received high-level political support for pioneering the use of paramedics to provide mini-laparotomy. In this context, even though there were little data to indicate that non-physicians could safely and effectively perform MR procedures, The Pathfinder Fund was able to convince officials at the Ministry of Health and Population Control and physicians from the medical colleges to allow paramedics to provide MR services (Ross, 2002).

In 1978, the year before the MR Policy was enacted, the Ministry of Health and Population Control and The Pathfinder Fund established large-scale MR training programmes in eight of the country's 13 medical colleges. The Population Control Division wanted two trained MR providers based in each of the country's 413 subdistricts. With support from within the government, and financial and technical support from The Pathfinder Fund, the MR Programme scaled up quickly. By 1995, MR services were reportedly available in all of the more than 4500 union-level primary-care clinics throughout the country, as well as secondary and tertiary facilities. The FWV paramedics are central to the scaling up of MR service provision in Bangladesh. Compared to doctors, paramedics are cost-effective, tend to come from similar social backgrounds as their clients, implying a higher level of accessibility; and are more feasibly retained in rural posts (Akhter, 2001).

Managing policy change

Since the circulation of a government memo authorizing MR services at the primary-care level of the health system in 1979, the MR Policy has not been significantly revised. There is a quiet consensus among high-level stakeholders that there is no urgent need to revise the MR Policy or to try to liberalize the abortion law as spotlighting risks a reversal of the existing relatively liberal policy. Within the current policy, MR NGOs have been able to develop standards and guidelines for NGO services, though these have not carried over to the government sector programme. With strong champions in the MR NGOs and a recent injection of donor funding, there are several initiatives to introduce new technologies, improve quality of care, and improve coordination between the government and NGO sector programmes. Thus, the widely accepted goal is to continue to make programme improvements within the current structure.

While there has been no organized domestic opposition to the MR Policy or Programme, a fear of formidable and well-organized opposition accompanies discussion of policy or programme change among MR Programme stakeholders. A careful political analysis investigating potential threats to the programme needs to be done. If a threat to the programme is identified, it might be possible for women's rights groups and civil society organizations to counteract potential opposition; however, this would require a shift from the prevailing presentation of MR as a medical intervention to MR as a basic right of a woman to determine the timing and spacing of her fertility. The current vertical structure of the MR Programme prevents integration with other reproductive health and rights issues such as addressing violence against women, adolescent sexuality, protection against sexually transmitted infections including HIV/AIDS, essential health services for the poor and ultrapoor, and broader issues. The 2007–2010 MR Programme funding from Sida promotes a broader health and rights approach, and may prompt the integration of MR into a broader reproductive health and rights strategy. Any advances in presenting MR as a reproductive right need to be carefully designed, implemented and monitored with an evidence-based awareness of potential domestic and international opposition.

Managing intersectoral processes

The MR Programme is vertical, housed within the MOHFW, Directorate of Family Planning, in the line of Maternal and Child Health. The programme continues with narrow political support and, within the substantial public sector, the programme has not moved beyond a predominantly supply-side approach. The health system approach of making services available at the primary-care level is critical but insufficient. A number of barriers, as discussed earlier, discriminately bar the poor and uneducated from accessing safe MR services. To reduce unsafe abortion more efficiently, the programme must tackle the demand side of service delivery – helping women and other household-level decision-makers to choose safe MR services over unsafe services that may initially seem more convenient and less expensive, but can lead to serious morbidity and death.

To address the societal barriers that prevent women from accessing safe MR services, the MR Programme requires a broader base of support. As yet, women's rights and civil society groups have not included defending a woman's right to safe MR services in their portfolios. Lawyers' associations, even the Bangladesh National Women's

Lawyers' Association, have not embraced a reproductive rights agenda that includes defending or modernizing the MR Policy.

In contrast to the MR Programme, HIV/AIDS programmes in Bangladesh receive broad multisectoral support. In recent years, 14 different government ministries have integrated HIV/AIDS programming into their annual planning processes. Though interventions are perceived as politically controversial, programme coordinators have been able to convince skeptics that controversial interventions are justified, and are in fact tenets of good governance that require multisectoral commitment (Faisel et al., 2004). This is reminiscent of the late 1970s when the Government of Bangladesh declared population control the country's main priority and the MR Programme received strong national and international political and financial support. Modern arguments that safe MR services, as part of broader reproductive health service delivery, are critical for national development and deserve broad multisectoral support would need to be framed in a reproductive rights agenda, perhaps acknowledging that, like HIV, unintended pregnancy "strikes" during the prime productive years, when a death has the most significant impact on the family, community and country.

The level of coordination achieved by the HIV/AIDS programme has been made possible by the uniquely high levels of international financial and technical support that the HIV/AIDS agenda receives. Nonetheless, the HIV/AIDS programming experience has important lessons for the MR Programme, including re-positioning the issue from politically controversial and health-specific to an essential element of broader good governance, and using this platform to engage widespread multisectoral government and civil society support.

Adjusting design

Donors, the government and NGOs have all played leading roles in the design of Bangladesh's MR Programme. While all three stakeholders are essential to the programme, the importance of direct donor financial and technical support to the programme and its design should be acknowledged.

Initially, the Pathfinder Fund (providing technical and financial support) and the Ministry of Health and Population worked together to create and gain stakeholder approval for an innovative, purely public sector programme design. When the programme shifted to a three-pillared MOHFW–NGO–donor programme design and donors provided support directly to the NGOs, the NGOs continued their programmes with high standards. The government programme continued but, without direct donor support, the level of technical and management support from the government diminished. In 1998, when under health sector reform donor funds were pooled and distributed by the government, the MR NGOs came very close to collapse. Eventually, with the support of key government stakeholders, the MR NGOs successfully appealed to the donors for continued direct support. Financial support was reinstated by the donor, Sida, as a reimbursement for services. As NGOs became more responsive to easily measurable and reportable indicators of the donor, such as "number of providers trained" and "number of MRs performed", the initial aim of providing equitably accessible quality services at the primary-care level became increasingly distant. At present, WHO and DGFP, with financial and technical support from the Netherlands, are managing a project to strengthen NGO–MOHFW collaboration within the MR Programme. This project is expected to raise the level of intersectoral collaboration and quality of care in the government and NGO sectors.

In recent years, two forces outside of the government are influencing the shape of the national MR Programme. Two international reproductive health and rights NGOs, Marie Stopes International and International Planned Parenthood Federation, have raised their visibility in Bangladesh as important stakeholders in the MR service delivery community. In addition, private sector MR providers are growing in number and influence. These forces mark opportunities to broaden the coalition of support for safe and accessible MR services.

Ensuring sustainability

The sustainability of the MR Programme is dependent on the government maintaining the policy and working to ensure the availability of high-quality services safely and equitably. This includes continued government and donor support to the MR NGOs for their key role in providing training, high-quality care and service delivery innovation. However, donors should rethink the payment per service scheme and consider one that reinforces programme efforts to ensure the quality and equity of services. Furthermore, a strong programme of monitoring and maintaining quality in public, NGO and private for-profit facilities is required in which the regulatory agency has the power to enforce service delivery standards and close facilities that do not meet

basic standards. This regulatory role lies solidly with the government.

There is a need for multisectoral partnerships in ensuring that women and other decision-makers know about and can access contraception to decrease unwanted pregnancies, and safe MR services as a back-up in the event of contraceptive failure.

Finally, in countries with inadequate tax bases such as Bangladesh, public health sector projects – particularly those that are seen as potential political risks – may require external donor support as well as strong national champions within and outside the government for sustainability over time.

2.5 Conclusion

The strategies of the Bangladesh MR Programme may have widespread applicability for reducing unsafe abortion. In terms of policy, countries with highly restrictive abortion laws, and high levels of morbidity and mortality from unsafe abortion should first consider liberalization of the abortion law. However, in some settings, an MR policy might be the only acceptable step to decrease reliance on unsafe abortion. Safe MR services in the context of a strict abortion policy are far better than no safe uterine evacuation services. The Bangladesh MR Policy could benefit from a serious review. In its present form, it represents a culturally and politically acceptable policy implemented in the 1970s to meet the nation's aims of reducing population growth. A revised policy would be more medically nuanced, call for the use of new and safer technologies, emphasize equitable access to care, and use stronger rights-based language.

Bangladesh is a global leader in the task-shifting strategy of having paramedics provide safe uterine evacuation services at the primary-care level. These cost-effective WHO-recommended practices of decentralization are fundamental for increasing access to safe services, and are as applicable in rural Bangladesh where the abortion law is highly restrictive as in rural USA where abortion is available on request but can be difficult to access.

In terms of structure, the three-pillared government–NGO–donor approach deserves credit for sustaining the programme. This analysis has shown that the programme has been strongest when the public, donor and NGO sectors worked in close coordination. Throughout the history of the programme, when the support of one sector has lessened, the support of another sector has strengthened. In this way, while the programme has not always been in perfect balance, it has been sustained.

Multiple entry points contributed to the development of Bangladesh's MR Policy and Programme in the 1970s: (1) Bangladesh was a new country identifying with secularism in which the political will to prevent births to women who had been raped during the liberation war was stronger than anti-abortion sentiment; (2) The international concern to limit population growth was punctuated by the Bangladesh famine of 1974: this yielded a sustained interest in uterine evacuation as a back-up method to contraception; (3) Manual vacuum aspiration technology had recently been developed; (4) A cadre of newly-trained and influential medical doctors advocated for abortion law reform; and (5) USAID, a leading donor, provided financial and technical support for the programme through the international NGO The Pathfinder Fund.

Several of these entry points are currently at play in many countries in the world – a population and rights agenda; the introduction of the medical abortion technology with mifepristone and misoprostol; and increasing levels of training of mid-level providers for basic health services. These provide an opportunity to develop coalitions to introduce life-saving reproductive health and rights policies and services. Another entry point – national, regional and global collaborations among advocates, service providers, policy-makers, researchers and donors – can be useful in sharing strategies and maintaining momentum to meet the reproductive rights agenda of ICPD in 1994, and to meet Millennium Development Goal 5, to reduce maternal mortality by 75% between 1990 and 2015.

Until the societal barriers to safe MR services are removed, clandestine abortion will continue to result in inexcusably high rates of abortion-related morbidity and mortality, particularly among the poor and less educated. Addressing gender and socioeconomic inequalities that limit women's knowledge of and ability to access the safe MR services to which they are entitled, will result in further reductions in abortion-related mortality. Broad-based, multisectoral partnerships between the government and NGOs are required to regain the innovative spirit of the early days of Bangladesh's MR Programme. This will enable a unified voice for gender equity that will support a call for reproductive rights, including equitable access among women to safe MR services.

Acknowledgements

The authors are particularly indebted to Gabrielle Ross who has carefully analysed Bangladesh's MR Programme in her professional career and academic work, and provided comments on an early draft of this manuscript; also to Trude Bennett, Shelley Goldman, and Reena Yasmin for their reviews of earlier versions of this paper. Any errors are the fault of the authors alone.

References

1. Ahmed J and Afroze D (2006). *BWHC: annual report 2005.* Dhaka, Bangladesh Women's Health Coalition (2006).

2. Ahmed MK, Van Ginneken J, Razzaque A (2005). Factors associated with adolescent abortion in a rural area of Bangladesh. *Tropical Medicine and International Health*, 10:198–205.

3. Akhter HH (1988). Abortion in Bangladesh. In: Sachdev P. (ed.) *International handbook on abortion.* Westport, Connecticut, Greenwood Press.

4. Akhter HH (2001). Midlevel providers in menstrual regulation care: the Bangladesh experience. In: Johnston HB, K Otsea (eds.) *Expanding access: advancing the role of midlevel providers in menstrual regulation and elective abortion care.* Chapel Hill, NC, Ipas.

5. Ali MS et al. (1978). *Report on legal aspects of population planning in Bangladesh.* Dacca, Bangladesh Institute of Law and International Affairs.

6. Amin R et al. (1989). Menstrual regulation training and service programs in Bangladesh: results from a national survey. *Studies in Family Planning*, 20:102–106.

7. Amin S (1996). Menstrual regulation in Bangladesh. IUSSP Seminar on Socio-cultural and Political Aspects of Abortion from an Anthropological Perspective. Trivandrum, Kerala, India.

8. Bangladesh Association for Prevention of Septic Abortion (2006). *Annual report of BAPSA: July 2005 to June 2006.* Dhaka, BAPSA.

9. Bates L et al. (2003). From the home to the clinic and from family planning to family health. *International Family Planning Perspectives*, 29:88–94.

10. Begum S, Kamal H, Kamal G (1987). *Evaluation of MR services in Bangladesh.* Dhaka, Bangladesh, Bangladesh Association for the Prevention of Septic Abortion.

11. Bhatia S, Faruque AS, Chakraborty J (1980). Assessing menstrual regulation performed by paramedics in rural Bangladesh. *Studies in Family Planning*, 11:213–218.

12. Bhuiya AU, Aziz A, Chowdhury M (2001). Ordeal of women for induced abortion in a rural area of Bangladesh. *Journal of Health and Population Nutrition*, 19:281–290.

13. Blair H (2005). Civil society and pro-poor initiatives in rural Bangladesh: finding a workable strategy. *World Development*, 33:921–936.

14. Blane J and Friedman M (1990). *Mexico City policy implementation study*. Arlington, VA, Population Technical Assistance Project Occasional Papers.

15. Brownmiller S (1975). *Against our will: men, women, and rape*. New York, Simon and Schuster.

16. Caldwell B et al. (1999). Pregnancy termination in a rural subdistrict of Bangladesh: a microstudy. *International Family Planning Perspectives*, 25:34–37 & 43.

17. Chakraborty N et al. (2003). Determinants of the use of maternal health services in rural Bangladesh. *Health Promotion International*, 18:327–337.

18. Chaudhury RH (1975). Attitudes of some elites towards introduction of abortion as a method of family planning in Bangladesh. *Bangladesh Development Studies*, 3:479–494.

19. Chaudhury RH (1980). Attitudes towards legislation of abortion among a cross-section of women in metropolitan Dacca. *Journal of Biosocial Science*, 12:417–428.

20. Chowdhury M et al. (2007). Determinants of reduction in maternal mortality in Matlab, Bangladesh: a 30-year cohort study. *The Lancet*, 370:1320–1328.

21. Chowdhury SNM, Moni D, Sarkar T (2003). *A situation analysis of the Bangladesh National Menstrual Regulation Programme*. London, Reproductive Health Alliance.

22. Crane BB and Dusenberry J (2004). Power and politics in international funding for reproductive health: the US Global Gag Rule. *Reproductive Health Matters*, 12:128–137.

23. Dixon-Mueller R (1988). Innovations in reproductive health care: menstrual regulation policies and programs in Bangladesh. *Studies in Family Planning*, 19:129–140.

24. Donaldson PJ and Tsui AO (1990). The international family planning movement. *Population Bulletin*, 45;1–46.

25. Drummond W (1971). Raped Bengalis called heroes. *New York Post*, 22 December, USA.

26. Ekwempu C (1990). Uterine aspiration using the Karman cannula and syringe. *Tropical Journal of Obstetrics and Gynaecology*, 8:37–38.

27. Faisel A et al. (2004). Strengthening HIV/AIDS prevention through multisectoral planning in Bangladesh. International Conference on HIV/AIDS. Bangkok, Thailand, 11–16 July 2004.

28. Germain A (1997). Addressing the demographic imperative through health, empowerment and rights: ICPD implementation in Bangladesh. *Health Transition Review*, 4:33–36.

29. Government of the People's Republic of Bangladesh (1976). *Bangladesh National Population Policy: an outline*. Dhaka, Government of the People's Republic of Bangladesh, Population Control and Family Planning Division.

30. Hossain A (2008). Why health and rights? *Health and rights: working for sexual and reproductive health and rights*, 1:1.

31. Islam A and Tahir M (2002). Health sector reform in South Asia: new challenges and constraints. *Health Policy*, 60:151–169.

32. Islam MM, Rob U, Chakraborty N (2004). Menstrual regulation practices in Bangladesh: an unrecognized form of contraception. *Asia-Pacific Population Journal*, 19:75–99.

33. Johnston HB (1999). *Induced abortion in the developing world: evaluating an indirect estimation technique*. Baltimore, Maryland, Johns Hopkins University, Department of Population Dynamics (unpublished dissertation).

34. Johnston HB (2004). *Evaluation of the Swedish support to the menstrual regulation programme of Bangladesh, June 2003 June 2004*, Dhaka, The Swedish International Development Cooperation Agency (Sida).

35. Karman H (1972). The paramedic abortionist. *Clinical Obstetrics and Gynaecology*, 15:379–387.

36. Khan AK (2002). Obstetric complications: the health care seeking behaviour and cost pressure generated from it in rural Bangladesh. *Mymensingh Medical Journal*, 11:110–112.

37. Khan AR (2000). History of menstrual regulation in Bangaldesh. In: *National reproductive health profile of Bangladesh*. New Delhi, World Health Organization, South-East Asia Regional Office.

38. Killingsworth J et al. (1999). Unofficial fees in Bangladesh: price, equity and institutional issues. *Health Policy and Planning* 14:152–163.

39. Lakshminaranayan R (2007). *Populations issues in the 21st century: the role of the World Bank. Health Nutrition and Population Discussion Paper*. Washington DC, The World Bank.

40. Lee K et al. (1995). *Population policies and programmes: determinants and consequences in eight developing countries*. London, London School of Hygiene and Tropical Medicine.

41. Maloney C et al. (1981). *Beliefs and fertility in Bangladesh*. Dhaka, Bangladesh, International Centre for Diarrhoeal Disease Research, Bangladesh.

42. Ministry of Health and Population Control (1978). *Bangladesh fertility survey: 1975–1976: first report*. Dhaka, Government of the People's Republic of Bangladesh and the World Fertility Survey.

43. Ministry of Law, Justice, and Parliamentary Affairs (1977). *The British Penal Code of 1860. First Edition, Volume 1, ACT 1836–1871, Modified 30/6/1977*. Dacca, Government of the People's Republic of Bangladesh

44. Mookherjee N (2008). Gendered embodiments: mapping the body-politic of the raped woman and the nation in Bangladesh. *Feminist Review*, 88:36–53.

45. National Institute of Population Research and Training (NIPORT), Mitra and Associates, et al. (2007). *Bangladesh Demographic and Health Survey 2007, preliminary report*. Dhaka, Bangladesh and Calverton, Maryland (USA), National Institute of Population Research and Training, Mitra and Associates, and ORC Macro.

46. Oliveras E et al. (2008). *Situation analysis of unsafe abortion and menstrual regulation in Bangladesh*. Dhaka, ICDDR,B.

47. Paulin F and Ahsan SK (2003). *Swedish support to the Menstrual Regulation Programme of Bangladesh*. Dhaka, Embassy of Sweden.

48. Piet-Pelon NJ (1998). *Menstrual regulation impact on reproductive health in Bangladesh: a literature review*. Dhaka, Bangladesh, Population Council.

49. Population Control and Family Planning Division (1979). *Memo No. 5-14/MCH-FP/Trg./79/M.R. Program*. Dhaka, Government of the People's Republic of Bangladesh.

50. Potts M and Diggory PEA (1977). *Abortion*. Cambridge, Cambridge University Press.

51. Rahman M, Davanzo J, Razzaque A (2001). Do better family planning services reduce abortion in Bangladesh? *Lancet*, 358(9287):1051–1056.

52. Reproductive Health Services Training and Education Programme (2006). *RHSTEP annual report: July 2004–June 2005*. Dhaka, Reproductive Health Services Training and Education Programme (RHSTEP).

53. Ross GC (2002). *Sustaining menstrual regulation policy: a case study of the policy process in Bangladesh*. London, University of London, London School of Hygiene and Tropical Medicine.

54. Schuler SR and Hossain Z (1998). Family planning clinics through women's eyes and voices: a case study from rural Bangladesh. *International Family Planning Perspectives*, 24:170–175, 205.

55. Schuler SR, Bates LM, Islam KM (2002). Paying for reproductive health services in Bangladesh; intersections between cost, quality and culture. *Health Policy and Planning*, 17:273–280.

56. Schurmann AT and Mahmud S (2009). Civil society, health, and social exclusion in Bangladesh. *Journal of Health Population and Nutrition*, 27:536–544

57. Singh S et al.(1997). Estimating the level of abortion in the Philippines and Bangladesh. *International Family Planning Perspectives*, 23:100–107, 144.

58. Warriner IK et al. (2006). Rates in complication in first-trimester manual vacuum aspiration abortion done by doctors and mid-level providers in South Africa and Vietnam: a randomised controlled equivalence trial. *The Lancet*, 368:1939–40.

59. White H (2007). The Bangladesh health SWAP: experience of a new aid instrument in practice. *Development Policy Review*, 25:451-72.

60. World Health Organization (2003). *Safe abortion: technical and policy guidance for health systems*. Geneva, World Health Organization.

61. World Health Organization (2007a). *Unsafe abortion – global and regional estimates of the incidence of unsafe abortion and associated mortality in 2003*. 5th edition. Geneva, World Health Organization.

62. World Health Organization (2007b). *Maternal mortality in 2005: estimates developed by WHO, UNICEF, UNFPA, and the World Bank*. Geneva, World Health Organization.

Youth for youth—a model for youth suicide prevention

3

Case study of the Assembly of Manitoba Chiefs Youth Council and Secretariat

Stephanie Sinclair,[1] Amanda Meawasige,[1] Kathi Avery Kinew[1,*]

[1] Assembly of Manitoba Chiefs

[*] Corresponding author: kathiaverykinew@manitobachiefs.com

Abstract

This case study describes the journey of indigenous youth in developing, implementing and evaluating a First Nations suicide prevention strategy in Manitoba. The method of analysis was based on the cultural teaching of First Nations people in Manitoba, that is, thoughts conceived within the traditional way of life by the Cree, Dakota, Dene, Ojibway and Oji-Cree peoples. The aim of the youth suicide prevention initiative was to reclaim and restore the identity, culture, language, history, relationships and spirit of self-determination that rightfully belongs to the First Nations of Manitoba. The theoretical and operational framework of the actual youth interventions and implementation were based upon the traditional First Nations values of restoring health as 'life in balance' in First Nations youth and communities. Four key periods of intervention, in which the 'youth-for-youth model' was pursued and tested included (1) organizing and expanding the youth network, and identifying suicide prevention as a priority, (2) training and adapting an effective intervention model through community development, cultural respect and youth leadership development; (3) building cultural identity and developing the community through youth workshops, and Elder and Youth gatherings; and (4) raising awareness among adult leadership within First Nations, federal and provincial governments as well as the private sector to build youth strengths and obtain resources. The themes that emerged were related to the youth-for-youth leadership model, which provided the strength to overcome barriers and a way to implement the changes the youth identified as needed. The youth worked on many levels simultaneously to achieve the goals, engaging with key stakeholders, leadership and government agencies, and advocating for what the youth wanted. The case study describes the processes involved in empowering youth, managing intersectoral processes and managing policy change. It demonstrates that youth suicide prevention strategies are successful when the youth are the leaders. The report is written from the perspective of the two youth suicide prevention coordinators.

3.1 Background

History and terminology

The First Peoples of Canada, or "Indians" as they were originally described, were constitutionally separated from the other citizens of the country in 1867 and came under federal government jurisdiction through the Indian Act of 1876. At this time, all of these peoples, some hunter-gatherers, some agriculturalists, were moved onto small tracts of non-arable land called reserves, which were and are far removed from the mainstream population. While most services for Canadians are provided under provincial jurisdiction, the First Nations remain under federal jurisdiction.

The term "indigenous" refers to First Nations, Inuit and Métis peoples; 80% of these are First Nations. The term First Nations citizens will be used throughout to distinguish them from First Nations which are separate and distinct Nations.

Inequity and suicide

Suicide was rare among the indigenous people of Canada before European contact (White and Jodin, 2003). However, suicide has become a major cause of death among First Nations youth in the past four decades. The suicide rate for indigenous people is three times that of the general Canadian population (Royal Commission on Aboriginal Peoples, 1996). The suicide rate for First Nations people aged 10–25 years is as much as eight times higher than that of non-First Nations youth (Health Canada, 2002). While there is much variation in suicide rates across First Nations, the overall rates are high. This immeasurable tragedy of the loss of youth and their future potential has had a ripple effect on families and communities, and also demonstrates a pronounced inequity in Canada. In the Province of Manitoba, the suicide rates have remained consistently high and have been increasing over the years (Office of the Chief Medical Examiner, 2003–2008).

Unfortunately, statistics do not provide an accurate picture of the problem of suicide among First Nations people due to the fact that in the Province of Manitoba, the Chief Medical Examiner does not determine race at the time of death. Therefore, many of the deaths by suicide in the rural areas and cities have not been classified as those of First Nations people. This is a fundamental point to consider, with urban centres having large First Nations populations. Furthermore, deaths may be classified as accidental rather than suicide, resulting in underreporting of cases. Beyond the actual deaths by suicide, there are no systematic and consistent means of data collection. Therefore, the number of suicide attempts and incidents of suicidal ideation are not captured.

First Nations people have the worst socioeconomic conditions in Canada and, hence, the poorest health status in the country (Assembly of First Nations, 2007). Indigenous people have a life expectancy that is approximately seven years shorter than the average Manitoban. The difference increases to over 10 years for on-reserve First Nations citizens (Martens et al., 2002). According to the United Nations Human Development Index (HDI), First Nations rank 68th among 174 nations. Canada has dropped from being the best country in the world in which to live to the eighth due, in part, to the housing and health conditions of First Nations (Assembly of First Nations, 2007).

Social determinants

Context and position

The history of Canada includes extensive attempts to colonize First Nations people, the results of which still continue to dominate their lives today. The intent of the Indian Act, 1876 was to assimilate First Nations citizens into society, and was pursued at many levels. First Nations land was appropriated and reserves were established, residential schools were developed through a collective effort between the church and the Canadian government, and cultural and spiritual practices were outlawed. The Indian Act, 1876 controlled and still controls many aspects of the lives of First Nations citizens, including health services, social services, taxation; livelihood such as hunting and fishing rights; citizenship including voting rights; and organization and governance structures (Indian Act [RSC, 1985, c. I-5]).

The government's designation of "Indian" became one of the most divisive aspects of the Indian Act, 1876. First, it divided the Canadian indigenous peoples – the First Nations, Inuit and Métis – into an arbitrary but devastating class structure. The Act also created divisions

based on urban versus reserve residence and gender. Further, it created a divide between level of government – federal and provincial – which resulted in a continued jurisdictional debate over who has the responsibility for the social and health concerns of First Nations people (Smye, 2008).

Differential exposure

The history of First Nations people is marked by cultural oppression and forced assimilation since the point of European contact, and can be regarded as one source of the high rates of mental health and social issues present among First Nations people (Kirmayer et al., 2003). The cultural changes resulting from assimilation practices have impacted the genders differently in terms of continuity of roles. There has been more continuity in the social roles for women, who focus on child-rearing, as well as work and school. In contrast, First Nations men have experienced a profound disjuncture between traditional roles and the opportunities in contemporary society, in that traditionally men were involved in protection and subsistence activities for the community. The role of First Nations men has failed to be recreated into one that promotes a positive identity. The high suicide rate among young men can be related to this loss of valued status within First Nations communities (Kirmayer et al., 2000).

Labour force participation of First Nations citizens is 47% compared to 68% for non-First Nations citizens in Canada. In Manitoba, the non-First Nations unemployment rate is 6%, while it is 31% among First Nations citizens (Health Canada, 2009). In addition, average income and home ownership rates among First Nations citizens are considerably lower than those in the general population (Health Canada, 2009). More than half of on-reserve First Nations youth aged 20–24 years have not graduated from high school. In Manitoba as a whole, the rate of First Nations youth who did not graduate is 71% compared with 16% for all Canadians (Mendelson, 2006). This is of significant concern as indigenous people make up 12% of the total population of Manitoba and 20% of the school-aged population.

Residential schools have been the most cited cause of mental health concerns of First Nations citizens (Smye and Mussell, 2001). Residential schools were meant to separate First Nations children from their parents and assimilate them into the mainstream population. Children as young as three years of age were forcibly removed from their families and placed in these institutional environments. The residential schools were located in isolated areas and the children were allowed little or no contact with their families and communities; there was a strict regime of discipline and constant surveillance over every aspect of their lives. The children were forbidden to look or act like a First Nations person, which included speaking First Nations languages, dressing in First Nations clothes, eating First Nations foods, and practising First Nations spiritual beliefs. Physical, sexual, emotional and spiritual abuse was rampant in residential schools. Many First Nations children died, usually from starvation or tuberculosis and, in most cases, their families were never notified and these children were buried in unmarked graves. In 1953, at the height of the residential school era, there were over 11 000 students attending these schools (Kirmayer et al. 2003). The majority of residential schools ceased to exist by the 1980s but, since the beginning of the 1960s, a new wave of assimilation practices had been developed. For 30 years, large numbers of First Nations children were taken from their families and communities and placed in state care or adopted to non-First Nations families (International Conference on Ethics, 2007).

Intergenerational or historical trauma is a phenomenon that occurs when a trauma is not dealt with in previous generations but has to be dealt with in subsequent generations, and becomes more severe each time it is passed on. First Nations healers have observed and treated this condition, while referring to it as unresolved grief over generations (Kinew T, personal communication, 1989).

There are several indications that historical trauma affects the psychological, social, economic, intellectual, political, physical and spiritual aspects of First Nations people, and is linked with health, social issues and mental health problems, hypertension, heart disease and diabetes (Bullock, 1999). Psychosocial issues resulting from historical trauma include poverty, crime and violence, addiction to alcohol and other substances, depression, suicide and overeating (Nebelkopf and Phillips, 2004). Recent research has documented "cultural continuity as a hedge against suicide", noting that in the province of British Columbia, for instance, First Nations populations with more self-governance and activity in living their culture have few or no suicides (Chandler and Lalonde, 1998).

Differential vulnerability

Some wonder what makes today's First Nations youth so much more vulnerable to suicide than mainstream youth in Canada. First Nations youth feel the burden of oppression every day and experience domestic violence, death, suicide and poverty at an early age. Many are raised in single-parent homes, by grandparents or other family members; or they are raised in the state Child and Family Services system and are moved frequently. Many First Nations youth grow up without a sense of cultural identity and spirituality, without ever realizing that the deep roots of what they experience lie within the history of colonization, and government policies and actions. Lacking this historical knowledge and understanding, many First Nations youth find themselves helpless and without hope (National Aboriginal Youth Strategy – Manitoba Youth Consultation [2004], unpublished report).

The separation of children from their families and communities has had a devastating, long-lasting effect on the First Nations people. Generations of First Nations people did not learn family and community values. Individuals often feel stuck between two worlds, not belonging to either, causing identity confusion, frequently leading to depression, substance abuse and sometimes suicide. The intergenerational effects of residential school can be seen within families; the legacy of the children who had little to no memories of parenting from their birth families but instead grew up in institutions. This has resulted in a generation of First Nations citizens with no knowledge of child-rearing but who knew instead the punitive experiences of residential schools—lack of warmth and intimacy; repeated physical and sexual abuse; and systematic devaluing of First Nations identity (Kirmayer et al., 2003).

Many First Nations citizens in Manitoba live in Third World conditions with lack of adequate housing, employment and educational opportunities. The First Nations youth on-reserve have very little access to recreational facilities or organized sports. In urban settings, First Nations people face poverty, racism, discrimination, gangs, violence, and very few complete their education (National Aboriginal Youth Strategy – Manitoba First Nations Youth Consultation [2004], unpublished report).

Differential health-care outcomes

One of the most prevalent issues facing the indigenous people in the field of mental health is the lack of knowledge about the type of treatments and services that best meet the needs of indigenous clients (Thomas and Bellefeuille, 2006). The belief systems of indigenous people regarding mental health and healing have been largely ignored and often rendered invisible in developing policies, programmes and services. The result is that the mental health-care needs of indigenous people have not been recognized and met (Smye and Mussell, 2001).

Mental health services that are based on western concepts of mental health and illness have been identified as largely ineffective in responding to the needs of indigenous people (McCormick, 1998; Warry, 1998). Therefore, it is not surprising that indigenous people tend to not use the mental health services provided (McCormick, 1996; Pederson et al., 1990) and, once services are accessed, approximately one-half of the clients drop out of treatment (Sue, 1981; Duran and Duran, 1995). One of the consequences of this cultural blindness is that many indigenous people do not receive adequate mental health services and instead end up in correctional institutions (Waldram, 1997).

Institutional framework

The Assembly of Manitoba Chiefs (AMC) is an organization of the leaders of 64 First Nations across the province of Manitoba, situated in the middle of Canada, including prairies, parklands, boreal forest and tundra in the far north. Formed in 1989 as a reorganization of earlier First Nations political advocacy organizations, the AMC is dedicated to strengthening, securing and implementing the Treaty and inherent rights of the First Nations people, and to improving the socioeconomic status of the people's everyday lives (www.manitobachiefs.com).

The AMC adult leadership passed a resolution in 1998 to establish a Manitoba First Nations Youth Advisory Council (MFN YAC) to ensure a voice for the youth at the decision-making table, and to undertake initiatives focused on the youth and, in 1999, to establish a Youth Secretariat. Jason Whitford, an Ojibway from Sandy Bay First Nations, became the first Regional Youth Coordinator at AMC.

The MFN YAC is made up of First Nations youth throughout the province, representing the five language groups: Dene, Oji-Cree, Ojibway, Cree and Dakota. From the beginning, the Regional Youth Coordinator ensured that the AMC Youth Secretariat and the MFN YAC followed the traditional cultural ways of First Nations people. Each meeting begins with a prayer, smudging with indigenous plants of sage or sweetgrass, reading of the Traditional Code of Ethics based on the traditional cultural teachings of values, and with roundtable

introductions before starting any discussions. Regional youth gatherings are three-day events where Youth Representatives from throughout Manitoba assemble to discuss common topics. Each gathering is attended by 150–200 First Nations youth from the 64 First Nations and elections are held for the positions of Regional Youth Leaders and National Assembly of First Nations Youth Representatives, who participate in committee meetings and make presentations to provincial and federal politicians to urge action on First Nations youth concerns. For many, this is their first engagement in a political process.

Key interventions

The essential aim of the Youth Suicide Prevention Initiative is to reclaim and restore the identity, culture, language, history, relationships and spirit of self-determination that rightfully belongs to the First Nations of Manitoba.

Leadership development

From the beginning, the programme emphasized, encouraged, supported and trained young leaders "not for tomorrow – but for today" to promote and revive traditional roles, cultural values and to work with the Elders in rejuvenating the traditional approaches to healing, as well as to provide a voice in the wider political debates on issues related to First Nations youth. The early experience was used to formulate the Youth Leadership Development Curriculum, an eight-week training programme with four components: cultural, economic, political and social (CEPS) piloted in 2005 and continued thereafter with on-and-off funding from the federal department of Health (Health Canada).

The Youth Suicide Prevention Strategy

The AMC Youth Secretariat staff developed a culturally specific programme with four components, leaving communities with a positive plan of action.

1   *Interagency communication and coordination*
- Bringing together the various key agencies and programmes within a geographical area to facilitate a coordinated response. The process usually entails mapping and activation of formal and informal community resources as well as guidance for the actions of all local agencies following, for example, a youth suicide or suicide attempt.

2   Applied suicide intervention skills training (ASIST) for community caregivers developed by Livingworks Inc., Calgary, Alberta

- This workshop provides information to prevent the immediate risk of suicide with emphasis on suicide first-aid, helping a person at risk to stay safe and seek further help, including how to link people with community resources.

3   Grief and loss of cultural awareness and tradition focusing on healing after suicide and dealing with grief and loss

- A meeting with youth and Elders from the community to discuss their deep feelings and learn how traditional healing and teaching can help them. Depending on the community, the Elders may lead ceremonies grounded in traditional First Nations cultures and history, which can assist individuals in moving toward a state of mental well-being.

4   Developing a community suicide prevention strategy for "planning alternative tomorrows with hope" (PATH)

- Taking a community development approach, residents identify strengths and beauty in their community, as well as problems that need to be resolved, and work together on a plan of action. These plans can take broad upstream approaches, e.g. evolving around making improvements to the quality of life for community members. The aim is to leave the community with a sense of hope and empowerment, as well as the responsibility to act.

Each of the First Nations that the AMC Youth Secretariat has worked with is different in terms of its infrastructure, religious and spiritual beliefs, language and community support. The usual process is that a First Nation contacts the AMC Youth Secretariat who discusses the needs of the community, the current situation and what they would like to accomplish. The Secretariat then works with the identified community liaison person to organize the events, recruit participants and coordinate on-site activities. This preparatory process is an important and integral part of the programme in order to ensure that the First Nation has the ownership before, during and after the interventions.

Objective of the case study

The objective of this case study is to document and analyse, from a social determinants and community perspective, the *experience of implementing* the suicide prevention programme. Its aim is to draw lessons that could be useful to other communities trying to address situations similar to those faced by the First Nations youth in Canada, as well as for those who want to provide financial, moral or political support to First Nations and all Indigenous peoples. Of the broad WHO priority public health conditions (PPHC) case study themes, special emphasis is paid to scaling up, adjusting design, managing policy change and sustainability.

3.2 Methods

The focus of this single-case explanatory study (Yin, 2003) is on the experiences of implementing the programme with particular emphasis on the "how" and "why" processes of the four themes, i.e. scaling up, adjusting design, managing policy change and sustainability.

The data for the analysis comprise the analysis of social determinants at play, as presented in the introduction to this chapter, and process data from the period of implementation.

To present the process data, a life-history approach (Taylor and Bogdan, 1998) has been taken, organized around four distinct periods of the programme's life, i.e. the beginning, reaching out, the uphill path, and speaking truth to power. To support the memories of the authors, annual reports of activities, evaluations by participants in workshops, databases of trainees, surveys, minutes from various meetings and briefing notes were consulted. This "first-person" approach has been taken rather than the conventional approach of presenting the raw data as extracted directly from the sources in order to emphasize the dynamics and continuum over time of the events that shaped the evolution of the programme. The life-history approach also provides a more readable and cohesive presentation of the events.

A critical issue in taking such an approach is its construct validity, i.e. whether it provides a correct account of the reality (Yin, 2003). In order to validate the findings, i.e. the life history and the analysis, the draft report of the study was reviewed by the MFN YAC members as well as the AMC, and their feedback incorporated into the final study report, on the basis of which this chapter is prepared.

3.3 Findings – life history

"The beginning"

Youth suicide became a priority for the AMC Youth Secretariat when the federal government rolled out its National Aboriginal Youth Strategy and funded consultations across the country. In 1999, the AMC Youth Secretariat staff, led by Jason Whitford, interviewed over 900 First Nations youth throughout Manitoba. These youth overwhelmingly identified youth suicide as their number one health concern. They were tired of being consistently devastated by losing another brother, sister, cousin or friend to suicide, week after week, in what seemed like an endless stream, from community to community. Further ideas on how to develop a youth suicide prevention initiative came from the MFN YAC and youth attending the regional youth gatherings. Evaluations from these gatherings revealed a desire to learn more about the history of First Nations people by examining traditional roles and cultural values, and working with the Elders in rejuvenating the traditional approaches to healing. Thus, the Youth Secretariat hosts annual summer gatherings in partnership with a First Nation on traditional territory, often sacred ceremonial land. Elders from each of the five language and cultural territories share their traditional ecological knowledge and science with the youth, and train them to become leaders, "not for tomorrow, but for today".

The Youth Suicide Prevention Initiative (YSPI) became a reality in October 2002, when a YSPI Coordinator, Stephanie Sinclair, was hired to work with the AMC Youth Secretariat and AMC Health Department. The YSPI Coordinator researched different intervention models and found that the ASIST programme best suited the needs.

In 2003, the Chiefs formalized an agreement that the youth were the leaders of the YSPI. Then, Grand Chief Dennis White Bird ensured that the youth took the lead in any negotiations and discussions to address youth suicide, allowing for the empowerment of the Youth Secretariat. Much effort was involved in gaining the Chiefs' understanding and support. While the Grand Chief and some leaders and Elders recognized the leadership role of the youth, others were reluctant to have the heavy burden of suicide prevention placed on young shoulders. It seemed that such adult leaders did not realize that the youth already felt the burden, and that they needed to take action to help their brothers and sisters before any more tried this escape route.

In addition, government funding agencies were unsure of the ability of youth to take leadership responsibility. Initially, Health Canada's First Nations and Inuit Health Branch (FNIHB) funded the position of the YSPI Coordinator for six months only, to undertake a limited project to examine FNIHB data related to suicide attempts and completed suicides, to review the system, and make recommendations for improving the response. As a result, the YSPI Coordinator position was funded by FNIHB during 2003–04, and the AMC Youth Secretariat was able to conduct three ASIST training sessions with hired consultants.

"Reaching out"

Momentum was gained after the Regional Youth Coordinator, Jason Whitford and the YSPI Coordinator, Stephanie Sinclair became certified ASIST trainers in November 2003. This reduced the costs of the training, allowing more communities to be covered. The youth suicide prevention strategy at this stage focused on training youth and people who worked directly with youth. All evaluations were overwhelmingly positive, but recommended that the training materials and programme be more culturally appropriate.

In March 2004, the Youth Secretariat organized a youth conference in a Manitoba First Nation with a suicide prevention focus. This community had suffered the loss of a 15-year-old boy just days earlier. During the opening, the boy's aunt spoke. She shared her feelings of the inconceivable loss of her nephew and the reality the family now faced in going through life without him. She encouraged the youth to seek out help in times of need, to look after one another and recognize that suicide was not the answer. Her willingness to speak set the tone for the conference and gave permission to everyone to openly and honestly talk about suicide. The conference had Elders as resource people, ensuring that Ojibway, Cree, Oji-Cree, Dakota and Dene cultures and ceremonies were integral parts of the meeting.

The youth present provided feedback on what they believed were the causes and possible solutions for the problem of suicide among their peers. The causes identified included: the impact of colonization on First Nations families including Indian Residential Schools as a main contributor; loss of one or both parents; loss of parental communication skills with children; loss of culture and identity; lack of support for children and youth in the family and community; and dysfunctional family environments. The solutions identified focused on identity and culture, reclaiming control and relationships for themselves within their family and community.

This, together with experiences from conducting the three-day ASIST training, led AMC youth to develop a five-day expanded programme to include healing based on culture and tradition, and to leave First Nations with a positive development plan for a better future. These additions were aimed at not only providing helpful tools for the participants but also as an important way to empower the community, and to debrief the Youth Secretariat staff from their role as facilitators. Amanda Meawasige from Migizi Sagai'gan Nation, YSPI Worker (2004–2008) together with Jason began to roll out the expanded programme.

The expanded training was piloted in May 2004 in a First Nation which had high rates of death by suicide and numerous attempted suicides, and was now facing a group of young girls who had formed a suicide pact. FNIHB provided emergency crisis funds for the AMC Youth Secretariat to provide suicide prevention services to this First Nation. Unfortunately, just days prior to the arrival of AMC youth and guests to attend the gathering, one of the girls followed through on the suicide pact and died.

The atmosphere in the First Nation was heavy, but later evaluations showed that the expanded, culturally based programme provided relief to the community, and an ability to plan and take ownership. During the community development phase of the programme, community needs and strengths were identified and an action plan to address all concerns was prepared. The discussions and planning revolved around making basic improvements to the quality of life for community members, including ideas such as community by-laws to control dogs and prevent dog pack attacks, erecting street lights and planning a day for a communitywide clean-up.

At a meeting organized later by a Tribal Council and FNIHB, the Elders presented the AMC Youth Secretariat with an eagle feather for its work on suicide prevention. This is a high honour in all indigenous cultures as it is believed that the eagle flies the highest to speak with and take the people's collective thoughts and prayers to the Creator. The Elders honoured the youth for taking ownership of their issues and working toward solutions for their communities, creating hope for future generations.

As word about the programme began to spread, a waiting list started growing. In response, the Youth Secretariat hosted a "train the trainers" session in partnership with Livingworks Inc. in June 2004. Participants came from urban, rural and isolated communities throughout Manitoba, and included Youth Secretariat staff and MFN YAC members. Twelve First Nations people become certified ASIST trainers, expanding the network of trainers and the reach. As a related strategy to empower First Nations youth, AMC youth Stephanie Sinclair and Kathleen McKay successfully bid for a contract with the Assembly of First Nations to create a youth leadership development curriculum. Their success was largely due to their suicide prevention work as well as their work in the MFN YAC and the inner city Keewatin Youth Initiative (KYI) in Winnipeg. (This programme has been noted by the Senate Committee on Urban Aboriginal Youth as a "best practice" in Canada.) The contract allowed the Youth Secretariat to hire additional staff, including a second youth suicide prevention coordinator to develop an eight-week course comprising CEPS areas. The goal was to develop the next generation of leaders armed with a strong sense of cultural identity and pride. Funded by Health Canada, the CEPS curriculum was piloted in 2005 with 30 participants from across Canada. Evaluation of the pilot was positive and feedback was used to refine the curriculum.

"The uphill path"

The AMC Youth Secretariat had developed a database to keep track of all participants of the suicide prevention programme and proposed to hold a meeting entitled "Caring for the caregivers" to review how the programme had benefited communities and to allow for networking to share experiences. The Youth Secretariat sent its proposal to the FNIHB – Manitoba Region. However, the proposal was rejected and instead, two years later, the FNIHB used the idea and sponsored a conference with the same name and theme, hiring Stephanie Sinclair to coordinate it. The YAC approached the psychiatry department of a local university which was not interested in First Nations-led research, but instead a long-term, positive partnership was formed with a world-renowned psychologist at the University of Victoria in British Columbia.

In September 2004, Health Canada announced funding in the area of Youth Suicide Prevention entitled, "Upstream investments" to reflect and implement the National Aboriginal Youth Suicide Prevention Strategy (NAYSPS).

The goal of this strategy was to increase resilience and reduce the risk of suicide among Indigenous youth by undertaking activities in prevention, early intervention and crisis response. The AMC asked the MFN YAC to review the NAYSPS. The Council found that while most of its own initiatives and philosophy had been adopted and integrated into the national plan, no acknowledgement had been given. Despite the MFN YAC bringing this information to the federal department's attention, no additional citation was made and there was no funding for the AMC Youth Secretariat's suicide prevention work for the fiscal year 2004–2005.

In January 2005, an isolated Manitoba Cree community, accessible only by air, requested the AMC Youth Secretariat to deliver the youth suicide prevention programme and to provide informational presentations at the school level. Because they lacked resources aimed at elementary school-level youth, the AMC Youth facilitators provided workshops only for the middle school level. A letter was sent from the Principal seeking permission from parents to engage their children in discussions around youth suicide and to provide informal intervention training. Once their initial feelings of discomfort dissipated, the youth were very receptive. This first attempt at integration with the education system provided promise for positive interaction between the community health staff and schools in establishing joint action to prevent youth suicide.

Many requests for YAC's services came from various social organizations. While requests from within the city of Winnipeg, where AMC is located, were easy to accommodate, there were requests from non-First Nations schools and organizations outside the city. This is when the Secretariat ran into jurisdictional barriers.

Suicide prevention funding to date, whether for the programme or travel expenses, comes from Health Canada, as a federal obligation to First Nations, but it only funds projects for on-reserve First Nations citizens. Numerous letters and proposals have been sent to the Province of Manitoba requesting travel assistance at the very least, but to no avail. Despite benefiting from the YSPI Coordinator participating in the provincial prevention committee, the province has to date refused to offer any funding for the Coordinator's position or to the AMC Youth programme. The Youth Secretariat does its best to provide services to those who request it, regardless of jurisdiction or ethnic origin. However, again for the fiscal year 2005–2006, core funding for the work was not available.

The NAYSPS funding was managed regionally by FNIHB to develop a process of distributing funding to First Nations and organizations. A working group was created of community representatives, tribal councils, the federal department of Indian and Northern Affairs (INAC), the federal Royal Canadian Mounted Police, FNIHB, Manitoba Health, Manitoba Aboriginal and Northern Affairs, and the AMC Youth Secretariat. The group held its first prioritization meeting in November 2005. The meeting primarily focused on reviewing and familiarizing participants with the NAYSPS, including the objectives, funding breakdowns and discussion on the development of a community-initiated process to distribute resources.

It was clear that there were not enough resources for all communities to receive a meaningful allocation. Therefore, the group proceeded with discussing how to develop a fair process for communities to access the funds and determine which type of activities would be considered for suicide prevention. The NAYSPS criteria stated that communities must demonstrate capacity to develop and deliver suicide prevention programming. This was antithetical to the belief of the Youth Secretariat because the communities with the least capacity were the ones who suffered the most from the epidemic of youth suicide.

However, the meeting supported renewed funding for the AMC Youth Secretariat in 2006–07 to continue with: *creating awareness and understanding on the topic of suicide; research and consultation; resource development; and the work of the First Nations Envisioning Committee and visiting First Nations to facilitate the work necessary to envision a future without suicide.*

The second regional prioritization meeting took place in December 2005 with the same participants. Issues that arose included: proposal process versus application process, the pros and cons associated with each; the establishment of a community-based peer review; determining whether there would be a call for proposals or whether proposals would be accepted on an ongoing basis; budgetary impacts and flexibility; the feasibility of multi-year funding projects; developing a scoring system that would identify community needs; and developing an effective evaluation framework. As several participants voiced concern over the Youth Secretariat's capacity to be a partner in a project of this magnitude, it was suggested that they update the Chiefs' resolution to support their full and meaningful involvement in the delivery of the NAYSPS for First Nations in Manitoba.

"Speaking truth to power"

It looked like a promising time. However, although the national CEPS programme was viewed as a success by all involved, no funding was provided in 2006 and 2007 by Health Canada. Further, government officials opted for frameworks by consultants rather than building on experience gained in community-based programming or recommendations by the youth. The youth, however, accessed funding through another federal department specific to Manitoba and the programme continued. Then, through the advocacy efforts of the youth, Health Canada's regional office notified the Assembly of First Nations Youth Council that it would fund the MFN YAC to revise, edit and enhance the CEPS programme and develop a training of trainers programme. In the meantime, the AMC Youth Secretariat had incorporated the CEPS programme into its KYI. The AMC Youth Secretariat also made it known that the CEPS programme would not be dropped, and that plans to incorporate the training in Manitoba First Nations were a high priority.

The Manitoba First Nations Envisioning Committee was established at the AMC to develop a five-year action plan on suicide prevention with funding from INAC. The work involved the YSPI Coordinator and the Regional Youth Coordinator, Elders and experienced youth suicide prevention counsellors. They developed a five-year plan for educational resources for children and submitted it to the INAC, but it was not approved for funding. INAC instead offered to fund a pre-existing theatre project by Tina Keeper, a famous First Nations actress (later a Member of Parliament). Keeper declined the offer as more was needed than continuing to raise awareness. The Youth Secretariat was frustrated. Every agency contacted to support the Youth for Youth approach, including Manitoba Health, the Winnipeg Regional Health Authority and FNIHB developed paper strategies. Not one would support the ongoing daily activities of the AMC Youth Council and Secretariat.

In January 2006, the YSPI made a presentation to the Chiefs in Assembly, highlighting the work that had been initiated and produced long before the existence of funding. Several Chiefs again questioned the ability of youth to tackle such a massive issue, and the wisdom of placing such a burden on the youth. One prominent Chief of a southern First Nation advised the Assembly to listen to the youth before judging. The YSPI Coordinator and Regional Youth Coordinator then recounted their years of training youth and adults in the ASIST, expanded ASIST and CEPS programmes, as well as their experience in research, policy and proposal development. This illustrated how the youth could be engaged in political processes and also deliver tangible solutions for youth suicide. The Chiefs in Assembly unanimously passed a resolution for the MFN YAC and AMC Youth Secretariat to take a regional and national lead in youth suicide prevention and to support community-based First Nations initiatives.

The YSPI was not funded by the FNIHB Manitoba Region in the fiscal years 2004–2005 and 2005–2006. Funds had to be carried forward from the CEPS contract in order to retain the YSPI Coordinator in 2004–2005. In 2005–2006, the YSPI Coordinator was employed through the KYI, and through sporadic contracts provided by the FNIHB when a community experienced a suicide. Finally, in 2006–2007, funds from the Upstream Investments in Health programme agreed upon in 2004 by First Ministers (Federal, Provincial, Territorial), were made available through FNIHB. The YSPI Coordinator position was funded once again. However, since 2002, the role of the YSPI Coordinator had expanded beyond training and capacity building to include: policy analysis, government relations, advocacy, research projects, and membership in numerous national and provincial suicide prevention committees. Continued lobbying by the AMC Youth Secretariat and Council led Health Canada in 2008 to support on- and off-reserve delivery of the CEPS. It has now been offered several times and further developed

The Manitoba First Nations Youth Suicide Prevention Strategy meaningfully involves youth at all levels of planning and delivery, and has been replicated by two other provinces.

3.4 Discussion

The YSPI has had a significant effect in the time described in this case study, often against difficult odds. While its impact on suicide rates might be difficult to measure, it has had an impact on the ways that youth suicide and its causes are viewed by communities as well as the mainstream Canadian systems. The following discussion will focus on four themes, i.e. adjusting design, managing policy change, scaling up and sustainability.

Adjusting design

One of YSPI's main strengths is its responsiveness and ability to evolve with input from the youth and communities, which is important because First Nations are not a homogeneous group. Although they share some cultural traditions, they also have diverse linguistic, social, economic and geographical conditions, requiring different approaches to prevent suicide. What the youth share is their commitment to youth leadership to find the ways out of suicide – for youth, by youth.

The suicide prevention programme has grown to become, at its core, an open intervention built around the ASIST, complemented by modules specifically tailored to each community. Over time, it has become clearer that the root social determinants of suicide and suicide attempts lie, and must be addressed, not at the individual level but upstream at the community, society and historical levels. This realization has led to the addition of a leadership development programme aimed at equipping young First Nations with the skills and qualities required to influence these upstream social determinants.

The ability to adjust and quickly respond to diverse needs is probably grounded in First Nations' youth ownership of the issue, youth empowerment, and the fact that the YAC cared enough to not give up. Further, the funders of the various activities over the years have allowed the youth secretariat to juggle funds between projects, and the senior AMC management has defended the right of the programme to be judged on results rather than on penny accounting.

Managing policy change

The original objective of the intervention was to "*prevent the immediate risk of suicide*" and "*help a person at risk stay safe*", focusing on the individual rather than on policies. However, the role of the programme and thereby the YSPI Coordinator has evolved over time: "*… beyond training and capacity building to include: policy analysis, government relations, advocacy, research projects, and membership of numerous national and provincial committees …*". The programme has successfully pushed borders for explicit and implicit policies at different levels and fields.

First, it has pushed both the norms and policies regarding where and how the question of suicide can be addressed. It has provided a public forum for families and others to raise and debate their concerns not just to get relief for their grief but also to start taking ownership, and thus feel empowered. A major policy change that might have the most significant impact was to allow suicide to be addressed in schools.

Second, it moved the issue from the micro level – dealing with actual suicides, suicide attempts or "at-risk youth" – to the macro level, encouraging all levels – community, the public, economic and political – to address the social determinants that lead to youth suicide.

Third, it empowered youth to address the issue affecting them. This did not come without difficulty and the battle has not yet been completely won. There was and continues to be resistance both within the established hierarchies of First Nations as well as within mainstream Canadian officialdom towards giving responsibility to the youth. Change would not have been possible without the support of some wise Elders and Chiefs who advocated for the youth.

The strength of the programme in influencing policy processes is that it is rooted in the community and integrates cultural traditions, while at the same time acknowledges some realities of mainstream Canada. It has incrementally moved forward, always based on concrete action and achievements, combined with responsiveness and vision – constantly pushing and advocating. Ideas and approaches have been adopted not only by replication, but also conceptually in strategies and official Canadian approaches to First Nations suicide prevention efforts, although due recognition is not always given.

Scaling up

Since the first ASIST, the programme has considerably increased in volume in terms of both scope and reach. However, demand has continued to exceed capacity. Although additional ASIST facilitators were trained, there were no resources or structures to systematically follow up what they actually did after training. Growth is restricted not only by limitations of financial resources, and by infrastructure and management structures, but also due to the fact that size may distance the programme from the community. To attract additional resources, the programme had to participate in more extra-community relations, for example, with government funding agencies. This will inevitably lead to increased bureaucratization as was obvious during the NAYSPS negotiations. The leadership's attention was diverted from directly addressing community concerns towards "*policy analysis, government relations, advocacy, research projects, and membership of numerous national and provincial committees regarding suicide prevention*".

The scaling-up potential of this type of programme probably lies in learning and adapting best practices.

A strong potential for accelerated scale-up exists in the close ties between the suicide prevention and leadership training (CEPS) programmes. The CEPS programme provides skills and tools and the YSPI provides practice. This basis, grounded in community and tradition, will help young leaders to tackle the upstream social determinants that can only be resolved with the support of mainstream society.

Sustainability

The YSPI has, since inception, received project support from various sources with very little infrastructure funding, barely covering minimum staff salaries. Specific project funding has had to be stretched to cover gaps in core funding. The experience has been that the communities with the greatest needs are also those with the least capacity to address them. A continued inflow of financial resources, encouragement and impetus from outside the concerned communities is required, together with dedicated leaders of all ages from within the community.

The question of sustainability appears to hinge on establishing a functioning interface between an informal and flexible community-based approach and officialdom with its needs for rules, transparency and accountability. The AMC Youth Secretariat could be a model to illustrate the usefulness and feasibility of having one or more intermediaries between the community and the bureaucracy.

While in the short term it is important to sustain some basic organizational structures, sustainability of interventions and impact is important in the long term. For this, the hope is that the new generation of leaders being trained in the CEPS programme will take on the long-term and comprehensive upstream efforts required to repair the damages caused by history.

Limitations of the study

The main limitation of the study lies in it being a single case design that builds on the personal experience and views of the authors. However, while this might be a limitation, it is also its strength, as it provides insight into processes and feelings that are likely to be common in many cases where oppressed people take ownership to change their future. The personal perspective is particularly relevant where there is a fundamental difference in beliefs, values and ways of viewing the world between the community and the mainstream society, including the research community.

3.5 Conclusion

The YSPI provides an example of oppressed peoples who take things in their own hands and make a difference. The case also shows that it is a hard struggle before the efforts pay off. Many battles have to be fought to overcome barriers in both internal and external resistance to change. Sacrifices have to be made at a personal "job-security" level and goodwill has to be mobilized, in particular, at the interface between the community organization and the official system. Suicide is just one symptom of the deeply rooted problems and historical trauma underlying the heavy social problems of today's First Nations. Interventions to prevent suicide among First Nations youth can only scratch the surface, even if they address the social determinants at the levels of differential vulnerability and exposure. However, the question of suicide can be used as an entry point for addressing the far-reaching social problems that exist among the First Nations people. In the longer run, the CEPS youth leadership programme may prove its worth in making the changes required at the level of context and position to effectively address the root causes of youth suicide among the First Nations people of Canada.

References

1. White J and Jodoin N (2003). *Aboriginal youth: a manual of promising suicide prevention strategies.* Calgary, Alberta, Center for Suicide Prevention.

2. Royal Commission on Aboriginal Peoples (1996). *Report of the Royal Commission on Aboriginal Peoples.* Ottawa, Ontario.

3. *Acting on what we know: preventing youth suicide in first nations. The report of the Advisory Group on Suicide Prevention* (2002). Ottawa, First Nation Inuit Health Branch, Health Canada.

4. Office of the Chief Medical Examiner (Deaths by suicide in the Province of Manitoba). 2003–2008. Data shared with AMC Youth Council with permission of the CME.

5. *Assembly of First Nations, Making Poverty History Campaign (2007). The 9 billion dollar myth exposed: why First Nation's poverty endures.* Ottawa, Assembly of First Nations. Available at: www.afn.ca (accessed on 13 March 2010)

6. Martens PJ et al., Health and Information Research Committee (Assembly of Manitoba Chiefs) (2002). *Health and health care use for registered First Nations' people living in Manitoba, a population study.* Manitoba, Manitoba Center for Health Policy.

7. *Indian Act (R.S., 1985, c. I-5)*. Government of Canada. Available at: http://www.canlii.org/en/ca/laws/stat/rsc-1985-c-i-5/31743/rsc-1985-c-i-5.html#history (accessed on 13 March 2010).

8. Smye V (2008). *Access issues for aboriginal people seeking primary care services in an urban center.*Ottawa, Canadian Institutes of Health Research.

9. Kirmayer L, Simpson C and Cargo M (2003). Healing traditions: culture, community and mental health promotion with Canadian Aboriginal peoples. *Australian Psychiatry*, 11:S15–S23.

10. Kirmayer L et al. (2000). Psychological distress among the Cree of James Bay. *Trans-cultural Psychiatry*, 37:35–36.

11. *A statistical profile on the health of First Nations in Canada: determinants of health 1999 to 2003* (2009). First Nations, Inuit and Aboriginal Health Branch, Health Canada. Available at: http://www.hc-sc.gc.ca/fniah-spnia/pubs/aborig-autoch/2009-stats-profil/index-eng.php (accessed on 13 March 2010).

12. Mendelson M (2006). *Aboriginal peoples post secondary education in Canada.*] Ottawa, Caledon Institute for Public Policy.

13. Smye V and Mussell B (2001). *Aboriginal mental health: what works best. Discussion Paper.* Vancouver, BC, Mental Health Evaluation and Community Consultation Unit, University of British Columbia.

14. Assembly of First Nations, National Chief Phil Fontaine: presentation to the International Conference on Ethics (2007). Gatineau, Quebec, AFN Policy Forum/Special Chiefs Assembly, May 22, 2007. Available at: http://www.afn.ca/article.asp?id=3639 (accessed on 13 March 2010).

15. Yellow Horse Brave Heart and Brave Heart J. In: Nebelkopf E and Phillips M (eds) (2004). *Healing and mental health for Native Americans: speaking in red.* New York, Altamira.

16. Chandler MJ and Lalonde C (1998). Cultural continuity as a hedge against suicide in Canada's First Nations. *Transcultural Psychiatry*, 35:191–219.

17. Thomas W and Bellefeuille G (2006). An evidence based formative evaluation of a cross cultural Aboriginal mental health program in Canada. *Australian Journal for the Advancement of Mental Health*, 5:1–14.

18. McCormick R (1998). Ethical considerations in First Nations counseling and research. *Canadian Journal of Counseling*, 3294:284–297.

19. Warry W (1998). *Unfinished dreams: community healing and the reality of aboriginal self government.* Toronto, University of Toronto Press.

20. McCormick R (1996). Culturally appropriate means and ends of counselling as described by the First Nations people of British Columbia. *International Journal for the Advancement of Counselling*, 18:163–172.

21. Trimble JE and Flemming CM (1990). Providing counselling services for Native American Indians; client, counselor, and community characteristics. In: Pederson PB et al. (eds). *Counseling across cultures.* Third edition. Honolulu, University of Hawaii Press: 177–204.

22. Sue DW (1981). *Counseling the culturally different: theory and practice.* Toronto, ON, John Wiley & Sons.

23. Duran E and Duran B (1995). *Native American post-colonial psychology.* Albany, NY, State University of New York Press.

24. Waldram JB (1997). *The way of the pipe: aboriginal spirituality and symbolic healing in Canadian prisons.* Peterborough, ON, Broadveiw.

25. www. manitobachiefs.com

26. Yin RK (2003). *Case study research – design and methods.* Thousand Oaks, California, Sage Publications Inc.

27. Taylor SJ and Bogdan R (1998). *Introduction to qualitative research methods – a guide book and resources.* New York, USA, John Wiley & Sons, Inc.

Food and vegetable promotion and the 5-a-day programme in Chile for the prevention of chronic noncommunicable diseases

Across-sector relationships and public–private partnerships

4

Irene Agurto,[1,]* Lorena Rodriguez,[2] Isabel Zacarías[3]

[1] Consultant, Pan American Health Organization
[2] Chilean Ministry of Health, Food and Nutrition Department
[3] Institute of Nutrition & Food Technology, University of Chile
* Corresponding author: iagurto@yahoo.es

Abstract

Utilizing a social determinants of health framework, we analysed intersectoral/interagency collaboration and public–private partnerships for fruit and vegetable consumption to prevent noncommunicable diseases in Chile. Our analysis was based on interviews with key informants and reviews of documents and reports Combining state and market forces could enhance both the scope and the resources for public health. Working together also helped to overcome the potential conflicts between commercial and social interests. For example, clear political direction led to a successful private–public partnership, while weak policy leadership might result in not achieving the desired population outcomes despite considerable investment. While equity concerns are included in some of the specific programmes, it is unclear if general policies can actually target specific inequities in the country, e.g. ethnic minorities, those living in remote areas, etc. Despite the potentially common goals, more attention needs to be paid to institutional and organizational interests and arrangements, as well as different ways of implementing interventions and policies at all levels. Balanced participation, focused particularly at the local levels, clear leadership and shared vision will help to ensure that each organization's interest is considered while ensuring that population health is safeguarded. Stronger involvement of civil society organizations is needed.

4.1. Background

The growing burden of chronic noncommunicable diseases (CNCDs) worldwide, including in the developing world, as well as the current international food trends make it imperative to develop broad alliances and partnerships between the health and agriculture sectors, and the private sector and community to tackle preventable risk factors for CNCDs in an equitable manner.

Non-pharmacological measures to prevent CNCDs, such as consuming a healthy diet, exercising regularly and stopping the use of tobacco have been documented by the World Health Organization (WHO) Global Strategy on Diet, Physical Activity and Health (WHO, 2004), the WHO Fruit and Vegetable Initiative (WHO, 2003), and the joint WHO/FAO expert consultation on Diet, Nutrition and the Prevention of Chronic Diseases (WHO/FAO, 2003). Increasing individual fruit and vegetable consumption to up to 600 g daily would reduce the worldwide burden of ischaemic heart disease and ischaemic stroke by 31% and 19%, respectively. For stomach, oesophageal, lung and colorectal cancer, the potential reductions are 19%, 20%, 12% and 2%, respectively (Lock et al., 2005).

CNCDs – cardiovascular diseases, cancer, diabetes and chronic pulmonary obstructive diseases – cause two out of every three deaths in the general population of Latin America and the Caribbean, and almost half of all deaths in the under-70 years' age group. In addition to causing premature deaths, these diseases cause complications and disabilities, limit productivity and require costly treatments. Together with genetic disposition and age, risk factors contributing to these diseases include poor diet, physical inactivity, smoking and alcohol abuse; other factors range from hypertension, to high cholesterol, to overweight and obesity (PAHO, 2007).

Chile ranks fortieth in the 2009 United Nations Development Programme (UNDP)'s Human Development Index, with 13.7% of the population below the poverty line, and 3.2% indigent. The ratio of the richest 10% to the poorest 10% is 26.2. The per capita expense on health is US$ 792 (UNDP, 2009). However, deep inequities persist, particularly among women, children, ethnic minorities, those in isolated regions and underemployed workers.

Of the Chilean population, 33.7% have hypertension, 35.4% have high cholesterol levels, 22% are obese, 38% are overweight and 54.9% have a high or very high risk for developing cardiovascular disease. The prevalence of disease and risk factors is consistently higher among those with less education: the prevalence of diabetes is 10.2% among those with basic education, 2.7% among those with high school education and 1.2% among those with university education (Ministerio de Salud de Chile, 2006). Obesity affects 7.4% of children below six years of age; it increases to 17% in first graders and is about 25% in adults and the elderly. If overweight is considered, over half of the national population falls into this category. According to the National Health Survey, 2003, it is estimated that there are 3.4 million obese people in the country and it is expected that this number will exceed 4 million in 2010 if the current trend continues (Ministerio de Salud de Chile, 2006). There is an inverse relationship between obesity and school education, which increases from 16.8% in people with a university education to 31.1% among those with a basic education.

Fruits and vegetables are widely available in the country – 146 kg per person per year are available (Jacoby and Keller, 2006). Around 80% of these are supplied by local producers and account for 2.82% of the cost of living index in Chile (Instituto Nacional de Estadísticas, 2010). However, though Chile is also an important fruit exporting country, consumption of fruits and vegetables is low: in 2005, 48% and 64% of the population ate fruit and vegetables daily, respectively, 31% and 28% ate these twice a day, 15% and 4% three times a day, and 6% and 4% ate four or more times a day. In 2006, 52.7% of the population ate vegetables daily, and 47.4% ate fruit daily (Encuesta IPSOS, Santiago, agosto 2005 [unpublished technical report]).

Key interventions, which include promoting fruit and vegetable consumption, are given below:

Health-led interventions:[1]

Global Strategy against Obesity (Estrategia Global contra la Obesidad, EGO), a national policy since 2006 focusing mainly on child obesity, uses the "Guidelines for a healthy life" of the Ministry of Health. This promotes the increased consumption of water, fish, fruits, vegetables and low-fat dairy products; a decrease in the intake of saturated fat, sugar and salt; and promotes physical activity, active recreation, sports practice and 30 minutes of moderate exercise on a daily basis. It is implemented through the public service network and includes the involvement of public schools, industry, and academic and scientific organizations for the development of nutritional guidelines, their implementation, recommendations, research, social marketing and communications.

Nutritional intervention through the life cycle for prevention of obesity and CNCD: This national programme has been in existence since 2004 and focuses on pregnant women and children below 6 years of age. It provides nutritional counselling and promotes exclusive breastfeeding; introduces new health controls for postpartum women and children

up to 3.5 years of age. It also identifies and monitors newborn children with risk factors for CNCDs, and low birth weight and macrosomic infants. Training of health staff is included.

Health promotion: Established in 1998, this national programme promotes healthy lifestyles, develops psychosocial and environmental health protection factors, and prevents CNCD risk factors through social marketing and communications. Nationally, it convenes a broad array of public and civil society institutions. Locally, social marketing activities are carried out by specific health promotion committees, mainly involving health, education and the community.

Education-led interventions

Food served at school and day-care facilities: Three organizations deliver meals to vulnerable infants and children attending public and semi-public schools and day-care facilities nationwide; one of these organizations covers almost 3 million students from public schools. Vulnerability is determined on a case-by-case basis and meals are served according to the children's needs. These three organizations have different scopes of work, but coordinate the food programme among them. Healthy diet and physical activity is promoted at school by other supporting programmes.

Public–private interventions

The 5-a-day Consortium: Following WHO's suggestion, the international 5-a-day fruit and vegetable promotion campaign was established in Chile and involves academia and the private sector, with the technical support of the health and agricultural sectors. The organizational scheme suggested by specialized agencies is a public–private cooperation. The private sector includes agricultural exports firms, supermarkets, distribution chains, fresh produce markets, among others. Media awareness, distribution of educational material, social marketing at points of sale, and community and academic activities are carried out nationally and locally. This Consortium also leads a Healthy Diet Committee within the agricultural public sector's exports-oriented strategy.

[1] All programmes are locally adapted at the regional and municipal level.

Private sector

Fruit and vegetable-related private sector associations carry out national and point-of-purchase campaigns, corporate social responsibility activities, and community involvement focusing on customers, associate members and business partners.

A social protection system, not addressed in this case study, is currently being set up, which targets mainly vulnerable children and their families through sets of social policies.

This case study focuses on the fruit and vegetable consumption policies for the prevention of noncommunicable diseases (NCDs) in Chile and the interagency relationships across the public–private divide to analyse how challenges are addressed and how they influence processes and outputs.

4.2 Methods

Utilizing the social determinants of health (SDH) framework, we analysed intersectoral/interagency collaboration and public–private partnerships. The study includes the challenges encountered by interagency relationships and across the public–private divide, ranging from the architecture of partnerships to different organizational settings and cultures, as well as interests. The way these challenges are addressed may affect the overall effectiveness of policies, particularly in terms of influence, scale and sustainability.

The chosen units of analysis are as follows:

- *The interventions themselves*, described and classified according to a structural interventions framework (Blankenship et al., 2000);

- *Intersectoral/interagency and inter-programme relationships*: analysis of the links between different organizational and programme settings working towards a common purpose;

- *Public–private partnerships*: analysis of the links between institutional settings with different purposes and missions working towards a common end;

- *Capacity to influence policy*: how these initiatives and actors were influenced by others, and how they can expand their influence to shape policies.

Information was collected through a review of documents and interviews with key informants representing relevant fruit and vegetable initiatives at the national and regional levels. These included high-ranking individuals from the private, public, international and nongovernmental organization (NGO) sectors. Small projects were not considered, given the policy focus of this study. Sixteen interviews were conducted. Private sector interviewees included representatives from supermarket associations, fresh produce markets and distributors, agricultural producers and communications firms. Public sector interviewees included representatives from four different fruit and vegetable-related programmes pertaining to the educational sector; four representatives from the health sector at the national and regional/municipal levels; and one representative of the agricultural sector. The 5-a-day Consortium and a representative from an international health organization were interviewed. It was not possible to conduct five interviews corresponding to regional initiatives of the health sector. Consumers' views were not considered in this case study, given the public policy focus of this case.

The interview guide covered a brief history of each programme or initiative, including the main drivers, persons or organizations that were influential for this purpose; the SDH that were addressed; funding; formal and informal institutional relationships (public/private and intersectoral); programme changes over time; key interests at stake and ways of addressing fruit and vegetable consumption. As this case study focused on process analysis, most of the information provided in the interviews was not documented and thus difficult to verify. Document review included background information, programme documents, visits to websites, and to supermarket and fresh produce markets. A literature review was also conducted.

Information obtained from the interviews was organized according to content, intially by the types of interventions, and then according to the processes they entailed, focusing on the nature of formal and informal relationships. Specific examples that allowed or inhibited intersectoral/interagency relationships between different organizational settings were also examined. Categories for organizing and qualifying the interventions were in accordance with the SDH framework.

An unexpected situation occurred while conducting the study; inclement winter weather resulted in very high fruit and vegetable prices. However, as actual consumption or consumers' views were not considered in this study, this factor would not have altered the results.

Table 1. Interventions organized according to structural categories

SOCIAL DETERMINANTS/PATHWAY	Intervention categories		
	Availability	Acceptability	Accessibility
Deep inequities between income levels; ethnic groups; regions affecting mainly women, children and underemployed workers			Food served at school for vulnerable children (Ministry of Education [MOE])
Cultural food intake patterns affected by global trends in fast-processed foods, particularly among the younger population	National guidelines updated to include a specific number of portions of fruits and vegetables	Awareness, promotion both by the private sector and the Ministry of Health (MOH)	
Value of locally grown, fresh and seasonal produce are not mainstream ideas in the country	Guidelines for fruit and vegetable portions being modified in schools		
Healthy food alternatives are not easily available in the market	Private sector activities to increase availability and quality of fruits and vegetables		
School food composition not healthy enough			

Source: Blankenship et al. 2000

4.3 Findings

Interventions

Based on the background information and interviews, the current interventions are mapped against structural categories and social determinants. It is striking that, with two exceptions, the maximum emphasis is on availability interventions (Table 1).

Most of the governmental interventions, as the interviewees pointed out, are based on the assumption that the price of fruits and vegetables is too high, particularly for the poorest among the population. However, as noted earlier in this chapter, the cost of fruit and vegetables consumed accounts for 2.82% in the cost of living index in Chile; for example, 1 kg of lemon costs $100 pesos, while a single can of a soft drink beverage costs $500 pesos.

It is apparent that implementation processes face challenges in addressing both equity and vulnerable populations, particularly across sectors with different approaches. As depicted in Table 1, interventions to improve the availability, acceptability and accessibility of fruits and vegetables and address equity are still inadequate. Inequities as identified by the current government's programme do not appear to be addressed through these interventions.

Accessibility has been addressed through slow improvements in the fruit and vegetable content of school meals, by trying to follow the dietary guidelines which include the number of fruit and vegetable portions. For provinces in the extreme south, where the availability and accessibility of fresh produce is scant, the health sector has decreased the recommendation to four portions. As pointed out by an international health representative, the dietary guidelines do not offer recommendations to consumers according to age, gender and type of activity. School meals are provided according to "extreme poverty and equity criteria, according to calorie needs", as the educational sector representatives pointed out, and not under a healthy diet scheme as "the purpose [of the rations] is not nutritional, food is meant to attract families [to school]", as another educational sector interviewee mentioned. Another interviewee from the same sector said that "there is a need for a common framework as the health sector focuses on energy consumption and food intake, and the educational sector focuses on conditions for development".

The 5-a-day Consortium carries out academic and technical support activities to improve acceptability, as well as private sector activities to improve quality and access. The Consortium focuses on lifestyle interventions, using a health promotion framework under the assumption that most of the Chilean population "may be classified as belonging to the middle- and low-income groups" (*the Consortium's board member*). There are some 5-a-day committees at the local level, mostly working with the health sector or within the health sector structures.

Lifestyle interventions are conducted mostly by the health sector. They focus on children and pregnant women, and address childhood obesity. Health education is provided through promotional programmes, which are currently "undergoing a restructuring process to incorporate the social determinants of health" (*policy-maker, health sector*).

Intersectoral/interagency and inter-programme relationships

At the central level, public social sectors converge at the Social Cabinet and, at the intermediate level, interactions are mostly driven by the initiative of technical government officials. Health sector officials participate in the experts' groups formed by the educational sector, and the dietary guidelines are "one of several criteria used by the educational sector to establish the terms of reference for the tendering process", as stated by a policy-maker in the educational sector.

The health and education sectors interact frequently at the municipal level, since they are both under this administration and are technically supervised by the vertical programmes on health and education, respectively. For instance, obesity prevention and control programmes are carried out in schools, and children referred to the health centre for follow up and individual counselling. They also interact through the

health promotion, EGO or 5-a-day committees driven by the health sector. The structure, capacity and mix of interventions may vary from one locality to another, depending on the local leadership.

At the central level, interactions between the agricultural and health sectors are not regular, except for food safety. According to an agricultural sector policy-maker, the agricultural sector's involvement in promoting a healthy diet and intake of fruits and vegetables is grounded in "positive externalities such as promoting an industry fostering adequate nutrition, and avoiding negative externalities such as obesity and deepening inequities in the country which may discredit exports, and damage the national image abroad".

At the local level, private producers and distributors, as well as supermarkets are involved in activities that are mostly spearheaded by the health sector.

Public–private relationships

Two broad types of relationships between public and private actors were identified, i.e. occasional and regular.

Occasional relationships are frequently seen at the municipal and regional levels, as in the local health promotion committees, "mostly initiated by the health sector seeking the financial support of the private sector" (*a municipal-level health interviewee*). Other committees, e.g. through their 5-a-day activities, develop a more balanced, albeit occasional partnership, where public and private partners engage in common activities, beyond providing sole financial support (*another health interviewee*).

An example of a public–private partnership led by the health sector is the one used to foster milk consumption, where all partners share the same motto "*I drink*" and pay directly for their publicity expenses, thus allowing for all private firms, regardless of their particular milk product, to participate in the initiative (*a national health sector policy-maker*). However, the health sector strictly regulates the use of its logo, resulting in occasional rather than regular relationships with the private sector (*a health sector interviewee*).

Regular relationships between public and private partners around fruits and vegetables are less frequent and the 5-a-day Consortium constitutes the best example. Health sector interviewees stated that they officially endorse the organization, perform an advisory role and provide in-kind support. The agricultural sector representative, however, stated that the sector participates fully, as it has a long tradition in public–private partnerships, and provides financial support on a case-by-case basis. Private sector interviewees stated that they engage actively, pay dues and provide other financial support, also on a case-by-case basis.

The main benefits of this public–private collaboration, as identified by the Consortium, are "being linked to the agricultural exports promotion committee, availability of healthy and safe food, corporate social responsibility, having had prior successful experiences in public–private partnerships, and promoting the country's image in light of exports".

One of the direct benefits of participating in the Consortium is the use of the internationally renowned 5-a-day logo. However, one supermarket chain targeting high-income customers developed a similar logo for its own corporate use and provided financial support to the Consortium. This image association, while helping to promote the 5-a-day concept through expensive TV advertising, also deterred some public agencies and other supermarket chains from being more involved, according to the Supermarkets Association representative interviewed.

The tendering process for the delivery of school meals is another example of regular public–private relationships. However, the new terms of reference are shifting to "frozen, prepackaged meals (cook-and-chill technology) due to quality and cost-saving" (*an educational sector interviewee*). This requires infrastructure and technology that the small, local producers do not have and thereby reduces their capacity to participate in tenders, according to an interviewee who was a fresh market producer.

Capacity to influence policies

The concept of fruit and vegetable consumption for CNCD prevention was initially promoted by international health agencies. The private sector founding members of the Consortium, such as the National Agricultural Association and the Fruit Export Association, pointed out that they were acquainted with this concept through their commercial activities abroad and were already sponsoring 5-a-day programmes in one of their main export markets. A wholesale distribution centre for internal markets was also aware of the initiative due to its involvement in international associations.

The Consortium and its associates have influenced other corporate actors, produced synergies and promoted fruits and vegetables from different angles, benefiting from the opportunity created by the international health trend in the subject, a positive convergence of interests, and the value assigned to prevention and public health, as was stated by the president of the National Agricultural Association.

The health promotion focus used at the time emphasized health education through the mass media and social marketing based on the view held at the Consortium's board that most of the Chilean population can be classified as belonging to the middle- and low-income groups. The Consortium's activities are currently being redefined from this general approach to a more specific one, targeting population groups through selected media channels, as pointed out by the communications interviewee.

Collaboration between the Consortium and the health sector to influence policies and strengthen technical capacity is ongoing, including technical support to the health services network, as well as for academic activities.

4.4 Discussion

Managing intersectoral relationships

The architecture of partnerships for fruit and vegetable promotion, both intersectoral and public–private, involves State and market actors, which might contribute to optimizing the overall setting for policy building. However, it could also benefit from including civil society and consumers as part of the general policy framework.

The particular key interventions and how the intersectoral relationships are managed may affect both the process as well as its outcomes. Potential conflicts as well as the potential synergies between the health, education and agricultural sectors at the central level coexist as follows.

Managing collaboration between the health and education sectors

Given the high volume of food served at schools by the special agencies of the educational sector, a mutually beneficial collaboration is crucial. Despite the progress that has been made over time, there is still room to improve the synergy between the two sectors, as they share a common focus and target group, namely, vulnerable children at risk for overweight and obesity. According to the educational sector, food is meant to attract children to school while the health sector focuses on a healthy diet. However, as healthy food appeals equally to school attendance, the potential conflict could be resolved. The way the composition of food is discussed within the convening experts' groups in the educational and health sectors, and considering the national health guidelines as only one of the criteria used, could be modified. Greater responsibility could be shifted to the health sector, using the nutritional guidelines as the main framework and possibly convening the same expert groups. This could fast-track the move to a focus on a healthy diet.

Should this happen, the current potential conflict between the small local producers who cannot meet the terms of reference of the tendering process for food delivery based on the "cook-and-chill" technology could be turned into new synergies. This would expand the choice to include fresh, locally available produce and adhere to the required food safety standards.

It is worth highlighting, however, that the three educational institutions responsible for food delivery to schools have agreed to common terms of reference for tendering, which facilitates relationships with private providers, as well as the quality control process.

This could also allow the educational sector to devote more resources and time for overseeing the process of delivery and quality control, which is already under way, as well as promoting a healthy diet and exercise at schools more intensively. Other supporting initiatives could be more extensively applied in schools, such as the Healthy Schools concept and targeting vendors inside and outside schools to make fresh snack options available and acceptable to children.

Creating a common conceptual framework – "conditions for development" within the educational sector and "social determinants of health" within the health sector – could create a very strong foundation for collaboration, as these are complementary and have many elements in common.

Managing collaboration between the health and agricultural sectors

These sectors primarily interact through the 5-a-day Consortium for fruit and vegetable matters, the exports' committee, and the recently formed food safety office. Both the Consortium and the exports committee convene mostly at the large agro-industrial export businesses; while links to small producers, who supply almost 80% of the fruits and vegetables of the internal market, are carried out through other less formalized fora. Although the Consortium framework of collaboration serves well the purpose of promoting exports and channelling corporate social responsibility campaigns, the internal markets and producers, as well as the health sector itself, appear to be placed in a weak position for promoting public health issues.

On the one hand, the health and private sectors, both large and small, could improve their collaboration. The big agro-industrial representatives expressed their will to further support public health policies, and the small producers even asked for further support from the health sector. However, the public and private sectors need to learn how to better work together, and overcome mistrust and potential conflict between commercial and social interests. A possible obstacle may be competition issues within the private sector itself, as happened with the emulation of the common logo by an individual supermarket chain described in the findings. However, it would appear that private sector associations and orientation to corporate responsibility could offer common ground both within the private sector and between this sector and the health sector. It could also be in the interest of the private sector for health officials to review their stringent rules on the use of their logo or establish other ways of endorsement and support for certain products.

On the other hand, the health sector should expand its approach to food safety, and its regulatory and supervisory functions to include a broader concept of public health, e.g. a healthy diet. This would offer a more comprehensive basis for the development of policies, guidelines and legislation.

Managing policy change

Chilean fruit exporters and distributors became acquainted with the 5-a-day international campaign fostered by international health organizations in their foreign markets and were most willing to support local initiatives. They consistently financed and promoted activities around fruit and vegetable consumption, demonstrating a positive effect of globalization both in their own best interest and for the good of public health. However, with respect to public health policy change, there have been some avoidable pitfalls.

—Implementing activities mainly through a private agency, i.e. the 5-a-day Consortium, which does not have regular financing and has a limited capacity for significant upstream interventions in particular, and where the participation of public agencies is not regular, may have had limited or detrimental effects on policy. However, the institutional design of the Consortium, involving the private and public sectors around common strategies, may offer a promising setting for policy change, should the public sector consistently support this initiative to help build capacity for policy implementation and take advantage of the interest of and financing by the private sector.

—As the array of interventions within the partnership is limited in this case, being restricted to mainly communication and sales-point marketing, it is important to ensure an appropriate branding of the whole spectrum of actors and over time. Although branding has actually had a very limited scope in the fruit and vegetable policy, the one devised for the dairy products partnership, i.e. "I drink" allowed for a broad and consistent identification of the intervention. The political leadership by the health sector in the latter case was instrumental in building a common ground between different commercial interests, which did not happen in the fruit and vegetable partnership.

—Last, but not the least, the underlying assumption that the poorest sections of society do not consume fresh fruits and vegetables because their prices are too high needs to be verified. According to the data collected in this case study, this is not true (except in sparsely populated far-flung areas of the country), especially when compared with unhealthy snacks and beverages. In fact, it is not known why consumption is low. Nevertheless, policy-makers across sectors appear to share this assumption and this might favour availability over acceptability interventions, put pressure on lowering internal prices and thus squeeze out the small producers and deepen their already aggravated situation of poverty.

Limitations of the study

The widely varying nature of the interventions makes it difficult to make a comparison across interventions. Although all interventions have written documents and background materials, the lack of comprehensive

evaluations, with the exception of the health promotion programme, may have led to the omission of some process issues. Further, the overall embedding of the fruit and vegetable initiative into broader healthy diet programmes makes it difficult to precisely determine the success of these particular initiatives.

4.5 Conclusion

The health, education and agricultural policies devised for tackling key risk factors for CNCDs, among them ensuring a healthy diet, evolve mostly around State and market forces. Building and managing relationships across sectors and public–private partnerships needs careful involvement of key players in the right settings and with the right leadership.

- The only body specifically devoted to promoting the 5-a-day fruit and vegetable recommendation in the country was built around and financed mostly by the agricultural exports business and in close relationship with the agricultural sector exports strategy, instead of around internal market producers and with a strong leadership from the health sector. The export businesses would also have been willing to participate in this policy setting and the outcomes would have had more impact on reducing inequities.

- The leadership for nutritional guidelines for meals served to vulnerable children at school lies within the educational sector at the technical, intermediate level, where the main criteria is the attractiveness of the food. The health sector plays only an advisory role. Both actors would benefit more from transferring more responsibility to the health sector and shift the focus to a combination of attractiveness and nutritional value.

- Combining State and market forces could enhance both the scope and the resources for public health when these work together to overcome the potential conflicts between commercial and social interests. Clear political direction led to a successful private–public partnership around dairy products, while weak policy leadership led to restricted use of endorsement in the area of fruits and vegetables. Endorsements are valuable assets for the private sector and, naturally, care has to be taken to grant them, yet building around common ground and respective interests may lead to further impact on public policies.

- Equity is embedded in the vertical health programmes – combating childhood obesity and nutritional assistance for pregnant mothers and their children, and in the educational sector – food programmes that serve food at school for vulnerable children. It is unclear, though, if general policies can actually target specific inequities in the country, e.g. ethnic minorities, those in remote areas, etc. Appropriate structures would be required for reaching and working with such populations. Current structures provided both by the health and education sectors could have this capacity if the policies are appropriately implemented at the local levels. However, these local levels would also require assistance in developing their own partnerships and intersectoral relationships, as has happened in some local provincial experiences.

Despite common goals, as is the case in promoting fruit and vegetable consumption for CNCD prevention, more attention needs to be paid to institutional and organizational interests and arrangements, as well as different ways of implementing interventions and policies at all levels. The architecture of partnerships and sustained funding are key issues to ensure effective interventions, and policies would require to be fleshed out in detail, ensuring not only balanced participation, but also a clear leadership with a shared vision so that each organization's interest is considered while the public health concern is safeguarded. One way to ensure the latter would be to involve civil society associations, as they may potentially provide the knowledge base, advocacy, and possibly help ensure appropriate depth of change and sustainability of interventions.

Acknowledgements

The authors wish to acknowledge Helia Molina for her support, Tito Pizarro, Francisca Infante, Fernando Vío and Claudio Bifani for their most helpful comments and reviews, and all interviewees for their time and commitment to the topic. Special thanks to Erik Blas for his contributions.

References

1. Blankenship KM, Bray SJ, Merson MH (2000). Structural interventions in public health. *AIDS*, 14 (Suppl 1):S11–S21.

2. *Diet, nutrition and the prevention of chronic diseases. Report of the joint WHO/FAO expert consultation* (2003). Geneva, WHO Technical Report Series, No. 916 (TRS 916). Available at: http://www.who.int/dietphysicalactivity/publications/trs916/download/en/index.html (accessed on 11 November 2010).

3. *Health in the Americas 2007* (2007). Washington, DC, Pan American Health Organization. Available at: http://www.paho.org/hia/homeing.html http://apps.who.int/gb/ebwha/pdf_files/WHA57/A57_R17-en.pdf

4. Instituto Nacional de Estadísticas. *Indice de precios al Consumidor Metodologia* (2010). Available at: http://www.ine.cl/canales/chile_estadistico/estadisticas_precios/ipc/metodologia/metodologia.php (accessed on 11 November 2010).

5. Jacoby E, Keller I citing a FAO Report (2006). Revista Chilena de Nutrición, 33 (Suplemento 1).

6. Lock K et al. (2005). The global burden of diseases attributable to low consumption of fruit and vegetables: implications for the global strategy on diet. *Bulletin of the World Health Organization*, 83 (2):100–108.

7. Ministerio de Salud de Chile (2006). *Segunda Encuesta calidad de vida y salud*. Available at: http://epi.minsal.cl/epi/html/sdesalud/calidaddevida2006/Informe%20Final%20Encuesta%20de%20Calidad%20de%20Vida%20y%20Salud%202006.pdf (accessed on 11 November 2010).

8. *UNDP Human Development Report 2009. Overcoming barriers: human mobility and development* (2009). Available at: hdr.undp.org/en/reports/global/hdr2009/ (accessed on 20 November 2010).

9. World Health Organization (2003). *Fruit and Vegetable Promotion Initiative: a meeting report*. Geneva, WHO.

10. World Health Organization (2004). *WHA57.17. Global strategy on diet, physical activity and health*. Geneva, WHO.

Dedicated delivery centre for migrants in Minhang District, Shanghai

5

Intervention on the social determinants of health and equity in pregnancy outcome for internal migrants in Shanghai, China

Su Xu,[1] Jia Cheng,[1] Chanjuan Zhuang,[2],* Shaokang Zhan,[3] and Erik Blas[4]

[1] Health Bureau, Minhang District, Shanghai, China
[2] Pujiang Township Health Centre, Minhang District, Shanghai, China
[3] Fudan University, Shanghai, China
[4] World Health Organization, Geneva
* Corresponding author: lyxie@shmu.edu.cn

Abstract

Since the early 1980s, the economic transition in China has led to differentials in economic growth between various parts of China and has resulted in more than 150 million rural-to-urban migrants. Migrants in the cities face a number of social, legal, insititutional and economic challenges, which manifest in marked inequities in health outcomes, particularly with respect to maternal health. These inequities have caused public concern over the past more than one decade and led in 2004 to the establishment of the first dedicated delivery centre for migrants. The concept was expanded to a total of 25 centres in the following years. To provide insight into the associated policy formulation and programme implementation processes, a review of mostly unpublished documents, and programme and official statistics was undertaken. This was supplemented by interviews with health managers in Minhang, other districts of Shanghai as well as at the Shanghai city level. This case study examines the processes behind the successful establishment of a pilot centre in Minhang District to provide safe and acceptable antenatal and delivery services to pregnant migrant women at an affordable price. It shows that the intervention is a feasible option for the health sector to redress inequities created by upstream structural social determinants. However, the case study also shows that there are important constraints and challenges in replicating the pilot model to other districts, and that some of these obstacles are related to transferring the values underpinning concerns about equity. The case study finally points to ways by which to increase the chances of successful replication and sustainability of institutional changes to address social determinants.

5.1 Background

Over the past three decades, China has experienced dramatic changes in both social and economic structures. Market-oriented economic reform has sustained an average growth of about 10%. While the overall population growth rate has slowed due to the effective family planning policy since the mid-1970s, the urban population has increased significantly due to migration. The disparities in social and economic development between urban and rural areas, between the eastern and western regions, and between the rich and the poor have grown rapidly since the economic reforms were launched in 1979 (Meng, et al., 2002; Walder, 1989).

Such differentials often lead to massive population movements. In China, a further complication is the existence of the *hukou* or household registration system, originally introduced during the "great leap forward" in the 1950s as a key policy instrument during a period of strict central planning (Wang et al., 2005). According to *hukou*, people are required to live and work only where they are officially permitted to. During the economic reform process of the past decades, the number of surplus workers in rural areas has increased, as has the demand for workers in the industries and construction sites in the cities. Together with a relaxation of the strict central control, this has offered an incentive for workers to migrate to cities in search of a better livelihood. However, since the *hukou* is still in place, they face significant challenges in the cities. More than a dozen certificates and approvals are required to get permission to live and work in the cities, a process that can take several months and involve considerable costs – and before they complete the process, they may find that the first certificates have expired.

Many migrants, therefore, chose to live and work without legal documentation. They find work at construction sites, small factories and rubbish collection – work that not only has low status and low pay but also excludes them from benefits such as health insurance and other social services of the legal workforce (Zhan, 2002). The monthly salary for an employed migrant worker in the city in the early 2000s was typically in the range of RMB 600–1200 (US$ 100–200). However, one month's salary in Shanghai could correspond to what they would earn from a full year's production in their home village. It is currently estimated that there are more than 150 million internal migrants in China who constitute about 30% of the total population in Shanghai. In one district (Minhang) almost 60% of the inhabitants are migrants.

Several studies have shown worse maternal health outcomes among migrants compared with residents in China (Gao, 1994; Jiang and Liu, 1997; Zhang, 2007;

Jiang, 2007. Analysis of 19 maternal deaths, unpublished paper). A review of the hospital medical records from 1993 to 1996 and interviews with mothers in Minhang district showed lower utilization of antenatal and delivery services as well as systematically worse pregnancy outcomes for internal migrants compared with permanent residents (Xie, 1997). The data demonstrated that insufficient antenatal care is one of the main reasons for the poor maternal health outcomes among migrants. Migrants were found to face a "package of obstacles", ranging from lack of legal status, low social status, lower income and education, lack of insurance, as well as discrimination by health service staff and other officials. Migrant women, therefore, often avoided using the antenatal care services and sought illegal delivery services (Zhan, 2002). All places providing delivery services outside of hospitals and specifically authorized health centres in China are deemed unsafe and illegal, and are closed down when found by the government. Their attractiveness to migrant women is related mainly to their relative cheapness, i.e. RMB 500 for the birth of a boy and RMB 300 for a girl, compared with RMB 3000 for a normal delivery at a hospital.

The increased market orientation of health services in China during the economic transition has in many hospitals led to 10–15% of the income coming from the government budget and 85–90% from service fees. Staff has been shown to employ a variety of strategies to generate extra revenue and increase individual bonuses through overprescription, unnecessary high-cost medical examination, overuse of expensive medicines, unnecessarily long hospital stays, delayed referrals, etc. (Zhan et al., 2004; Bian et al., 2004). Thus, migrant women in cities either do not seek care or seek it from alternative, illegal providers.

The Chinese government has gradually realized these problems and is moving towards their solutions. A policy issued in February 2009 offers a possibility for migrants to achieve resident status when they have lived in Shanghai for seven years, have contributed to the development of Shanghai and paid tax. Work is also ongoing to provide migrants with a social and health insurance system, equal right for their children to attend normal schools and setting of minimum wages. All these are signs of concern about the inequity between urban residents and rural-to-urban migrants. The Chinese government has further launched a long-term plan for the development of rural areas. However, even if such upstream measures represent moves in the right direction, achieving more equitable health outcomes is likely to take a long time.

A series of specific measures have been taken in order to improve maternal care for pregnant migrants. A city-level policy on registration of migrant deliveries in Shanghai came into force in 1994. Research on maternal care for migrants has been conducted and policy suggestions made since 1995, followed by a broad public dialogue, including on the social determinants of the differential outcomes. Studies have also been carried out in other districts, cities and provinces with similar results. The first concrete city-level policy in Shanghai on strengthening the management of maternal and child health care, including fee control and service quality assurance for rural-to-urban migrants, was issued in 1999. After further discussions among policy-makers, health managers and researchers, a dedicated delivery centre for migrants was launched as a pilot project in Minhang district in 2004, expanded to nine more districts at about the same time, and a further 13 in 2007. The pilot in Minhang and the concurrent scaling up have been generally considered successful in improving the maternal health of migrants and reducing inequities.

This case study explores the lessons learned from the pilot in Minhang and the scale-up across the city of Shanghai with the specific aim of providing guidance on how downstream interventions can be implemented to reduce inequities originating from more upstream social determinants.

5.2 Methods

The study was undertaken as an explorative case study (Yin, 2004) with the aim of finding out how the changes came about and why some of the interventions turned out more successful than others. The study has four subunits of analysis: policy formulation, pilot programme, replication in other districts of Shanghai, outcome of the policy. The study was carried out using a combination of qualitative and quantitative data collection instruments.

The initial data collection was carried out during July to September 2007 in Minhang district and Shanghai city. However, during the data analysis and interpretation phases of the study, it became necessary to go back to update data according to time-series as well as to gain further insight where the triangulation of different data and sources of data revealed inconsistency or directly contradicted information. The final data collection and verification of data thus continued up till September 2009. Information on policy formulation and implementation in Minhang district and the process of scaling up was collected mainly by interviewing managers of the Minhang District Health Bureau and the Maternal and Child Health (MCH) Department of the Shanghai Health Bureau. Data on assessing the outcome of this programme were provided by the MCH Department, both in the Shanghai Health Bureau and Minhang District Health Bureau. The main secondary data sources are the daily service records of all women accessing the hospital obstetrical services. Policy and programme documents relevant to the topic were provided by the Minhang District Health Bureau. All the data have been complemented by interviews with city- and municipal-level managers and decision-makers, as well as programme staff. City-level health managers and district government leaders and managers, including the Director of the District Maternal Care Centre and Director of the Pujiang Township Health Centre were interviewed to provide background information about the policy formulation processes.

A final interpretation was done with respect to the four themes that emerged from the initial analysis – impact of policy change, values, incentives and replication.

5.3 Findings

Policy formulation and decision

Around the year 2000, tragic cases of maternal death and delivery complications among migrant women frequently made it to the headlines of the mass media in Shanghai. Statistics from hospital service reports as well as research documented the significant magnitude of this public health problem. Improving maternal health for migrants became an important demand of the whole society. Almost all the suggestions at that time were about banning and eliminating illegal delivery services and enhancing migrants' health knowledge and changing their behaviours in seeking antenatal care and safe delivery services. However, no concrete proposal for how this might be done and what effect it might have were forthcoming and the Shanghai city policy-makers kept waiting for someone to come up with a promising solution. Consultative meetings were held with leading obstetricians to analyse each maternal death to establish the cause and what could be learned from the case. This group came up with an idea of creating a "PINMING YIYUAN" (*hospital for low-income people*) to receive

migrant women for delivery. However, health managers did not immediately respond to this idea.

Therefore, when a request from the Minhang District Health Bureau was made for approval to establish the Pujiang dedicated delivery centre, this was welcomed and a series of discussions and negotiations started. Officers in the Minhang District Health Bureau recalled that: "*Serious events of maternal death, emergency treatment and bad experiences from illegal delivery provision were reported from the hospitals' obstetrical departments almost every week. We decided to prevent these problems by establishing safe delivery services rather than dealing with the problems once the damage is done.*" Their initial idea was shared with all departments of the Minhang district government and a request to the City Health Bureau to establish a dedicated migrant delivery centre in Pujiang Township was supported by the entire district government.

While welcoming the request, the city-level officials were concerned about the feasibility of the proposal and asked the Minhang District Health Bureau to answer two questions: first, "*how to ensure quality and safety?*" and second, "*how to achieve lower effective fees at the same time as reaching a financial balance?*"

In response to the first question, the Director of the Minhang District Bureau promised that the district would create a dedicated place to host the service, buy the necessary equipment, invite a senior obstetrician to reinforce the service team and reorganize the team to provide safe delivery services. Further, a reliable referral system would be set up for defined complications. Concerning the second question, the district clarified that they would define and restrict the service items provided to avoid the temptation of overcharging as well as to contain costs. They would also reduce the length of stay for normal deliveries and finally shift resources within the health bureau's budget. Finally, they asked a district charity organization as well as all the other bureaus within the district government to support the programme. These answers, together with having mobilized the whole society within the district regarding the new maternal service model, convinced the City Health Bureau, which approved the model as a pilot project. The first policy on "Establishing a dedicated migrant delivery centre" jointly made by the nine departments of Minhang District government was issued on 22 December 2003 (Minhang District Health Bureau, 2003).

The pilot in Minhang District

Low income, lack of medical insurance, high cost, discrimination and negative staff attitudes towards migrants were the main obstacles to using maternal and child health-care services. The pilot programme included seven key components:

1. To change the policy so that uncomplicated deliveries would take place at the Pujiang township health centre rather than at a hospital, as was the case before. Complicated deliveries would be referred to one of the three hospitals in the district. However, this component was modified during the course of the pilot. As a senior obstetrician who had been working in the Fifth Hospital was assigned to the health centre, it began to handle more complicated cases, including performing caesarean sections.

2. The Health Bureau set a fixed ceiling for the total amount of fees for each normal delivery at RMB 800 in the centre against RMB 2500–3000 in the hospitals. A list of essential items of service was defined and measures were taken to eliminate institutional overcharging (Shanghai Health Bureau, 2004).

3. To rationalize procedures in order to cut costs and thereby price, women were to stay in the Pujiang centre for only one or two days after delivery compared with four or five days elsewhere.

4. To dedicate the service to migrants in order to create an environment where migrant women would feel safe and comfortable with other patients as well as staff

5. To modify staff behaviours through changing the incentive system, providing education and information, and changing monitoring and evaluation systems to focus on outcome rather than process

6. The District Health Bureau reprioritized and shifted budgets to establish a special budget both for institutional development costs and to compensate for the discounted service fee.

7. To undertake a public information campaign, advertising the availability of the service as well as to convey the values enshrined in the new service (*Shanghai Evening Post*, March 2004; *Jiefang Daily*, April 2004).

Shanghai city, in approving the dedicated migrant delivery centre in Pujiang township health centre, wanted to show that it cared about its migrant citizens and test whether the model worked and would be applicable in other districts as well. The Minhang District government took full responsibility for the preparation and running of the centre, as well as identifying problems and improving performance. The Vice-Mayor of Shanghai and the Director of the Shanghai Health Bureau participated in the opening ceremony and made several follow-up visits, thus indicating that the city attached importance to the problem of migrant maternal health and establishment of the centre. The Pujiang dedicated migrant delivery centre was the first such centre for rural-to-urban migrants in China and started operations on 27 July 2004 after seven months of preparation.

Working on perceptions and attitudes

The Director of the Minhang District Health Bureau was the active leader in the whole process, from policy formulation to programme implementation and follow up. The Director realized the importance of informing the public and ensuring conducive staff attitudes and behaviours. A protocol for implementing the policy was made by the Health Bureau (Minhang District Health Bureau, 2003).

A centre-piece of this protocol was the concept of "*helping the vulnerable*" and that doing so was not just about financial and material support but equally about respect for people, including those who are vulnerable and with low income, and avoiding discrimination. An evaluation scheme for staff attitudes and performance was set up and the meaning of improving maternal care for rural-to-urban migrants was explained to every manager and staff to encourage better service performance.

Managers from the District Health Bureau made regular visits to the Pujiang delivery centre to its check performance, including adherence to the low-fee policy. Information on the maximal fee was widely disseminated to both staff and service users. Written public announcements were also distributed in all communities, workplaces and institutions where migrants lived, worked or gathered.

Further, the District Health Bureau "marketed" the service in all the mass media. For example, a report on the opening of the centre was published on the first page of the *Shanghai Evening Post* on 28 March 2004, i.e. four months ahead of the official opening ceremony. It said: "*Cheap delivery costing RMB 800 all-in-all,*" "*RMB 200 government subsidy for normal delivery and RMB 400 for caesarean birth.*"

Fee collection and incentives

It is common in China for the take-home income of health staff to be determined by the fees they collect from clients. This mechanism encourages unnecessary and expensive medicines and medical examinations, and is detrimental to ensuring equity of access and use. To improve delivery outcomes for migrants, the Minhang District therefore had to develop new concepts for service delivery and incentive schemes for health workers, which focused on results rather than process.

An important determinant of pregnancy outcome is the access to and use of antenatal care. Many pregnant women had no antenatal care leading to lost opportunities to avoid a variety of pregnancy complications. To overcome this problem, a policy named "*Scheme for systematic maternal care for migrants in Minhang District*" was issued (Minhang Health Bureau, 2005). The policy introduced the concept of whole-course maternal care.

The "whole-course maternal care" scheme makes the township and village health workers responsible for promoting and organizing maternal care for all pregnant women from early pregnancy to 45 days after delivery. Health workers identify and contact every pregnant woman in their area and distribute a written announcement and a booklet to the woman. The announcement states the services that will be provided and that the service fees are fixed at RMB 150 for three antenatal visits and RMB 800 for a normal delivery. The booklet guides pregnant women on what to do, where to go, and provides other information about maternal care. A contact card, free of charge, is used for keeping a record of the woman's health status and the care received. These data are entered into a computer system. In the second week after registration and again in the eighth to ninth month of pregnancy, the woman receives a phone call and is asked "*Have you been to an antenatal care clinic?*" or "*Have you been visited by any village/township health worker and if so, who?*" The township and village health workers do not collect any fees at all but are responsible for helping the pregnant woman complete the whole-course maternal care including antenatal care, delivery and postpartum care till 45 days after delivery. The health worker will receive a bonus when she is verified to have helped the pregnant woman to complete the whole-course maternal care, i.e. distribute the booklet, fill in the contact card, and ensure all antenatal and postpartum visits, and neonatal physical check-up. The bonuses add up to RMB 23 for each pregnant woman and an additional RMB 22 if the woman is a migrant.

Service quality assurance

Realizing that the price and quality of providing delivery services were critically important technical challenges to the programme, the District Health Bureau took direct responsibility not only for the establishment of the dedicated migrant delivery centre but also for running and continuously improving it. Key leaders of the District Health Bureau visited the centre every one or two weeks to observe the functioning and assist in resolving identified problems. No complaints about the services being "too expensive", a popular criticism in contemporary China, or "the hospital is earning too much money" have been received up till now in Pujiang.

Much effort went into selecting and developing a competent team of staff and providing them with the materials and equipment to perform their duties. Standard operating procedures were set up, including when to start running the emergency procedure, a higher-level host hospital was identified for each type of complication and emergency, depending on the kind of specialty and advanced facilities required. For each emergency case, the District Health Bureau undertakes an ex-post analysis of the case and provides feedback for strengthening the procedures. In this way, the Pujiang delivery centre is supported by the whole district as well as the city MCH system. This could explain why not a single serious medical incident has been experienced in Pujiang since the inception of the programme in 2004, thus adding to the good reputation of and the increase in the number of deliveries at the centre.

Replicating in other districts

The Shanghai City Health Bureau was involved in the key preparations that led to the establishment of the Pujiang centre. Further, the Vice-Mayor of Shanghai and other municipal dignitaries visited the centre several times. They were satisfied with what they saw and found it to be a promising solution to an important problem in Shanghai. Therefore, nine other districts were asked to establish a similar centre each, through issuing a policy "Establishment of dedicated migrant delivery centres" in June 2004 with effect from August the same year.

The centre in Chonming was later replaced by two others due to the high volume of resident deliveries in the first. Although there have been some differences in development of the 10 centres, the dedicated migrant delivery service has in general been welcomed by migrant

Table 1. Number of migrant deliveries with fee reduction by district, centre and year.
The centres in bold started official implementation in 2004 and the rest, with the exception of number 25, in 2007.

District	Number and name of Centre	2006	2007	2008
Chang Ning	1. Central	0	0	0
Yang Pu	2. Central	0	2	2
	3. MCH	33	0	0
Baoshan	4. **Luo Dian**	992	318	493
Minhang	5. **Pujiang**	5176	9412	9293
Jiading	6. Nanxiang	699	371	613
	7. Anting	26	98	215
	8. **MCH**	854	510	876
Nanhui	9. **Xinchang**	651	126	121
	10. Datuan	200	0	0
Pudong	11. People's Hospital	41	13	59
	12. Seventh Hospital	2	5	19
	13. Punan	5	16	18
	14. **MCH**	52	0	40
Fengxian	15. **Qixian**	0	617	398
Songjiang	16. Central	194	32	139
	17. Sijing	6	41	81
	18. **MCH**	291	105	195
Qingpu	19. **Zhujiajiao**	283	275	478
Jinshan	20. Fengjing	0	48	187
	21. **Jinwei**	154	62	59
	22. Tinglin	0	123	120
Chongming	23. Miaozheng	379	104	77
	24. Changxing	105	4	14
Hongkou	25. Jiangwan	na	na	3
Total		10143	12282	13500

Source: Service report data from Shanghai Health Bureau. Recording started only in 2006.

women. It was soon found that, particularly at the outskirts of Shanghai, the coverage was deemed insufficient and an additional 13 centres were established in 2007. However, eight of these appear to have had a fee reduction practice prior to being designated for implementing the policy (Table 1). Although all these centres are established under the same policy, they operate in different ways: some centres are located within the district town, others are located in townships; some receive financial support from the district government (mostly RMB 200 per delivery), others receive nothing; some provide services to both migrants and residents,

others to migrants only; some do everything in their power to develop the centres while others do little; and some have involved charity organizations, while others have not.

There are clear differences between those centres that started implementing the policy in 2004 (bold in Table 1) and those that started later. With two exceptions, i.e. Pudong-MCH and Jinshan-Jinwei, the early starters have all reached and sustained a three-digit number of "fee-reduced" deliveries. This was the case for only five of the centres that started later. It is noticeable that of these, two (Jiading-Naxiang and Songjiang-Central) appear to have started implementing the policy in a substantial way already before they were told to do so in 2007. However, among the early starters, the Pujiang centre stands out as being particularly successful and popular. Government offices and health managers in different districts ascribe different reasons as to why this is the case. The first group of explanations relates to values. The perception in Minhang District is "*both residents and migrants should have equal rights of access to health services and the government should help those who cannot use or afford safe delivery services*". Responses to the interviews in other districts revealed a range of views among managers, such as: "*Why we should spend money on the migrant population? The target population of our health service should be local residents*," "*Migrant women are extra population*," "*District finance would serve our local residents only*" and "*The government should control the number of people moving from rural areas to*

Shanghai." Such views could explain the reluctance to take responsibility for the problems. Similar views also prevailed in Minhang at the beginning – but were proactively addressed by the Health Bureau Director in the public room as well as in private with key opinion-makers and health staff.

According to a health manager in the Shanghai Health Bureau, a second group of explanations might relate to psychology. According to him, the main difference between Pujiang and the other centres was that the Minhang District Health Bureau actively asked the Shanghai City Health Bureau to approve of its application to establish the centre. The other district health bureaus were asked to establish centres. That is, as he expressed it, the difference between "*I request*" and "*I am requested*", which might explain why Minhang Health Bureau did much more than the others to develop, improve,

Table 2. Number of deliveries at Pujiang Township Health Centre during 2008 by location of the mother

Living location		Number of deliveries
Mothers living in Minhang District		**4015**
Residents		43
Migrants		3972
Living in Pujiang township	1567	
Living in other townships	2405	
Mothers living in other districts		**5278**
Total		**9293**

Figure 1. Average monthly institution-based migrant deliveries in Minhang district from 2004 to 2008, by institution

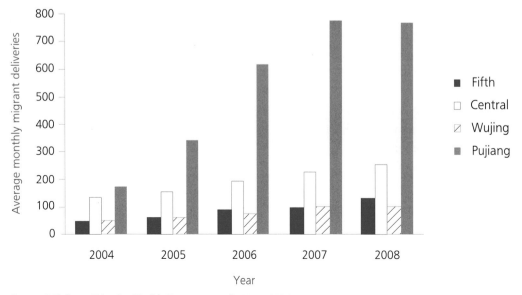

Source: Minhang District Health Bureau records 2004–2008

overcome problems and sustain its centre. A third explanation offered by the same manager as well as others is that the Pujiang Centre is almost exclusively for migrant women while the other centres are for both migrants and residents. Being a "migrants only" centre makes the Pujiang Centre much more famous and migrant women delivering in Pujiang feel less discriminated against. This might explain why half of the women who delivered in Pujiang are from other districts and provinces/cities (Table 2). One woman said it was cheaper to take a taxi to get to Pujiang for delivery than being delivered at her home hospital. Because the other delivery centres accept both residents and migrants, staff explained that they found it very difficult to arrange for a resident woman paying RMB 3000 to stay next to a migrant woman paying RMB 800. Staff working in the other districts reported that doctors would not necessarily inform migrant women about the fee reduction programme and they would thus end up paying the full fee.

Concerning the broader financing, the Minhang Health Bureau staff interviewed indicated that visiting health managers often suggested that "*Minhang district is so rich that you can afford the cost to support these policies*". They responded by saying that financing the dedicated delivery centre as well as other programmes (e.g. tuberculosis) targeting migrants was done largely through re-prioritizing and redistributing the existing budget rather than increasing the overall budget and that "*where there is a will, there is a way.*"

Outcome of the policy

The number of migrant women delivering at the Pujiang township health centre has risen significantly. Since starting to offer dedicated delivery services in July 2004, the number of deliveries increased from about 120 cases in the first month to almost 800 per month in 2007 and 2008, a number which is comparable with that of the largest hospital in Shanghai. However, in terms of the rate of increase in the number of migrant deliveries under the policy, the Pujiang centre stands out from dedicated delivery centres – some of which have conducted very few deliveries (Table 1).

In addition to the Pujiang township health centre, there are three hospitals – Shanghai Fifth Peoples Hospital, Minhang District Central Hospital and Wujing Hospital – providing delivery services in Minhang District. All these four institutions have experienced an increase in the number of migrant deliveries from 2004 to 2008

(Figure 1). In 2004, about 4000 out of a total of 6700 health facility deliveries in Minhang district were those of migrant mothers. In 2008, these numbers were 15 500 migrants out of a total of 18 000 facility-based deliveries within the district.

The service records of the four institutions providing delivery services in Minhang District show that since the opening of the Pujiang dedicated migrant delivery centre in 2004, the number of migrants choosing to deliver at the three non-dedicated facilities within the District has grown steadily without a change in fee policies (Figure 1). While the growth in the number of deliveries at the Pujiang centre was faster during the period from 2004 to 2007 compared with the other three hospitals, it appears that this growth could have levelled off. The number of migrant deliveries at the three hospitals might still be growing.

During 2008, more than half of those delivering at the Pujiang centre were living in districts other than Minhang. Within Minhang district, about 60% of those who gave birth at the centre were living in townships other than Pujiang (Table 2).

5.4 Discussion

Outcome

It is known that the use of antenatal care services is a strong predictor of pregnancy outcome, both in China and elsewhere (Zhan, 2002). Therefore, the change in incentive system from one based on charging for individual procedures to one based on completing the whole-course maternal health schedule, i.e. a system encouraging rather than being an obstacle to the use of services, would be a major contributor to a reduction in maternal mortality.

The increased focus on maternal and migrant health through the publicity by and attention from policy-makers and officials might have led to increasing awareness among migrants and contributed to changed norms and service use patterns even among those who can afford the higher costs at non-dedicated services. There is no indication in the data to suggest that the cheaper dedicated delivery services have replaced the higher-cost services in the three hospitals in Minhang, as there has been an increase in service utilization in all four facilities. It is more likely that the cheaper dedicated delivery service has catered to a segment of the migrant population that hitherto did not use facility-based antenatal and delivery services.

The improved quality of services and standardized referral procedures and practices would lead to a reduction in maternal mortality for the migrant population as a whole and particularly for the more vulnerable segment that had not previously been reached by the health services.

Values

The disparity in maternal health between migrants and residents was obvious from the beginning. While the initial focus might have been on individual tragic cases, researchers soon pointed out that the systemic differences, i.e. inequities between the two population groups, could be avoided by relatively simple means. Further, it was recognized in the media that it was a moral obligation for the society as a whole to reduce these inequities. However, while the health sector was called to act in the absence of interventions targeting the root cause of the problem, nothing happened for a long time to operationalize this obligation.

The Director of the Minhang Health Bureau saw from the beginning that successful reduction of the inequities between the two population groups would, in addition to health, technical and finance administration solutions, require addressing underlying values both in the society and within the service. He also realized that these values would have to be lived and constantly stimulated to grow and thrive – otherwise they would wither. From the results, it appears that there were three key pillars on which the approach to dealing with the values rested, i.e. respect, information and control.

Respect for the individual constitutes not only the right of access to safe delivery services but also the right not to be discriminated against or made to feel inferior. At the dedicated centre in Minghang, migrants are not an additional or marginal group from which lower fees are collected but the focus, the very *raison d'être* for the service. Although the initiative and the immediate answer in Minhang for improving pregnancy outcomes for migrants was with the health department, the application to Shanghai City was supported by all the departments of the District government. This could be taken as recognition of the multifaceted source of the problem,

that the situation was thought to be unjust and avoidable, and that the longer-term solution to this ethical challenge rested with the society at large.

Throughout the process of establishing the Pujiang dedicated delivery service, information played an important role. The public was informed through advertisements about the purpose and availability of the service. Further, the media and dignitaries were used to convey and legitimize the values behind the services and stress that the City of Shanghai has and takes responsibility for the health of migrants – even if they do not have a formal legal residential status in the city. Finally, the Minhang district took on the role of explaining to colleagues from other districts and parts of China that everyone can afford to be more equitable. To make the point, the Pujiang township centre provides delivery services to a very large number of mothers who are not within its natural catchment area. This might have led some of the other centres to adopt fee-reduction practices before they were instructed to do so.

The institutionalization of these values, however, did not rely only on "soft" persuasion, but included several control measures. Before the launch of the service, a protocol for its implementation was developed and intensive supervision and follow up took place over a long period. The formally defined expectations of performance combined with individual, group and institutional follow up from the District Health Bureau no doubt helped in changing the perceptions and attitudes towards migrants which prevailed initially in Minhang district. A further institutionalization of new ways of doing business was through the introduction of the new outcome-based incentive scheme.

Incentives

There are many examples documented in China of fee and incentive systems working against public health objectives (Zhan et al., 2004; Bian et al., 2004). Providers might even shape services and procedures to produce a higher income, including preventing or delaying patients from getting the correct treatment and benefiting from free services (Zhan et al., 2004).

An incentive system is a trade-off with three players – the individual patient, the service provider and the public. The individual patient's interest is in getting as much and as good a service with as low a payment as possible. The provider's interest is, within ethical bounds, to maximize the pay-out from the system. The public's interest is to attain, again within ethical bounds, as much population health as possible with a finite resource envelope. The challenge, from a systems perspective, is to define the package of basic services to be provided and pay a reasonable amount to achieve the desired outcome – an outcome that it is feasible to measure and cannot be easily altered.

The incentive system for township and village health workers based on the concept of "whole-course maternal health care" cuts across several providers and individual services as well as time, and is thus geared to address the full range of obstacles to effective access as defined by Tanahashi (1978). The system is not related merely to the use of services provided by the recipient of the incentive. The incentive is paid for identifying pregnant women in the community, and encouraging, guiding and assisting them to use the services from the early antenatal stage, through delivery and postpartum care. It is in the interest of the township and village health workers to provide services that are effective and easy to use.

In implementing the incentive scheme based on whole-course maternal health care, the Minhang District Health Bureau has come up with a number of innovative solutions to increase the use of services in general and to level up the use among migrants. The scheme puts the beneficiary rather than the provider or the procedure at the centre. It is not the number of procedures that determine the pay-out, but the number of target population members who have benefited from completion of the whole course of procedures undertaken by a range of providers. The scheme has two tiers. There is a base incentive for bringing a pregnant woman to complete the whole course and an additional incentive if the woman is a migrant. Further, the scheme uses a third party verifier who, independently of the township and village health worker as well as the service provider, contacts the mother to follow up and verify what services have been received. In doing so, advantage is taken of new technologies, including computerized databases and mobile telephones.

Finally, in China, providing fee exemptions or services at a reduced cost to correct inequities have frequently been a disincentive for institutions because they would lose money (Meng et al., 2002). In order to overcome this problem, the services at the Pujiang township delivery centre were rationalized and defined as being less costly

and further, the Centre was compensated for the loss of income from fees through reallocation of resources within the district health budget.

Replication and sustainability

Expanding the number of dedicated delivery centres for migrants to a total of 24 across Shanghai city by 2007 was successful. The expansion in dedicated migrant delivery centres and the associated community interventions have most likely contributed to a reduction in inequity. Further, the results show that many migrants prefer to deliver at the Pujiang township centre rather than in their own districts. This could indicate that in the eyes of some migrants, services elsewhere are still wanting. It was probably in replication and sustainability that the least success was achieved. The performance varied across centres with many centres performing well, and several others hardly showing an increase in the number of migrant deliveries. Some even showed decreasing numbers of migrant deliveries with fee reduction. There are also accounts of the lack of internalization of equity values. Some staff at these centres still see migrants as second-class citizens who should have stayed at home rather than drain city resources. Five years after the start, Minhang district still stands out as a shining example. To better understand this, it is useful to look at the role of the pilot, the approach to expansion and the leadership functions.

By all accounts, Minhang district fulfilled its role as a pilot. It transformed ethical principles of equity into practical action. It sorted out implementation problems and found innovative ways of reaching migrants, motivating staff, providing services, monitoring, etc. It provided proof of effectiveness, and showed that it is possible to improve equity in real-life circumstances without additional resources from outside the normal budget of a district. Further, it willingly opened its doors to visitors and colleagues from other districts in Shanghai and elsewhere to explain how it worked. Then, how is it that the model has not been equally successfully replicated throughout Shanghai city?

There were two major differences between the establishment of the centre in Minhang and the subsequent centres in the other districts. First, the wish or drive to create the Pujiang dedicated delivery dentre came from within the district itself. The idea and concepts were developed locally and the full district then requested Shanghai city for permission to start. The city, in turn, challenged the proposal before accepting it. The other districts were requested by the Shanghai City Health Bureau to establish similar centres through issuance of a policy. Second, the scale-up set in motion by instructions from the central Shanghai City Health Bureau transcended the societal ethical concern about migrant health into an administrative health sector-only concern.

When a model is developed in one setting or institution and, *prêt à porter* transferred to another, there is always a need for some adaptation both to the model and the institution in which it is to be applied. However minor this might be, it becomes particularly challenging when a model is meant to modify the functions of the institution, and the attitudes and behaviours of its staff. In Minhang, leadership was available for the values as well as the administrative and managerial transformations. This was not the case for all of the other 25 dedicated centres. At some centres, the old perceptions and attitudes towards migrants as an "extra population" or undue burden on the district prevailed long after the launch, and some showed no increase in the number of migrant deliveries. Sustaining a dedicated migrant delivery centre is likely to have impacts on budgets and service financing, which go beyond the individual institution to the district in general. This was the case in Minhang, where the district health budget was reprioritized in order to finance the fee reduction and reallocation of other resources. Unless there is a buy-in from the whole health sector and probably beyond, the model is unlikely to be sustainable, even if the management of the individual institution is in favour of the policy.

There was overall support for the equity objective in Shanghai city. However, the proactive leadership for value transformation that had driven the process in Minhang was not present at the city level to support those districts that were slow in implementation or where resistance to change prevailed. The comprehensive and omnipresent leadership that is required for a pilot and, indeed was present in case of Minhang, is different from what is required to roll-out the piloted model across multiple districts. In most cases, the technical know-how will either be available on-site or can be called upon by the local management. This is less likely to be the case with respect to a values transformation, which has to start with changing the mind-set of the local management in the individual institution and the health department

as well as the district government as a whole. While the policy and the different tools of the pilot model certainly helped, changing institutional attitudes and behaviours was unfamiliar and demanding for most managers. Further, the Minhang pilot benefited from the close attention of both Shanghai city dignitaries and the media, indicating to the staff that they had an important task to do on behalf of the whole society. In a roll-out, political and media attention will inevitably fade and the impetus they provide will have to be replaced, possibly by a professional values transformation support team.

Such a team should have some technical insight, but should primarily be skilled and equipped for supporting attitudinal and behavioural change. It should operate under the authority of the highest relevant level of multisectoral authority; in the case of Shanghai, the City Council. The team should be able to draw in dignitaries at critical points for each district or centre to boost morale and stress on societal values and the importance of reducing health inequities between migrants and residents.

Limitations of the study

This case is a study of a real-life situation that has evolved over almost two decades with all the complexities that policy processes have. There are many more elements of interest than there are data points (Yin, 2003). Further, there are difficulties in data availability and quality, some of which are intrinsic to the subject being studied – illegal services and non-registered populations. In China as well as elsewhere, there is a tendency to shape reporting as well as opinions to fit official agendas. We have, through combining qualitative and quantitative data and returning to data sources for more clarification, tried to go beyond the surface to explore what really took place. This has revealed a picture that is much more complex and nuanced than the one on the surface showing that things are going well.

5.5 Conclusion

The case described in this study from Shanghai demonstrates that it is possible to improve utilization of maternal health services in order to reduce the inequity between migrants and residents. It shows that additional resources are not necessarily needed. What is needed is an analysis of the main drivers of the inequity. Then, with an open mind, find out what can be done about these drivers, starting from where managerial control is the most direct, i.e. the individual service, followed by the sector and the wider society. The concept of dedicated delivery centres played some role in this; however, it might just have provided a much-needed "laboratory" for innovation. There are at least three key lessons to be learnt from the establishment of dedicated delivery centres in Shanghai.

First, the strength of the pilot project in Minhang was that it was internally driven and did not come about as a result of injection of external pressure or additional resources. It used local resources, commitment and innovation to develop, test and implement new ways of doing business. Financial sustainability of the pilot and subsequent replication was therefore not an issue. Second, one of the most innovative features of the pilot with respect to improving equity is probably the incentive system for township and village health workers. This system puts the focus on the beneficiary and the desired outcome rather than on procedures and health-care providers. This idea could be used independently of the dedicated service to also address inequities originating from other social determinants, in particular, those relating to population group vulnerability. Third, moving from a pilot to scale-up and replication is a critical transition. It is important to realize that it is as much about values as it is about systems and, if sufficient care is not taken, the risk is that only the systems and rhetoric get replicated. Conscious efforts, planning and management are required for the process of transforming values. The pilot project cannot provide much guidance on this. Phasing the expansion process and deploying a professional scale-up management team should be considered. Such a team needs to be able to draw on political and other societal leaders to keep up the encouragement and momentum after the immediate media and political attention have faded.

Most of the lessons learned from the dedicated delivery centres in Shanghai are also applicable to other settings and social determinants. However, it must be noted that while a health sector-based, even if multisector-backed, intervention can help to reduce the inequity in health outcomes, it does not remove the underlying social determinants of the inequity which, in the case of China, are rooted in geographical and economic imbalances, and a legal system that does not allow transfer of citizen rights from one part of the country to another.

Acknowledgements

The researchers are grateful to the World Health Organization for financial support (Project ID: EQH E50-370-6).

This study was mainly carried out in Minhang District. Mr Jian Yongzhi of the District Health Bureau helped in organizing document collection, sorting and arranging in-depths interview, Dr Zhang Xiaohua from Minhang District MCH Centre provided several years of reporting data on maternal health, Director Hu Yutang provided daily service data and routine report tables. All these greatly helped in completing the study.

Dr Zheng Pin from the Division of Maternal Health of the Shanghai Health Bureau provided city-level data on the 25 dedicated delivery centres that enabled the study group to have citywide information.

References

1. Bian Y et al. (2004). Market reform: a challenge to public health – the case of schistosomiasis control in China. *International Journal of Health Planning and Management*, 19 (S1):S79–S94.

2. Gao X (1994). Analysis of 24 maternal deaths in migrants in Shanghai, Shanghai. *Journal of Preventive Medicine*, 6:22–23.

3. Jiang H and Liu Z (1997). Study on maternal and child death of migrants in Shenzhen in 5 years. *Public Health in China*, 13:550–551.

4. Meng Q, Sun Q, Hearst N (2002). Hospital charge exemptions for the poor in Shandong, China. *Health Policy and Planning*, 17(suppl 1):56–63.

5 Minhang District Health Bureau (22 December 2003). MWB[2003] 127. *Announcement on establishing special delivery center for migrants in Minhang District*. Minhang District Health Bureau, Minhang District Population and Family Planning Commission, Minhang District Women Society, Minhang District Public Security Bureau, Minhang District Bureau of Administration Industry and Commerce, Minhang District Finance Bureau, Minhang District Civil Affair Finance Bureau, Minhang District Bureau of Culture, Broadcast and Television and Minhang District Office of administration of migrants.

6 Minhang Health Bureau (22 December 2003) MWB (2003) No 127. *Implementation protocol on migrants delivery care in Minhang District*. Attachment 3.

7 Minhang Health Bureau (6 July 2005). MWB (2005) No 72. *Scheme of systematic maternal care for migrants in Minhang District*. Attachment 1.

8   Low price obstetric service available now in Shanghai. *Shanghai Evening Post*, 28 March 2004:1.

9.   Opening of first low price obstetric service—special hospital for migrants delivery, qualified equipment and services at half price. *Jiefang Daily*, 3 April 2004:1.

10. Shanghai Health Bureau (28 June 2004). SWFJ (2004) No 14. *Announcement of delivery fee limitation for migrants in special delivery centers*. Attachment 2.

11. Tanahashi T (1978). Health service coverage and its evaluation. *Bulletin of the World Health Organization*, 56:295–303.

12. Walder AG (1989). Social change in post-revolution China. *Annual Review of Sociology*, 15:405–424.

13. Wang F et al. (2005). Reproductive health status, knowledge, and access to health care among female migrants in Shanghai, China. *Journal of Biosocial Science*, 37:603–622.

14. Xie X (1997). Health care for migrants in Minhang District during economic transition (unpublished master's degree thesis).

15. Yin RK (2003). *Case study research – design and methods*. Thousand Oaks, California, Sage Publications Inc.

16. Zhan S et al. (2002). Economic transition and maternal health care for internal migrants in Shanghai, China. *Health Policy and Planning*, 17(suppl 1):S47–S55.

17. Zhan S et al. (2004). Revenue driven TB control – three cases in China. *International Journal of Health Planning and Management*, 19 (suppl 1):S45–S62.

Reviving health posts as an entry point for community development

6

A case study of the *Gerbangmas* movement in Lumajang district, Indonesia

Siswanto Siswanto,[1,*] Evie Sopacua[2]

[1,2] Center for Health Policy and Systems R&D, Ministry of Health, Republic of Indonesia
* Corresponding author: siswantos@yahoo.com

Abstract

The objective of this study was to document and elucidate the implementation process of the *Gerbangmas* movement in Lumajang district as an innovation within a decentralized health system. Using a qualitative approach, data were collected through key informant interviews and document review, and then analysed thematically. The study revealed that the policy change of the *Gerbangmas* initiative was not a radical but an incremental process, which took approximately five years. It started from "Conventional Health Posts" to become "Enriched Health Post Halls", and was then revived by the *Bupati* into the Gerbangmas movement. The health sector has successfully advocated to the *Bupati* to create a common vehicle for all sectors. The study identified that the key features of *Gerbangmas* movement were (i) a neutral vehicle (non-sectoral), (ii) having shared goals, (iii) that all sectors could be passengers, (iv) strong power of the referee, (v) the existence of government financial stimulants, (vi) self-management by the community, and (vii) the existence of non-sectoral volunteers as the implementers. The *Gerbangmas* movement has encouraged multiple sectors to set programmes for community empowerment. The study recommended that for conducting community empowerment to address the social determinants of health, it is of importance to use a non-sectoral vehicle that can accommodate multisectoral interests.

6.1 Background

It has been understood by public health experts that population health status, shown by life expectancy, morbidity rate and mortality rate, is the outcome of medical and non-medical determinants. Blum (1974) stated that population health status was influenced by four factors, i.e. environment, behaviour, health-care system and genetics (demography). Blum also stated that out of the four factors, environmental and behavioural factors were the most influential compared with the rest, i.e. health services and genetic factors. With the use of Blum's framework, it can be concluded that, to promote population health status, non-medical interventions or the social determinants of health should be geared towards the improvement of community behaviour and the environment.

Frankish et al. (2007) identified ten social determinants of health that influence population health status: (i) income and social status, (ii) social support networks, (iii) education, (iv) employment and working conditions, (v) social environment, (vi) physical environment, (vii) personal health practices, (viii) healthy child development, (ix) culture and (x) gender. To incorporate these determinants, intersectoral actions are required in a partnership principle with each other.

Health promotion experts have been aware that intersectoral action is the key to success in improving the social determinants of health. However, development actors perceive that intersectoral action is something that is "sweet to talk about" but "hard to implement". Many practical experiences have shown that, very often, programme planning for intersectoral action resulting from a coordination meeting stops at the "meeting note" and is not implemented in the field. The obstacles to implementation of an intersectoral action plan can be understood as each sector would undoubtedly promote its own goal and interests.

Indonesia launched a decentralized system in 2001. This has provided district/municipality governments with more opportunities to make innovations for community welfare. Lumajang district, one out of 38 districts/ municipalities in East Java, has shown innovation in empowering the community to improve the social determinants of health via intersectoral action. Such community empowerment is called *Gerbangmas*, standing for *Gerakan Membangun Masyarakat Sehat*, meaning a "movement for healthy community development".

Through the advocacy of the Lumajang District Health Office, in January 2005, the District Governor (*Bupati*) of Lumajang launched the *Gerbangmas* movement as a strategy for community empowerment by using Health Posts[1] (*Posyandus*) as an entry point. *Gerbangmas*

---

[1] Health Posts (*Posyandus*) are community-based organizations with the principle of "from, by and for" the community themselves. These run five activities, i.e. mother and child health (MCH), family planning, nutrition improvement, immunization and diarrhoea control. *Posyandus* were established by the health sector as a response to the 1978 Alma Ata Declaration, which made use of the *PKK* movement (Family Welfare Movement) members as health volunteers. Day-to-day activities of *Posyandus* are run by the health volunteers.

Health Posts, as community institutions established to implement the *Gerbangmas* movement, had three functions: (i) as the centre for community education, (ii) centre for community empowerment, and (iii) centre for community services (Local Government of Lumajang, 2005). As an innovative community empowerment movement in the decentralized system, the policy of the *Gerbangmas* movement is interesting. The objective of this study is to describe the policy process of the *Gerbangmas* movement in Lumajang District, Indonesia, focusing on the way the policy was set up and implemented.

6.2 Methods

The case study employed a qualitative approach. Data and information were collected by two methods, in-depth interviews with key stakeholders and review of related documents. The interviews with key informants were tape-recorded in order to maintain the integrity of the information (Mack et al., 2005).

Key informants interviewed were: (1) representatives from the sectors in the district (Health Office, *PKK*, Development Plan Body, Legislative, Agriculture Office, Family Planning Office, Education Office, Community Empowerment Office, Religion Office, and Cooperative, Industry and Trade Office), (2) representatives from subdistrict levels (Head of Subdistrict administration, Head of Health Centre), and (3) representatives from the community levels (Head of Village Administration, Health Volunteers and informal leaders).

The documents reviewed included: (1) documents/secondary data related to the process of setting up the *Gerbangmas* policy (District Health Office and District Local Government), (2) documents/secondary data related to the *Gerbangmas* policy guideline (*PKK* office and District Health Office), (3) documents/secondary data related to the implementation of the programme (realization of the action plan, community resource mobilization, programme financing, human resources/volunteers, coverage, etc.) (District Health Office and Health Posts). Data were analysed qualitatively according to the various themes. The study was exempted from research ethics review as interviewees were interviewed in their official capacity only.

6.3 Findings

Gerbangmas policy structure

After a long political process to accommodate the interests of the stakeholders involved, the concepts of *Gerbangmas* were agreed upon. These concepts were documented in the form of the "*Gerbangmas* guideline for volunteers". The guideline consisted of (i) a background, (ii) framework of thinking, (iii) operational definition, (iv) goal and objectives, (v) organization, (vi) indicators to be achieved, (vii) programme implementation, and (viii) reporting system. As documented in the guideline, the concept of *Gerbangmas* is outlined in Table 1.

Table 1. The concept of *Gerbangmas* using Health Posts as a centre for community development activities (Lumajang *PKK* Team, 2006a)

Basic thoughts	Community addressed	Vehicle and priorities	Expected outcome
Healthy paradigm Environmental improvement Qualified family	People at sub-village level	Vehicle: Health Posts Priorities: MCH and health care Family endurance* Mental and spiritual building Healthy environment Clean and healthy behaviour Productive economy	The realization of Healthy Lumajang 2007 and Qualified Family in 2012

* Family endurance consists of four promotive health efforts, i.e. under-five growth stimulation, youth community activities in health, elderly community activities in health, and family planning.

The goal of *Gerbangmas* was the achievement of Healthy Lumajang 2007 followed by Healthy Indonesia 2010 and Qualified Family in 2012. The objectives of the movement were addressed at four segments, i.e. (i) the community, (ii) Health Posts, (iii) the government, and (iv) the private sector. The community objective was to increase the achievement of *Gerbangmas* indicators in the Health Post's areas, in order to support the achievement of Healthy Lumajang 2007 and Qualified Family in 2012. For Health Posts, the objective was to enhance their roles as centres for community education and training, and community empowerment and services. For the government, the objective was to increase coordination and synergy between development programmes. For the private sector, the objective was to increase the partnership of the government and private sector in the development of community health and welfare (Lumajang *PKK* Team, 2006a).

The *Gerbangmas* movement had 21 indicators to be achieved; 14 indicators for human development, one indicator for economy, and six indicators for household environment (Table 2). These 21 indicators accommodated the interests of all the sectors, i.e. *PKK*, religion, education, cooperative, industry and trade, health, family planning, agriculture and public works.

To understand the *Gerbangmas* concept, the following analogy is useful. The overarching goal of the *Gerbangmas* is Healthy Lumajang 2007 and Qualified Family 2012. The vehicle to achieve this is the *Gerbangmas* movement (assumed to be a non-sectoral vehicle). *PKK*[2] acts as the

Table 2. The indicators of *Gerbangmas* and targets in 2007 (Lumajang *PKK* Team, 2006a)

No	Indicators	Targets in 2007
1	Worship compliance	80% households
2	Literacy	100% population
3	Compulsory basic education	100% population
4	Poor people	<25% households
5	Use of iodinated salt	80% households
6	Under-five undernutrition (below red line)	<5% under-fives
7	Delivery by health staff	85% deliveries
8	Coverage of weighed/under-fives (W/U)	85% under-fives
9	Eligible couples with family planning	80% eligible couples
10	Under-five growth stimulation activity	100% Health Posts
11	Youth community health activity	100% villages
12	Elderly community health activity	100% villages
13	Productive economy group	60% villages
14	Health Posts with first or second strata (good and best)[3]	40% Health Posts
15	Early childhood education	100% villages
16	Clean, green and beautiful environment (green fences)	80% households
17	Use of house yard for productive plants	80% households
18	Use of healthy latrine	60% households
19	Use of safe water	70% households
20	Household waste management	80% households
21	Healthy house	60% households

[2] *PKK* is a semi-government NGO. Its members consist of government officials' wives and the community (mothers), founded in the New Order era (Suharto regime), whose function is to improve family welfare.

[3] Based on its performance, Health Posts were classified into four categories, i.e. poor, moderate, good, best.

driver of the *Gerbangmas* vehicle, while the passengers are all the sectors involved. The referee who prevents conflicts among passengers (sectors) is the District Secretary assisted by the District Planning Body. All sectors can therefore be on board at any time and for as long as required to support the goals of the *Gerbangmas* by implementing their development programmes. The *Bupati* demanded that all community empowerment programmes make use of the *Gerbangmas* as an entry point so that all development programmes at the community level could be integrated through the *Gerbangmas*.

At the village level, the *Gerbangmas* movement makes use of a four-cycle problem-solving approach: (i) problem identification, (ii) community dialogue to set up an action plan, (iii) execution of community programmes, and (iv) monitoring and evaluation. In the *Gerbangmas* movement, the management system was organized hierarchically from the level of Health Posts, to village, subdistrict and finally district level. The *Gerbangmas* management cycle was looked after by the *PKK* volunteers; the functions of multiple sectors were to provide funding and technical assistance with regard to their programmes. All programmes that enhanced community empowerment used *Gerbangmas* as a vehicle.

Above the Health Post level, hierarchical teams were established. At the village level, the Village *Gerbangmas* Team was formed. The head of the village was the governor of *Gerbangmas* at village level. At the subdistrict level, the Subdistrict *Gerbangmas* Team was formed. *Camat*, as head of the subdistrict government, was the governor of *Gerbangmas* at subdistrict level.

Gerbangmas initiative and its political process

The policy process of using Health Posts as the implementing institution of *Gerbangmas* occurred in an incremental manner. There has been intense interaction between the Head of the District Health Office, the *Bupati* and the chairperson of the District *PKK* (the *Bupati's* wife).

In 2001, the District Health Office wanted to improve "conventional" Health Posts (e.g. Health Posts that were conducted in the yard of a community leader with limited activities) to "Enriched Health Post Halls". The District Health Office succeeded in advocating to the *Bupati* to allocate IR 7.5 million (approximately US$ 800) to build Health Post Halls as a stimulant for the community movement. As a pilot project, each subdistrict had to propose one village for the allocation of IR 7.5 million to

build a Health Post Hall. This stimulant has encouraged community solidarity in working together to build more Health Post Halls, in terms of funding, workforce, materials and land.

As Health Post Halls were built, the activities of Health Posts were increased from five activities (i.e. MCH, family planning, nutrition, immunization and diarrhoea control) to include under-five growth stimulation and early childhood education. With the additional activities, Health Posts increased their operating schedule from once a month to twice a week, enriching Health Post activities. The sectors involved were expanding, from health and family planning to include education offices. Health Post Halls have therefore successfully improved Health Post activities and increased the number of sectors involved.

In 2005, the *Bupati* requested the Health Office, District Planning Body and Community Empowerment Office to establish the concept of community empowerment using Enriched Health Post Halls as an entry point. The Health Office then drafted the concept of community empowerment as *Gerbangmas*. Six meetings were held to discuss the concept of *Gerbangmas*. Each sector tried to include their indicators in *Gerbangmas*. Finally, with the commitment of the *Bupati*, 21 indicators of *Gerbangmas* were decided upon (*see* Table 2).

An interview with the chair of the *PKK* revealed that the initiative behind the *Gerbangmas* movement was the Head of the Health District Office.

"*In reality, the one who encouraged the PKK to be the motor of Gerbangmas is the District Health Office. District Health Offices acts as the think tank of Gerbangmas. PKK is the heart of the health sector. PKK and the health sector are united.*"

—Chair of District *PKK*

By using stakeholder analysis, the actors of *Gerbangmas* can be identified as follows. The head of the District Health Office, assisted by his staff, acted as the advocator; the key stakeholder was the *Bupati*; the partners of the advocator were the district *PKK* and other supporting sectors; and those who opposed the movement were sectors not involved in the shared indicators (the 21 indicators). The following statement was provided by the head of District Health Office:

"*We should realize that health is the outcome of all sectors' programmes. So, we need a neutral vehicle so that all sectors can be passengers. The interests of the health sector should be covered or blurred. The weakness of conventional village community health development – conventional Health Posts – is the fact that the vehicle claims to be multisectoral but the end goal is still the interest of the health sector. So, the coordination among sectors is easy to talk about but hard to implement.*"

—Head, District Health Office

The policy process of *Gerbangmas* was incremental (evolutionary) in nature. The evolution of "conventional" Health Posts to "*Gerbangmas* Health Posts" is shown in Figure 1.

Implementation of Gerbangmas from pilot project to districtwide scale up

Implementation of the *Gerbangmas* programme was divided into two steps: (1) pilot project and (2) escalation on a districtwide scale. In 2005, 34 Health Posts were selected to implement the *Gerbangmas* programme as a pilot project (Lumajang *PKK* Team, 2006b). The districtwide escalation of the *Gerbangmas* programme began in 2006 and continued in the following years. In 2006, the *Gerbangmas* programme was expanded to 500 Health Posts; in 2007 it reached 750 Health Posts. The escalation of the *Gerbangmas* programme within three years is shown in Table 3.

In the *Gerbangmas* movement, the Local Government provided IR 10 million[4] (about US$ 1135) to each Health Post for operational and interventional activities. The funding was divided into two: (i) IR 4 million was for operational activities (e.g. volunteers' incentives, administration, activity, data visualization, transport, meetings, etc.), and (ii) IR 6 million was for executing the community action plan. The community action plan was individualized according to the local needs. Every *Gerbangmas* Health Post was unique in terms of its community action plan. For example, in the *Gerbangmas* Health Post of Burno village, the community prioritized the development of latrines. In the *Gerbangmas* Health Posts of Ditotrunan village, the community priorities

Figure 1. The evolution of "conventional" Health Posts to "*Gerbangmas* Health Posts" in Lumajang District

Before 2001

Conventional Health Posts

- Activities: five health services: MCH, Family Planning, Nutrition, Immunization and Diarrhoea Control
- Population targets: mothers and children under 5 years of age
- Place of activities: house yard of community leaders
- Sectors involved: health and family planning
- No. of volunteers: five persons

2001–2004

Enriched Health Post Halls

- Activities: five health services plus under-five growth stimulation, early childhood education, health post for the elderly
- Population targets: mothers, children under 5 years of age and the elderly
- Place of activities: Health Post Halls
- Sectors involved: health, family planning and education
- No. of volunteers: five persons

2005 and after

***Gerbangmas* Health Posts**

- Activities: five health services plus family endurance, clean and healthy behaviour, education for under-five children and illiterate people, mental and spiritual building, productive economy
- Population targets: mothers, children under 5 years of age, the elderly and the entire community
- Place of activities: Health Post Halls, household and community groups
- Sectors involved: multiple sectors (all sectors)
- No. of volunteers: nine persons

[4] One US dollar (US$) is worth approximately 9000 Indonesian Rupiah (IR).

Table 3. Escalation of *Gerbangmas* Health Posts from 2005 to 2007

No.	Subdistrict	Number of *Gerbangmas* Health Posts (cumulative)		
		2005 Pilot project	2006 Escalation	2007 Escalation
1	Lumajang	8	57	87
2	Sumbersuko	3	23	39
3	Sukodono	3	36	49
4	Senduro	1	25	40
5	Gucialit	2	20	29
6	Padang	1	19	37
7	Pasrujambe	1	15	26
8	Klakah	1	25	37
9	Ranuyoso	1	23	34
10	Randuagung	1	25	37
11	Kedungjajang	2	30	42
12	Yosowilangun	1	28	40
13	Jatiroto	1	16	21
14	Kunir	1	23	34
15	Tekung	1	17	25
16	Rowokangkung	1	15	22
17	Pasirian	1	27	39
18	Tempeh	1	27	40
19	Pronojiwo	1	13	19
20	Candipuro	1	21	31
21	Tempursari	1	15	22
	Total Health Posts	34	500	750
	Total budget stimulant	IR 340 million	IR 5 billion	IR 7.5 billion

were household environment and productive economy. The budget from the government functioned as a stimulant and the community contributed half of the total budget at a minimum.

In *Gerbangmas* Health Posts, four volunteers were added, bringing the total from five to nine; the four additional volunteers were taken from local community leaders. The training of the *Gerbangmas* volunteers in 2005 for the pilot project was conducted in the Lumajang capital by the District *Gerbangmas* Team. The training materials consisted of (1) basic materials, (2) core materials and (3) supporting materials. The basic materials included the general policies and organizational structure of *Gerbangmas*. The core materials included (a) education (i.e. basic compulsory education, illiteracy alleviation, early childhood education), (b) health (i.e. under-five undernutrition, delivery by health staff, coverage of weighed under-fives, Health Post's strata, healthy house, healthy latrine), (c) family endurance (i.e. under-five growth stimulation, youth community activities in health, elderly community activities in health and family planning), (d) environment (i.e. green fences, use of house yard for productive plants and waste management), (e) productive economy, (f) mental and spiritual improvement, (g) *Gerbangmas* management cycle, (h) administrative matters of *Gerbangmas*. The supporting materials comprised management tools: (a) technique of community dialogue, community empowerment, writing proposals and reporting results, (b) guideline for filling the forms of the *Gerbangmas* management cycle.

In 2006, as the programme was expanded districtwide, training was done in a hierarchical manner. The District *Gerbangmas* Team conducted a "training of trainers" (TOT) for the Subdistrict *Gerbangmas* Team. The Subdistrict Team assisted by the District Team trained the Health Post's volunteers and village staff. This hierarchical method provided effective organization of *Gerbangmas*, starting from the district level to the Health Post level. After training, the volunteers were expected to be able to perform community surveys, facilitate community dialogue, propose and implement action plans, evaluate the results of those action plans, and to keep account of the money spent. The same method of training was used for escalation of the *Gerbangmas* project in 2007.

Operationalization of the *Gerbangmas* at Health Post level

The first activity done by the volunteers after training was a community survey to identify community problems with regard to the 21 *Gerbangmas* indicators. Using a *household form*, the volunteers conducted house-to-house surveys to identify problems according to the 21 *Gerbangmas* indicators in each household. From the household form, the data were transferred to a neighbourhood community form (forms for Neighbourhood Community[5]). From the neighbourhood community form, the data were entered in the Health Post's form. From these forms, the volunteers were expected to make a map to show the gaps between the reality and the target of *Gerbangmas* for each of the 21 indicators. From this, the volunteers could identify a list of community problems.

The next activity was community dialogue. The list of community problems identified was then discussed in a community dialogue forum to determine priorities and an action plan. The process of identifying the type of activities and the people who would receive stimulants needed a long discussion, negotiation and consensus among community members. Some Health Posts needed one meeting, others two, three or more, depending on the dynamics of community members. The results of the community dialogue were written up as a proposal for the community action plan, comprising two types of activities, e.g. operational and interventional activities. The stimulant of IR 10 million was allocated; IR 4 million for operational costs and IR 6 million for intervention costs. The household that got the stimulant contributed towards execution of the intervention.

To describe the use of the IR 10 million stimulant, one example of the community action plan in *Gerbangmas* Health Post Srikandi, Ditotrunan village, is elaborated. In 2007, the Health Post got the stimulant of IR 10 million. In its action plan document, allocation of the government's stimulant was divided into two. First, operational activities comprised volunteers' honorarium (incentive), meetings, administrative materials and other operational costs. Second, interventional activities comprised (i) communication, information and education (CIE) for compulsory basic education, (ii) CIE for under-five undernutrition, (iii) food supplements for children below the age of 5 years, (iv) CIE for family planning, (v) purchase of iodinated salt, (vi) purchase of appliances for under-five growth stimulation and early childhood education, (vii) productive economy, and (viii) village alley improvement. For interventional activities, the community was obliged to contribute additional funding to run the interventions.

The budget of IR 10 million was channelled to volunteers via the Health Post's bank account in a local bank. The transfer of money was divided into three steps: in the first step, IR 4 million was transferred for operational costs; in the second step, IR 3 million for the first intervention; and in the third step, IR 3 million for the second intervention. As the funding of IR 10 million was included in the local government budgeting system, the transfer of money was not always smooth, which in turn disrupted programme implementation. It could happen that the household that was to receive the stimulant was ready but the money from the government was not yet available.

Every quarter, the volunteers conducted monitoring to

---

[5] Neighbourhood Community is a group of 80–100 households. The community group is chaired by a person who is elected by the community members.

assess the progress in achieving the indicators. Supervision of the community action plan was done by volunteers assisted by the steering team. At the end of the year, the volunteers recapitulated the status of achievement of all activities and reported the results to the village authority. The results were then reported hierarchically to the Subdistrict *Gerbangmas* Team and finally to the District *Gerbangmas* Team. The gaps between achievement in the field and the target became new problems in the following year.

Multisectoral collaboration

The formation of the *Gerbangmas* Team in Lumajang District was clearly defined in the *Bupati*'s Decree No. 188.45/302/427.12/2005 and the roles of all the sectors in the *Gerbangmas* movement were clear (e.g. providing budget and technical assistance). In operating the *Gerbangmas* movement, the *Bupati* functioned as a policy commitment holder, the District *Gerbangmas* Team as implementer at the district level, the Subdistrict *Gerbangmas* Team as implementer at the subdistrict level, the Village *Gerbangmas* Team as implementer at the village level, and Health Post's staff (volunteers and community leaders) as implementers at the operational level.

During the district planning forum, the District Secretary together with the District Planning Body functioned as the referee for multisectoral planning. All the sectors were obliged to develop programmes for achieving the 21 shared indicators. Therefore, the priority problems identified through community dialogue were considered as a reference for all the sectors in developing their programmes. The District *PKK* also played an important role in providing inputs on community problems at the grass-roots level. Funding of the *Gerbangmas* movement was therefore not solely based on the IR 10 million for the Health Post's stimulant (from the Community Empowerment Office), but also from the multisectoral programmes which made use of *Gerbangmas* as an entry point for their programmes. However, the management of money from the other sectors (other than the IR 10 million from the Community Empowerment Office) was done by the respective sectors (not by the volunteers).

The power of *Gerbangmas* to direct multisectoral programmes in providing a budget for community empowerment was surprising. Table 4 illustrates the multisectoral programmes that supported the *Gerbangmas* movement in 2006. The *Gerbangmas*

encouraged all the sectors to compete for allocation of resources for community empowerment programmes at the grass-roots level.

The *Gerbangmas* movement was accepted by the people of Lumajang as a form of "social mobilization" and a means for improving multisectoral indicators of health and well-being. During field observations, a number of banners, logos and billboards related to the *Gerbangmas* could be seen along the city's roads, village alleys and rooftops. The campaigns, for example, were a plea for the success of the *Gerbangmas*, promotion of clean and healthy behaviour, stop smoking campaigns and other messages. Interestingly, all the campaign banners and billboards were made and put up by the communities. These demonstrated that the *Gerbangmas* movement was already accepted as a social mobilization tool for achieving a better quality of life.

The sustainability of *Gerbangmas*

A decentralized system that stresses on district autonomy would have advantages and disadvantages. A decentralized system encourages innovation, democratization, better community involvement and is based on local wisdom. However, a number of disadvantages emerged, notably with regard to the sustainability of the programme. It was common for a newly elected *Bupati* to replace their team (heads of sectoral offices) and set a new policy based on their own vision, as promised in their election campaign. Of course, the policy of the new *Bupati* could be very different from that of their predecessor. Based on general convention, a newly elected *Bupati* would make a district strategic plan for a five-year term. This strategic plan was usually in line with their vision and mission as promised in the election campaign.

In the case of the *Gerbangmas* programme, the threat of sustainability was therefore related to the succession of the *Bupati*. Even though all sectors were happy with the *Gerbangmas* movement, the future of the movement was dependent on whether or not the *Gerbangmas* programme would be continued by the succeeding *Bupati*. This fear was expressed during an in-depth interview with the Chair of the District *PKK* and Head of Community Health Promotion, District Health Office, as follows.

"To assure the sustainability of the Gerbangmas programme, the people of Lumajang should elect a Bupati who can continue Gerbangmas."

—Chair of District *PKK*

Table 4. Multisectoral programmes that supported the *Gerbangmas* movement in 2006

No.	Sectors (Sectoral Office)	Programmes related to community empowerment and services	Total budget (IR 1000)
1	Community Empowerment Office	Women's empowerment for family welfare, social support for the elderly, poverty reduction	5 205 136
2	Population, Family Planning and Civil Registration Office	Birth certificates for volunteers and poor families, family endurance (under-five growth stimulation, youth health, elderly health), family planning services	4 103 761
3	Education Office	Illiteracy alleviation, early childhood education, supply of educational tools for under-five growth stimulation	1 658 180
4	Health Office	Health Post revitalization, food supplementation for under-fives with undernutrition, supply of Health Post appliances, volunteers' jamboree, promotion of clean and healthy behaviour	1 216 844
5	Fishery Office	Promotion of sea and pond fishery, campaign for eating fish	132 300
6	Public Works Office	Village improvement	2 814 000
7	Cleanliness and Environmental Office	Supply of plants to the community, workshop on environment for volunteers, clean river programme, provision of garbage composter and garbage can, and other sanitation programmes	391 575
8	Labour and Transmigration Office	Rich labour project to decrease unemployment	359 880
9	Religion Office	Religious education for the community	2 415
10	Planning Body	Urban poverty alleviation by job training and productive economy programme	359 880
11	Agriculture Office	Yard intensification, supply of plants for productive farming	110 675
12	Cooperative, Industry and Trade Office	Training in productive economy for community groups and cooperative system	192 852
TOTAL			16 547 498

"With regard to the sustainability of Gerbangmas, the most crucial issue is top leader succession."

—Head of Community Health Promotion,
District Health Office

To address the issue of sustainability of the *Gerbangmas* movement, the local government of Lumajang, led by the District Secretary, decided upon two strategies. The first strategy was to make an official book on the *Gerbangmas* movement. The second strategy was to include the success story of *Gerbangmas* in the *Bupati*'s Accountability Report at the end of his term (in the year 2009) to a plenary local legislative meeting. An additional approach was to include the policy of *Gerbangmas* in the District Regulation, which was ratified by the District Legislative. If the *Gerbangmas* was already adopted in the District Regulation, there would be a better guarantee that the succeeding *Bupati* would continue the programme.

6.4 Discussion

The emergence of the *Gerbangmas* initiative as the Lumajang Local Government's policy was not a radical change but rather an incremental process, i.e. from an Enriched Health Post Hall to the *Gerbangmas* movement took about five years. This phenomenon was in line with Lindblom's (1959) theory of policy-making, which stipulated that policy change would occur in an incremental rather than a radical manner. The acceptance of the *Gerbangmas* initiative as a vehicle for accommodating the interests of multiple sectors required a process of advocacy, negotiation and compromise. In the case of *Gerbangmas*, the role of the Head of the District Health Office in continuously advocating for a multisectoral approach model of community empowerment was crucial. The role of the *Bupati* as a key stakeholder (decision-maker) in directing multiple sectors to have "shared goals" also played an important role. What really happened in the *Gerbangmas* policy set-up was a political process. As stated by Hill (1997), policy determination is not a rational process but a political process. Therefore, the set-up of any policy, including community empowerment, requires strong commitment from a key stakeholder or a top leader to direct multiple sectors in achieving certain goals.

The *Gerbangmas* initiative had an advantage in terms of "preventing the occurrence of sectoral egos" by establishing community development programmes

at the grass-roots level. What was interesting in the *Gerbangmas* movement was the nature of the policy. The *Gerbangmas* initiative has a number of outstanding characteristics as compared with the conventional primary health-care model (conventional Health Posts). Some examples include a more neutral and not a sectoral vehicle, shared indicators, stimulant budget from the government, self-management by the community and a neutral implementer (*PKK*). These characteristics of community empowerment were of importance in facilitating the coordination, synchronization and cohesion of multiple sectors and encouraging social mobilization (De Maeseneer et al., 2007). Therefore, the model of *Gerbangmas* could improve the concept of Alma Ata's Primary Health Care, which stresses on health sector indicators but tries to involve multiple sectors in achieving the health sector's goals (WHO, 1998). In the *Gerbangmas* model, none of the sectors were winners or losers; all the sectors were winners. The *Gerbangmas* can be seen as a model to address the social determinants of health (income, environment, education, nutrition, sanitation, housing, religion, etc.) through the efforts of multiple sectors and not by looking after the sole interests of each sector. Rather, all the sectors were committed to look after shared interests.

The tactic of the Head of the District Health Office to blur the health sector goals (health status improvement) with a common goal (family welfare) by using a neutral vehicle (*Gerbangmas*), a neutral implementer (*PKK*), top leader commitment (*Bupati*), shared goals (21 indicators of the *Gerbangmas*), and a neutral referee (District Secretary) was very important in terms of policy advocacy as well as health politics. In the past, in fact, even at present, the model of "each sector employing its own community programme by establishing its own vehicle" is still being used as a model for community development programmes at the grass-roots level. In this case, conflicts between the interests of different sectors are likely to occur as each sector wants to be the best. This situation would cause an unhealthy competition while recruiting volunteers from the community by each of the sectors, and there would be too many community-based institutions that would cause confusion in the community. In the future, health development actors should be smart in executing health interests without defeating other sectors, as stated by Degeling (1997) that "a smart political actor should be able to transform his/her interests to be others' interests".

The concept of *Gerbangmas* of including multiple sectors' interests (21 indicators of *Gerbangmas*) in a single vehicle (*Gerbangmas*) was a breakthrough approach in addressing the social determinants of health. The Mc Keown thesis (Szreter, 2002) states that the health status of a community is the outcome of the development programmes of multiple sectors. Raphael in Mouy and Barr (2006) defined the social determinants of health as "the economic and social conditions that influence the health of individuals, communities and jurisdictions as a whole". The shared indicators of *Gerbangmas* have proven to be an effective instrument in synchronizing multisectoral programmes at the community level. Other key factors for the success of *Gerbangmas* were self-management by the community and the provision of government stimulant. The delegation of all management processes from government staff to the community (volunteers) led to a better sense of belonging to the programme among community members, which in turn effected a kind of social mobilization. To be a successful community empowerment programme, social mobilization is a further important step to be taken (WHO, 2003). It seems that the stimulant model as implemented in *Gerbangmas* would improve the morale of volunteers, as they were entrusted to manage a "governmental budget" and get "money incentives" as well. This would improve the community's trust in the government.

The escalation of the programme from pilot project (34 Health Posts) to a districtwide programme (500 Health Posts) did not experience much difficulty. It seems that the high commitment of the *Bupati*, multiple sectors, and the local legislature were the factors that facilitated programme escalation. However, the assurance of money transfer in a timely manner was crucial for executing the programme smoothly. The problem of cash flow is a weakness of the governmental stimulant model as compared with a pure empowerment model. A pure empowerment model would be more sustainable if an income-generating model for funding is already established. Examples of a pure empowerment model are the Community-led Total Sanitation (CLTS) and the Water and Sanitation Programme East Asia and Pacific (WSP-EAP) (Kar and Bongartz, 2006).

A government policy that does not have the back-up of a high-level government regulation will possibly fail to maintain its sustainability. In the case of the *Gerbangmas* programme, which was backed only by the *Bupati*'s Decree, it was difficult to guarantee sustainability, particularly with the provision of IR 10 million as a stimulant for community programmes. Removal of the government stimulant could be detrimental to the programme. In

terms of sustainability, the *Gerbangmas* programme faced uncertainty due to the successive *Bupatis*' ability to change the policy of their predecessor. In order to ensure the sustainability of the *Gerbangmas* movement, a higher level of regulation should be established (i.e. district regulation), ratified by legislature, which would be a policy umbrella for the succeeding *Bupati*.

From the findings and the discussion of this study, a proposed prescriptive model of community empowerment for addressing the social determinants of health at the local government level can be outlined as follows: (i) the key role of the health sector in a local government is to advocate to key stakeholders in the local government (top authority and legislative) to change its political structure to support health development; (ii) the local government should establish a "neutral vehicle" with "shared goals" to look after multisectoral interests to achieve the social determinants of health; (iii) the rules of the game should be established, as this encompasses which players are on board, who is the referee, and how the game is played; (iv) the programmes should be community empowered in nature (horizontal rather than vertical programmes) so that they can be easily accepted by all the sectors; (v) management of the programmes should be done by the community themselves with technical assistance from the respective sectors; (vi) government financial stimulant is required to show government commitment in improving community living conditions.

6.5 Conclusion

From the findings of this study, it can be concluded that to carry out a community development movement in health at the grass-roots level, the health sector should be able to play an elegant game by creating a neutral vehicle in such a way that the other sectors involved would not lose their interests. It seems that the policy process of creating such a vehicle is incremental in nature, so the health sector needs to continuously advocate to key stakeholders (top leaders) and multiple sectors, and project the health sector's interest to be the interests of multiple sectors. To achieve this, "a single neutral vehicle of community empowerment" that can accommodate multiple sectors' interests as well as top leaders' interests needs to be developed. The vehicle is therefore characterized as (i) having shared goals, (ii) a means for all sectors to achieve their interests, (iii) having the support of top leaders, (v) having government stimulants, (vi) being self-managed by the community, and (vii) being implemented by neutral community volunteers (as opposed to sectoral volunteers). The government stimulant should be implemented in a cautious manner as there is a dilemma in terms of accelerating programmes versus ensuring their sustainability.

References

1. Blum HL (1974). *Planning for health: development and application of social change theory.* New York, Human Sciences Press.

2. De Maeseneer J et al. (2007). *Primary health care as a strategy for achieving equitable care: a literature review commissioned by the Health Systems Knowledge Network.* Geneva, World Health Organization.

3. Degeling P (2007). *Management of organization.* Sydney, University of New South Wales.

4. Frankish J et al. (2007). Addressing the non-medical determinants of health: a survey of Canada's health regions. *Canadian Journal of Public Health*, 98:41–47.

5. Hill M (1997). *The policy process in the modern state.* London, Prentice Hall.

6. Kar K and Bongartz P (2006). *Update on some recent developments in community-led total sanitation. Update paper on IDS Working Paper 257.* Brighton, England, Institute of Development Studies.

7. Lindblom CE (1959). The science of 'muddling through', In: Pugh DS (ed.) (1984). *Organization theory.* (2nd ed). Harmondsworth, England, Penguin Books.

8. Local Government of Lumajang (2005). *The Bupati's Decree No. 188.45/218/427.12/2005 about healthy community development movement (Gerbangmas) in Lumajang District.* Lumajang, Local Government of Lumajang.

9. Lumajang PKK Team (2006a). *Gerbangmas guideline for cadres.* Lumajang, Local Government of Lumajang.

10. Lumajang PKK Team (2006b). *The implementation of Gerbangmas in Lumajang District, 2005.* Lumajang, Local Government of Lumajang.

11. Mack N et al. (2005). *Qualitative research methods: a data collector's guide.* North Carolina, Family Health International.

12. Mouy B and Barr A (2006). The social determinants of health: is there a role for health promotion foundations? *Health Promotion Journal of Australia*, 17:189–195.

13. Szreter S (2002). Rethinking McKeown: the relationship between public health and social change. *American Journal of Public Health*, 92:722–725.

14. WHO (1998). *Health for all in the twenty-first century.* Geneva, World Health Organization.

15. WHO (2003). *Community empowerment for heath and development.* Cairo, World Health Organization Regional Office for the Eastern Mediterranean.

Child malnutrition: engaging health and other sectors

The case of Iran

7

Sara Javanparast[1],*

[1] Discipline of Public Health, Flinders University, Australia
* Corresponding author: sara.javanparast@flinders.edu.au

Abstract

In spite of impressive improvements in many health indicators, child malnutrition — particularly its unequal distribution — has remained a concern for Iranian health and nutrition policy-makers and practitioners. The *Meshkat Salamat* pilot project was the first comprehensive effort by the health system to overcome undernutrition among children in rural areas, based on cross-sectoral action. It commenced in 1996 for a period of three years. Following an evaluation that demonstrated significant improvement in anthropometric indicators among children, the project was scaled up to reach national coverage. This case study examines, through interviews with key players and review of documentation, the implementation of the project with particular emphasis on the processes of scaling up, managing multisectoral action and ensuring sustainability. The findings reveal both opportunities and challenges. The opportunities emerged from a well-structured and available primary health-care network. The challenges were particularly related to the expansion phase, when the project received fewer resources and less support. The nutritional outcomes were achieved in a pilot situation; moving from a controlled and somewhat protected environment to face the real world posed a different set of challenges and called for something in between a pilot and a roll-out phase to test the scalability of programme strategies and approaches before moving to a large-scale operation. An unstable managerial environment was shown as the single most limiting factor in programme scale-up and sustainability as well as for multisectoral action. Hence, broader actions at the organizational level are required to achieve and sustain nutritional objectives.

7.1 Background

Due to the multifaceted aspect of childhood undernutrition, a comprehensive approach, taking the social determinants into account, has been recommended to address this public health condition. In spite of a general agreement on the need for much broader actions to achieve a real change in the prevalence and unequal distribution of child malnutrition among and within countries, there have been limited practical recommendations on how health systems can contribute in undertaking a comprehensive approach. This gap can be filled by putting together experiences from different settings to examine how theories behind malnutrition reduction strategies are translated into effective programmes in a real-life context.

Iran is located in the Middle East region. After the establishment of a primary health-care system in 1979, and integration of many health programmes within the system, the country has made impressive improvements on many health indicators such as child mortality, immunization, breastfeeding and iodine deficiency elimination. However, the country still faces challenges associated with the nutritional status of children. The prevalence and distribution of child malnutrition has been a big concern for Iranian health and nutrition policy-makers and practitioners. According to the

Anthropometric Nutritional Indicators Survey (ANIS I) undertaken in 1998, 15.4% and 10.9% of Iranian children under the age of 5 years suffer from stunting and underweight, respectively (MOHME/UNICEF, 1999). Figure 1 demonstrates the distribution of childhood underweight in 1998.

There is an obvious disparity across provinces and between rural and urban areas, with rural children more than 50% more likely to be underweight than urban children (13.7% vs 9.6%) (FAO, 2002).

A wide range of nutritional interventions such as breastfeeding, growth monitoring and promotion, nutrition education, micronutrient supplementation and salt iodination have been implemented through the primary health-care system. The majority of these interventions were led and implemented by the health sector alone.

The *Meshkat Salamat* project was the first and one of the most comprehensive endeavours of the health system to improve the nutritional status of children in rural areas via a social determinants approach, and to narrow the rural–urban divide in childhood malnutrition.

The nutrition project, called *Meshkat Salamat* in Farsi, was designed to address the medical as well as underlying

Figure 1. Distribution of underweight among children below 5 years of age in Iran, 1998

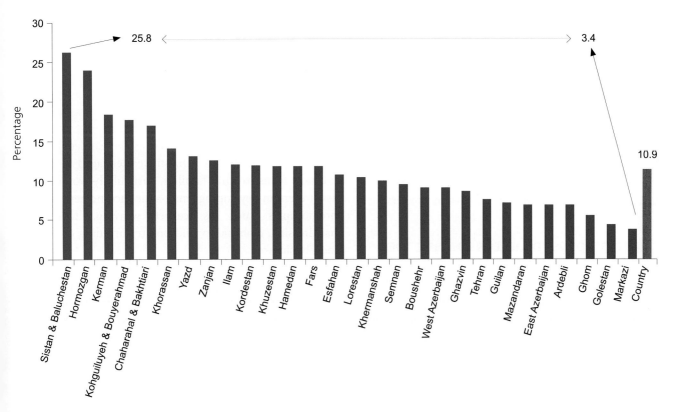

Source: ANIS I (MOHME/UNICEF, 1999)

and basic determinants of childhood undernutrition in rural areas of Iran, focusing on intersectoral collaboration and community empowerment. The core components of the *Meshkat Salamat* project are discussed below.

Nutrition education

Education committees were formed at the provincial and district levels comprising representatives from different sectors. These committees prepared training materials and conducted training workshops for people to play a crucial role in transferring information on nutrition, child feeding, growth monitoring, family planning and food safety to the rural population such as staff in health, education, agriculture and literacy movement organizations, teachers, child-care centres, and the Emdad Imam Relief Organization.

Strengthening literacy programmes for women

This task was undertaken by the Literacy Movement Organization and education sectors with the aim of improving women's literacy. A full list of illiterate women in each rural area was prepared by the community health worker and sent to the Literacy Movement Organization for enrolments in courses and follow up. Some hours of the literacy courses were allocated to issues around health and nutrition.

Improving sanitation and access to safe drinking water

Collaboration was achieved between the Environmental Health Unit, Water Resources and Wastewater Organization, Ministry of Jihad-e-Agriculture, Environmental Protection Organization at the local level in order to increase accessibility to safe water and sanitation. Distribution of chlorine and training of local communities to chlorinate drinking water manually, assessment of rural water pipe systems, and training of rural women to boil water before consumption were among the core activities.

With regard to sanitation, the expansion of sanitary toilets, building of septic tanks, and education for a healthy environment were supported by health workers as well as peripheral workers from all other sectors. Financial support was provided to families in need of building sanitary toilets.

Promoting home gardening

To encourage people to consume more vegetables, agriculture extension workers distributed seeds to health houses and schools. Practical training on nutrition and planting vegetables at home were conducted through the Rural Women's Unit of the Bureau of Promotion of Rural Women and by agriculture extension workers.

Enhancing physical access to basic food

Physical access to basic food was improved by implementing a variety of activities including: collaboration with local food shops to sell basic foods, e.g. dairy products, legumes, etc.; providing business loans by rural cooperations for the establishment of

local food shops; encouraging rural households to start rearing livestock and poultry to improve the availability of dairy products and eggs, with the involvement of the department of agriculture (animal husbandry unit); and providing food baskets to particularly vulnerable families.

Implementing small-scale income-generating programmes

Social welfare organizations such as the Emdad Imam Relief Organization and Behzisti were engaged to grant business loans to rural families, particularly women, to assist them in developing small-scale income-generating programmes such as carpet weaving, tailoring, hairdressing, embroidery and poultry breeding or other local businesses.

The implementation process of the above components was facilitated by the well-established primary health-care network in Iran. A high rate of coverage provided the opportunity to access all rural and remote areas for educational purposes and communication. All other

Figure 2. Comparison of childhood malnutrition in the pilot areas before and after the intervention

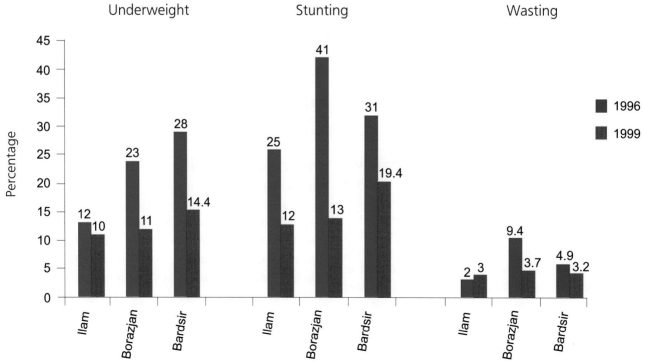

sectors used the structural capacity of the primary health-care network in order to implement their activities, For example, educating family members on child-feeding practices, introducing illiterate mothers to the Literacy Movement Organization, distributing vegetable seeds for home gardening and providing free food baskets as a safety net programme were all undertaken via the primary health-care network. Further, the involvement of *behvarzes* (community health workers who are selected by and live in the main villages) enabled the translation of identified policies into practice, and helped to connect programme planners with the community.

The project was implemented in two phases, i.e. a pilot in three provinces from 1996 to 1998, and a scale-up phase (from 1999 to 2006) during which the project was rolled out throughout the country. A cross-sectional study undertaken at the end of the pilot period demonstrated an almost 50% reduction in child underweight, stunting and wasting in the three pilot provinces (Sheikholeslam et al., 2000).

Another outcome of the pilot project was the development of a collaborative environment via building trust and friendship among different sectors and demonstrating that it was feasible to collaborate between the government and nongovernment sectors to impact the nutritional status of rural populations.

After three years, the results of programme evaluation were released, followed by the preparation of a national guideline.

Despite a positive outcome in terms of malnutrition reduction and the apparent feasibility of the strategy, the project faced several challenges when moving to scale.

This case study examines the implementation process of the *Meshkat Salamat* project with the aim of drawing positive lessons on scaling up, managing multisectoral action and ensuring sustainability, as well as identifying what could have been done differently so that similar programmes can achieve national coverage.

7.2 Methods

A single case study with two groups of study sites was undertaken: pilot provinces and non-pilot provinces, and with two subunits of analysis, i.e. the pilot and the scale-up phases (Yin, 2003). Ilam, Kerman and Boushehr provinces – the target areas in the original pilot project – were selected to investigate the opportunities and challenges they faced during the implementation of the pilot project. Four more non-pilot provinces were selected based on data availability and their interest in participating in the study to provide additional information on the scale-up.

To meet the objectives of the study, primary and secondary sources of evidence were pursued. Data collection was done mainly through review of available documents including proposals for the project, internal records and progress reports at the national and provincial levels. A standard tabular format was used in assessing the items under review. However, lack of accurate documentation was an issue of concern in collecting appropriate information. Document review was supplemented by interviews and focus group discussions to further elucidate the views of different stakeholders with regard to the study questions.

Two informant groups were selected in each province: (a) head of the provincial nutrition division as a "resource person" familiar with the project and engaged in the implementation process; (b) representatives from relevant social sectors (education, agriculture, social welfare, rural cooperatives and literacy movement) which were, or are, involved in the project.

All individual and group interviews were conducted in the Farsi language using an interviewer and focus group guide. In order to improve the accuracy of the transcribed materials, the transcripts were spot-checked by the principal researcher. After transforming the interview data into written documents, the following steps were taken for data analysis: (a) context description; and (b) data classification and interpretation via qualitative content analysis.

Throughout the study, data triangulation (Denzin, 1978) was employed by utilizing different methods in the collection of research data from various data sources, which helped to enhance the rigour of the case study.

Ethics approval was granted by the World Health Organization Ethics Research Committee and ethics committee in the Research deputy, Ministry of Health, Iran. Participants were fully informed about what they were being asked to participate in as well as confidentiality issues. Consent forms were signed by each participant.

7.3 Findings

The pilot phase

The rural areas of three districts (Eivan in Ilam province, Bardsir in Kerman province and Borazjan in Boushehr province) were selected as pilot areas based on a number of criteria including: high prevalence of childhood malnutrition, well-distributed primary health-care network, capable health management, and sufficient health personnel. All the rural areas in each district were covered, i.e. 139 in Ilam, 122 in Borazjan and 176 in Bardsir.

Review of the available documents at the national and provincial levels demonstrated that clear strategies underpinned the pilots in the three original provinces. These are discussed below.

Strong political commitment

Coordination between national-, provincial- and district-level politicians was clearly visible in the design and implementation process of the *Meshkat Salamat* project. Almost all provinces documented the development of a central project committee chaired by local governors in order to ensure political commitment and enhance the collaboration of other sectors with health. This was partly driven by the engagement of key players at ministerial levels.

Intra- and intersectoral action in project design, implementation, supervision and evaluation

Intersectoral action was the principal approach to tackling the socioenvironmental determinants of malnutrition and was considered as an influential factor in the success of the pilot project. Nationally, collaboration between the Ministry of Health and other relevant ministries was established to formulate policies, strategies and agreements. At the provincial levels, interaction between the health and social sectors including Agriculture, Education, Literacy Movement Organization, Imam Khomeini Relief Organization (a social welfare sector) and Rural Cooperatives was the cornerstone of the project. The Literacy Movement is a department within the Ministry of Education and is responsible for educating rural illiterate adults. Social Welfare is a governmental organization which covers poor people in rural areas in terms of health insurance, food aid, etc. The Rural Cooperatives Organization is under the Ministry of Agriculture and is responsible for distribution of food items and managing the rural market.

Working with other sectors within the provinces was facilitated mainly by the involvement of governors, existence of positive perception in some sectors with regard to the necessity of working with health for sustainable development, and informal relationships. The latter was particularly prevalent in local areas because complexity and bureaucracy were less than at the national level. Informal relationships were developed through building friendships among members of the different sectors.

Moreover, vertical alignment of the purpose, activities and support linked the different levels within the health system. Health staff in pilot areas were engaged in the original design of the project via attending the national meetings and discussions. The focal point of the project in one of the pilot areas attested: "*I was involved in this project from the first step. I attended the meetings held at national level with the representatives of other social sectors. We were able to comment on the initial design and implementation of the project in our province.*"

Clear job description

One of the strengths of the *Meshkat Salamat* project was that the roles and responsibilities of each organization were clearly identified in the central committees, taking their capabilities and resources into account. Clarification of the roles and responsibilities of and interrelationships between the wide network of various sectors encouraged planning, adherence to plans and priorities, and rigorous project monitoring and evaluation.

Organizational capacity

Staff training was one of the principal components of the pilot phase, and aimed to increase staff knowledge in order to improve the technical component of the project. A wide range of in-service training and workshops was developed with all sectors as well as retraining of health workers. Training courses for schoolteachers, agricultural experts and social workers are examples of organizational capacity enhancement.

Reviewing the relevant documents revealed that in many areas, incentive systems such as staff promotion were established to increase the attendance rate of staff members, particularly those from the non-health social sectors.

Public awareness and engagement

Educating the public on the problem of child malnutrition and raising awareness about health determinants were incorporated in the development of project policies and strategies. In many rural areas, volunteers among rural women were recruited and trained to transfer information and education.

Targeting

Targeting was considered in the programme design. The three pilot provinces chosen were areas with a high prevalence of malnutrition, and families with undernourished children were the principal project target group.

Rigorous monitoring and evaluation

Supervisory teams were formed and trained at the provincial and district levels with the active participation of representatives from all sectors involved in the programme. Supervision was scheduled once a month for provincial supervisory teams and twice a month for district supervisory teams. Supervisory checklists were developed to standardize monitoring activities in all pilot areas. The results of these regular supervisions were discussed in provincial meetings chaired by the Governors.

An initial situation analysis was performed before launching the project in the three pilot provinces. The socioeconomic status of households and anthropometric indicators of children were determined via a cross-sectional survey. The results were compared with the post-interventional situation after three years of implementation.

Internal and external technical and financial support

The pilot project was funded by the Ministry of Health, with financial and technical aid provided by the United Nations Children's Fund (UNICEF); the latter provided almost half of the project fund.

The scale-up phase

The findings described in this subsection give an overview of the expansion of the *Meshkat Salamat* project to the whole country. This reveals a number of challenges faced during the roll-out of the pilot to achieve national coverage in a real-life situation. The differences between the implementation process of this phase and the pilot phase are discussed below.

Continued supportive policy environment

The pilot phase of the project witnessed a strong and supportive policy environment with active engagement of politicians at national and local levels. One of the respondents who was involved in the pilot project described the role played by the local governors in the success of the programme: "*Meetings were held in the governor's office. Just in this way, representatives of other sectors would attend the meetings. We sent all invitations via the governor-general and tried to solve the challenges in working with other sectors via the governor's engagement.*"

The expansion phase of the programme, however, faced the problem of reduced support from local governments and managers. Accordingly, the level of collaboration among various sectors decreased. The representative of the health sector in one of the non-pilot provinces stated: "*Now, the governor's role is only to sign the invitation letters for meetings, which are prepared by health sector. In other areas, we do not have any sort of support. In the pilot period, the governor was actively involved and there was direct supervision.*" Consequently, project follow up weakened after the pilot phase.

Managerial problems

One frequent finding from stakeholder interviews was the existing challenge at the managerial level of rapid turnover and misperception. This problem was less apparent during the short time frame of the pilot period, and is more likely to affect programme effectiveness in the long term.

The rapid turnover of managers at different levels, leading to loss of continuity, was identified as a principal challenge to success. It was also identified as a factor that limits long-term interinstitutional relations. A respondent in a non-pilot province stressed: "*In our country, managers are changing every six months and the new manager may not believe in this project. The high turnover at managerial level is one of the most important obstacles.*"

Moreover, the lack of common vision between the managers in the health and other sectors with respect to nutritional goals was mentioned as a main challenge. A health representative in one of the non-pilot provinces mentioned: "*One of our main problems in implementing this project was that the managers in the other sectors had very limited knowledge regarding health and nutrition. We had to spend lots of time and energy to convince them."*

Another health staff stated that "*A misperception exists among managers in other sectors that health and nutrition issues are the responsibility of the health sector alone.*" A representative of the education sector also believed that "*working together in our country strongly depends on the perceptions and interests of managers in different organizations. For example, misperception exists in the education sector in our province as the manager does not believe in this project so doesn't advocate for teachers to attend the training classes.*"

Leadership

The project aims, strategies and activities were principally designed at the national level. This issue was expressed widely by respondents from different sectors. A respondent from the agriculture department said: "*The project was designed at a ministerial level and passed on to the provinces. Usually top policy-makers are not familiar with operational problems at the periphery, so we face problems in the implementation phase.*" A top–down approach was prominent in the expansion phase in which pre-determined strategies were advised and implemented.

Furthermore, the Ministry of Health was the principal designer and organizer with almost all social sectors believing in health as the coordinator. A representative of the provincial government stated: "*There is no nutritional goal within the local government. We can play our role via supporting health in facilitating its activities and bringing other sectors around a table.*" Interestingly, this belief was also present among health staff; they felt they needed to be the leaders, supporters and defenders.

This way of thinking was reflected in other aspects of collaborative work. For example, the majority of those interviewed believed that collaborating with the health sector posed extra work for staff in other sectors and, to ensure sustainability, an incentive system including financial or job promotion should be considered.

Financial scarcity

From the documents reviewed, there was evidence that funds allocated to the project within the health sector as well as funds for key activities were included in the budgets of other sectors. Nevertheless, the review highlighted that perhaps the biggest barrier to or lack of

opportunity for collaboration and sustainability of the project was constrained financial resources. This issue was particularly apparent in the expansion phase. The short-term financial assistance from external sources was considered a success factor in the pilot phase. The following statement by the health representative demonstrates this challenge in a pilot province: "*In the pilot phase, we had good support of financial and human resources. Unfortunately, when the programme was expanded to the whole province, all available resources decreased. For example, in the pilot phase, we had 16 cars in two districts in order to do regular supervision, but now we have 4–6 cars to cover the whole province.*"

It was frequently articulated that financial scarcity had a huge impact on the level of collaboration among different sectors. It was believed that intersectoral collaboration was difficult when finances were limited because organizations tended to "pare back" in order to ensure they achieved their core business. Resource scarcity also led to shortages in essential facilities such as transport, recruiting human resources for training, providing vegetable seeds for planting and cooking facilities for classes.

In order to overcome the financial scarcity, a few local initiatives were undertaken such as sharing facilities and resources among various sectors. A respondent from the Agriculture department mentioned: "*In our district, due to the lack of enough budget within the agriculture sector, the health centre purchased and distributed vegetable seeds among households or social welfare organizations accepted to allocate funds for renovating toilets in families with children under five.*"

Official bureaucracy

The existence of an inflexible and slow official bureaucracy was a barrier to the success of the project in relation to other sectors and coordinating activities. Within such an institutional environment, many activities had to be postponed till the long official process was finalized within the management or finance offices. Nevertheless, in some cases, this problem was solved by building intra- and intersectoral relationships based on trust and friendship.

Weakened project monitoring and evaluation

Reviews of documents and interviews with people in non-pilot areas revealed that, in contrary to the pilot phase, there was no systematic analysis done of the initial situation. A variety of methods and data collection instruments were used, including cross-sectional surveys, reports and data gathered regularly at district level. Furthermore, none of the non-pilot provinces used a standard methodology to evaluate programme components after almost six years of implementation.

Community participation

A review of the experiences demonstrated that the main emphasis of the *Meshkat Salamat* project was on education of the community to raise their nutrition awareness to better accept the information provided.

Table 1. Summary of the main items reviewed, the challenges and actions taken to address them, including the recommendations made by those interviewed

Items	Challenges	Actions taken/recommended
Managing intersectoral collaboration	Maintaining collaboration	Involving politicians (governors-general) as committee chairs and programme coordinators
		Identifying clear roles and responsibilities for each organization
		Using the capacities of the PHC network and community workers as an opportunity to integrate the activities of different organizations
		Establishing informal relationships among members of different sectors, based on trust and friendship
		Recommending incentive systems to maintain collaborative action
Project management	Unstable managerial environment	Recommending systems reform with respect to managerial selection and turnover
	Misperception	
	Official bureaucracy	
Adjusting design	Geographical/cultural issues	Decentralizing authority to the district level
	Local needs	Involving provincial-level staff in programme design
Ensuring sustainability	Financial scarcity	Sharing facilities and resources among different organizations
	Institutionalization	Redistributing funds
	Community involvement	Targeting and prioritizing areas with a higher prevalence of malnutrition
		Allocating a specific budget for the project within the MoH national budget
		Promoting community self-help
		Including nutrition in the political agenda
		Engaging community volunteers
Going to scale	Reduced resources	Sustaining support from the government and donors, particularly in terms of budget allocation and evaluation
	Reduced political support	
	Reduced follow up and supervision	

A health staff stated that, "*Educating rural women regarding child-feeding practices is our main job. We include nutritional topics in our training materials and educate mothers in classes.*" A member of the agriculture sector asserted that "*We have taught about nutritional issues and have transferred the information to rural people in our classes or meetings.*"

The project also incorporated broader strategies to promote community self-help such as the provision of cooking facilities by mothers for training classes, using community volunteers in educational activities or distribution of food baskets, and engaging well-off families to support families in need.

However, the provision of free food baskets as one of the components of the project was critiqued by the study respondents as a limiting factor to community development, empowerment and self-reliance, which led to community reliance on governmental donations. The focal point of the project in one of the pilot provinces stated: "*We always emphasize on the provision of free food baskets to poor families. I do believe that this strategy just makes people rely on donations… It does not help people's sustainable access to food. We can't provide free food forever.*"

To sum up, some of the challenges and remedial actions undertaken in the implementation process of this nutrition project on a large scale are discussed above. Some challenges were addressed through national or local initiatives, while a few other challenges seemed to be connected to the more sophisticated political context in which the programme was implemented, and required a broader approach.

7.4 Discussion

In this section, the findings are discussed with the aim of drawing lessons with respect to the three themes of priority public health conditions, i.e. scaling up, managing multisectoral action and ensuring sustainability.

The implementation approaches of a successful pilot project are not necessarily feasible on a large scale

Examination of the *Meshkat Salamat* pilot project demonstrated that the project was successful in achieving the desired outcome, i.e. reduced child malnutrition within the short period of its implementation. However, there could be three main reasons to believe that the success would not easily be replicated when rolling out to the whole country. First, the pilot districts within the three provinces were selected based on a high level of malnutrition, thus providing a great potential for improvement. Second, the districts were also selected based on a well-established PHC infrastructure, capable management and sufficient health staff, i.e. available capacity for improvement. The third reason was the significant additional technical and financial resources brought in by UNICEF for the pilot districts. However, the shift from a pilot project to a large- or full-scale operation moved away from intensive support in a fairly well-controlled environment to real-life challenges.

Comparing the pilot and scale-up phases of the *Meshkat Salamat* project reveals that the non-pilot provinces faced many more challenges in terms of political support, leadership, resources, and programme monitoring and evaluation. Hanson et al. (2003) have categorized the level of constraints in scaling up health interventions, which range from the community level to health system and policy, management and governmental levels. Expansion of the *Meshkat Salamat* project experienced various constraints related to inputs, process, system and values. Although some local initiatives were undertaken to facilitate scalability of the project such as decentralized management, fund-sharing or informal relationships with staff from the social sector, it seems that success in expanding the project requires solutions to system constraints and changes in norms and values, which are much more difficult to achieve.

Political involvement was a key success factor in the pilot phase. A political scale-up strategy which addresses national-level barriers to effective scale up is cited by Uvin and Miller (1996), who emphasize on strengthening government systems. Our findings suggest that strong leadership from a high level of government is required to coordinate the efforts of government sectors, including for establishment of performance standards for the other sectors at the periphery which oblige them to participate in, and comply with, the programme. However, as critical as government leadership is, this is possibly one of the most difficult factors to put into place.

Examination of the *Meshkat Salamat* project and its roll-out throughout the country revealed that, in spite of the positive impact of politicians' involvement on establishing collaborative action, political actors such as governor-generals supported the initiative with only minimal risk and resource investment, through invitations or offering the use of facilities, and therefore provided a different type of relationship to that required for joint and sustainable action, such as policy development. In other words, politicians' involvement was mainly through chairing the key committees, which did not translate into sustainable political commitment. As a consequence, political support was strongly dependent on the individual's perceptions and interests. Weakening political support after the transfer of managers or senior officials is an example of such an unstable policy environment.

In addition to politicians, health managers are considered essential contributors to effective scaling up (Green and Collins, 2003). The lack of management capacity was found to be a major constraint to attaining nutritional goals. Implementing comprehensive interventions and, more importantly, maintaining the positive outcomes of existing programmes are strongly affected by the health management system. As a part of health systems development, it is essential that attention be paid to providing appropriate consideration to the process of health managers' selection, their competencies and stability. The long-term aim should be to build the capacity of national and local governments to incorporate nutrition goals within their own domain. In other words, child nutrition needs to be mainstreamed into the political and sectoral agendas, so that nutrition initiatives can be implemented in any political circumstance.

The ability to manage cultural, economic and geographical diversity in which the programme is to be implemented is also an important issue in scaling up (Ismail et al., 2002). This issue is much more prominent in a heterogeneous country such as Iran with a diverse cultural, ethnic and socioeconomic population. Lack of attention to future scaling-up options in the original design of the project was also a potential weakness. Nevertheless, the local organizations were able to make minor changes to the initial programme design to address a greater perceived need. Changing the target groups or decentralizing authority to the periphery were remedies undertaken to facilitate the implementation process at local levels.

To ensure multisectoral participation, more emphasis needs to be placed on process rather than just health outcomes

Achieving success in nutrition programmes requires not only the achievement of certain desirable outcomes, such as reduced child malnutrition, but also that they be achieved by way of a good process. Gillespie and Haddad (2001) define a process-focused project as one in which participation, local ownership and empowerment are the driving forces, and argue that outcome and processes should be viewed as dual objectives.

Leadership of the project by the health sector may work in the short term with strong supervision, resources, support and follow up. However, it is critical for all involved sectors to have a sense of ownership and collaborate effectively to achieve the long-term goals. This implies that the vision, goals and objectives of the activity as well as its results and achievements (or failures) are fully internalized by the actor(s) concerned (Harris et al., 1995).

The findings of this case study demonstrate a lack of shared values and interests among the different stakeholders, which is an essential condition for success (PHAC, 2007). Instead, intersectoral collaboration was principally established via informal and personal relationships between members of different organizations, based on trust and friendship. Indeed, strengthening this aspect could positively impact on long-term collaboration with other sectors. O'Neill et al. (1997) argue that positive collaborative experiences build personal relationships between members and influence willingness to be involved in future actions. The ability of a programme to sustain collaborative action over large geographical and administrative areas is largely due to the ability to establish a sense of ownership from the start and to institutionalize and mainstream the programme into sectoral activities.

With respect to programme monitoring and evaluation, the project's main focus was on outcome indicators. It is argued that the use of evaluation data is a vehicle to gain incentive and support for programme continuity (Scheirer, 2005). In the *Meshkat Salamat* project, the impressive results of the pilot phase were useful in justifying expansion of the programme to policy-makers. However, in the scale-up phase, there was no common monitoring and evaluation framework and it is questionable if narrow health indicators such as nutrition are sufficient to engage other sectors when an external push and resources are no longer available.

Sustaining a scaled-up multisectoral programme requires the right mix of sectoral integration, targeted funding and community participation

Sustainability seems to be influenced strongly by factors related to people behind the project. In an environment of rapid turnover of managers, inability to sustain action is a serious risk. This is even more so when the results are dependent on simultaneous and complementary activities across several sectors and departments. In such settings, it is of paramount importance to institutionalize roles and functions, i.e. to get them integrated into job descriptions and performance criteria, including into the curricula of the relevant training institutions. Only by doing so can they become independent of who occupies a certain post at a given moment in time.

During the pilot phase, the programme benefited from substantial additional resource input. About half of the pilot project costs were covered by UNICEF. This allowed the provision of significant extra inputs in the form of equipment, supplies, training, technical expertise and supervision. It was not possible to sustain this in the scaled-up programme. However, the other half of the resources of the pilot came from government and local NGO sources, with which it ought to be possible to sustain the programme even on a larger scale. Apart from providing "additional" resources, the UNICEF input might also have been important in providing resources not tied to a particular sector and thus being locked into inflexible bureaucratic processes. Provision of government resources untied to individual sectors, for example, through the office of the Governor to facilitate required intersectoral action, might also be considered. This may also contribute to sustaining the interest and leadership of the Governor in the programme.

A sense of community ownership is achieved when the community becomes more self-reliant, has the capability to analyse its own needs and plan activities to address those needs. Moreover, community support can also help to secure resources and mobilize support for continuation. Self-reliance and a sense of ownership of the initiative by the community are said to be a prerequisite for the success and sustainability of collaborative actions (Gray, 2002; Shannon et al., 2003). Tartar (1996) believes that the level of participation varies from participation in the benefits of health policies and programmes, to a broader level of participation in planning, implementing and evaluating health programmes. Ismail et al. (2002) also classify the levels of community participation – from a passive form in which the community is the recipient of services to self-mobilization, in which people take the initiative independent of project staff and have control over decision-making. In spite of the fact that nutrition education to the rural community assisted in improving their nutritional knowledge and behaviour, there was little evidence of engaging community representatives in the processes of planning, implementing and evaluating the project, or control over collaborative action.

Limitations of the study

This case study had a limited number of sites. The non-pilot provinces were selected based on their interest in participating in the study. This would probably have excluded those with the most problems, e.g. in scaling up, collaborating between sectors and sustaining efforts. However, the objective of the study was to qualify, i.e. to understand the "how" and "why" rather than to quantify. Finally, Iran may differ from many other countries principally in two ways, i.e. the political situation is particularly complex and the primary health-care system is probably stronger and closer to the original primary health care concept than is the case in most other countries.

However, given these limitations, it is still believed that the findings and conclusions provide generic messages of value to all programmes attempting to address the social determinants of health through scaling up and sustaining multisectoral approaches.

7.5 Conclusion

The final thought, then, rests on the likely conclusion that intersectoral action to address the social determinants of malnutrition can work in the setting of Iranian primary health care. The experiences from the reviewed nutrition project justify this claim. There are many opportunities, such as a well-structured primary health-care network, availability and accessibility of health-care facilities, and a positive view of comprehensive primary health care among the health and social sectors. Moreover, the study shows that undertaking local initiatives such as building friendships and trust among members of different sectors can be an effective remedy for overcoming complex bureaucratic and other organizational constraints. However, the documented nutrition outcomes relate to the pilot phase and evidence collected for the expanded programme indicates several challenges encountered while moving from a controlled and somewhat protected environment to a large-scale, real-world situation. This would thus call for a phase in between a pilot and a roll-out phase to test the scalability of programme strategies and approaches before moving to large-scale roll-out.

An unstable managerial environment was shown to be the single most limiting factor for programme scale up and sustainability, as well as for multisectoral action. Hence, broader actions at the organizational level are required to achieve and sustain nutritional objectives.

Acknowledgments

The author gratefully acknowledges the cooperation of Dr Robabeh Sheikholeslam, Head of the Nutrition, Health and Development Institute in Iran, whose expertise has been of great value. Thanks also to Ms Zahra Abdollahi, senior nutrition expert in the Ministry of Health, Iran, for organizing field work, data collection and overseeing the document review process, and to Ms Saeedeh Valaie, who undertook the interviews and focus group discussions at a provincial level. The author also acknowledges the participation of provincial colleagues in the health and other sectors, who gave so generously of their time and shared their experiences. The draft report benefited from the review and comments received from Dr Hossein Afzali, and was edited by Ms Nina Vine.

Finally, the author would like to express her thanks to the World Health Organization for funding this project, without which this report would not have been possible and, in particular, Erik Blas for his valuable comments and input.

References

1. Denzin NK (1978). *The research act: a theoretical introduction to sociological methods.* New York, McGraw-Hill.

2. FAO (2002). *Nutrition country profiles – Iran.* Rome, Food and Agriculture Organization of the United Nations.

3. Gillespie S and Haddad L (eds) (2001). *Attacking the double burden of malnutrition in Asia and Pacific.* Manila, Philippines, Asian Development Bank.

4. Gray A (2002). *Integrated service delivery and regional coordination: a literature review.* New Zealand, Gray Matter Research Ltd.

5. Green A and Collins C (2003). Health systems in developing countries: public sector managers and the management of contradictions and change. *International Journal of Health Planning and Management,* 18:S67–S78.

6. Hanson K et al. (2003). Expanding access to priority health interventions: A framework for understanding the constraints to scaling-up. *Journal of International Development,* 15:1–14.

7. Harris E et al. (1995). *Working together: intersectoral action for health.* Canberra, AGPS.

8. Ismail S, Immink M, Nantel G (2002). *Improving nutrition programs: an assessment tool for action.* Roma, FAO.

9. MOHME/UNICEF (1999). *The nutritional status of children: October–November 1998.* Tehran, MOHME/UNICEF.

10. O'Neill M et al. (1997). Coalition theory as a framework for understanding and implementing intersectoral health-related interventions. *Health Promotion International,* 12, 79–87.

11. PHAC (2007). *Crossing sectors: experiences in intersectoral action, public policy and health.* Public Health Agency of Canada, World Health Organization, Regional Network for Equity in Health in East and Southern Africa. Available at: http://www.phac-aspc.gc.ca/publicat/2007/cro-sec/index-eng.php (accessed on 3 March 2010).

12. Scheirer MA (2005). Is sustainability possible? A review and commentary on empirical studies of program sustainability. *American Journal of Evaluation,* 26:320–347.

13. Shannon C et al. (2003). *Achievements in Aboriginal and Torres Strait islander health: final report.* Canberra, Office of Aboriginal and Torres Strait Islander Health.

14. Sheikholeslam R et al. (2000). *Multi-disciplinary interventions for reducing malnutrition among children in Iran.* Tehran, Ministry of Health, Iran.

15. Tatar M (1996). Community participation in health care: the Turkish case. *Social Science & Medicine,* 42:1493–1500.

16. Uvin P and Miller D (1996). Paths to scaling up: alternative strategies for local nongovernmental organizations. *Human Organization,* 55:344–354.

17. Yin RK (2003). *Case study research: design and methods.* Thousand Oaks, Sage Publications.

The Millennium Villages Project

Improving health and eliminating extreme poverty in rural African communities

Yeşim Tozan,[1,*] Joel Negin,[2] James Wariero[3]

[1] Department of International Health, Boston University School of Public Health, Boston, MA, United States of America
[2] Sydney School of Public Health, University of Sydney, New South Wales, Australia
[3] World Agroforestry Centre (ICRAF)/MDG Centre East and Southern Africa, Nairobi, Kenya, and The Earth Institute at Columbia University, New York, United States of America
* Corresponding author: tozan@bu.edu

Abstract

This case study reviews early experience with a multisectoral development project, the Millennium Villages Project (MVP), in rural African communities. The MVP puts the key recommendations of the UN Millennium Project into practice at the village level to achieve the Millennium Development Goals (MDGs) at a cost of US$ 110 per capita per year on an accelerated timeline of five to ten years as a proof-of-concept project. Of the 12 MVP sites, this case study has been carried out in the first MVP site in Sauri, Kenya, where routinization of the interventions is known to have occurred with documented outcomes over a period of three years. While the emphasis is on the distinctive aspects of the integrated development process based on implementation experiences in three mutually reinforcing sectors (i.e. health, agriculture and education), the case study reviews the local-level institutional and policy environment in which the MVP is executed. The MVP demonstrates that integrated interventions that target simultaneously the availability, acceptability and accessibility dimensions are feasible and can lead to high-impact programmes at the village level. While MVP's efforts to build community capacity and engagement in their own development challenges will be likely to persist beyond the project term, larger-scale public investment is necessary, for instance, in public sector staffing and roads, telecommunications, and input and output marketing systems to ensure the sustainability of project achievements within the project area and the scalability of the approach to other rural communities in Kenya. Governments and donors need to become more flexible and establish mechanisms to facilitate intersectoral synergies and increase their responsiveness to community priorities.

8.1 Background

Smallholder subsistence farming communities in rural areas of Africa are at the global epicentre of extreme poverty and hunger; these communities are often geographically isolated and live in areas with limited or no access to basic public services, and are burdened by disease, climatic shocks, environmental degradation and social exclusion. Rural development policies in developing countries have been shaped by the shifting investment patterns between the social and productive sectors, and the changing role of the government in development policies and activities (Ashley and Maxwell, 2001). Experiences are mixed, and most rural development programmes have proved unsustainable in the past five decades. Poverty reduction, a critical component of the Millennium Development Goals (MDGs), has been placed centre-stage in the revived debate on rural development (Ellis and Biggs, 2001). Overall, there is renewed commitment to promoting pro-poor growth policies and linking international-, regional- and national-level interventions among policy-makers, national governments and donor agencies; however, it is less clear how to deliver proven, practical interventions to well-known problems of the rural poor (Ashley and Maxwell 2001; Farrington and Lomax 2001; Cabral 2006).

A key recommendation of the United Nations (UN) Millennium Project – the official UN strategy on the MDGs formulated by development practitioners and experts from across UN agencies, governments, civil society, the private sector and academia – is that the interlocking dimensions of poverty require coordinated action and sustained investment in multiple sectors at an appropriate scale, with costs shared by communities, national governments and donor agencies (UN Millennium Project, 2005). In remote rural areas where food security remains a major concern, the UN Millennium Project recommends that public investment be targeted at agricultural food production, health, education and basic infrastructure to improve human, social and physical capital so as to trigger a structural transformation in rural livelihoods and productivity to promote poverty exits.

This case study reviews early experience with a multisectoral development project, the Millennium Villages Project (MVP), in rural African communities. Consistent with the long-standing Official Development Assistance (ODA) targets, the MVP aims to put the key recommendations of the UN Millennium Project into practice at the village level to achieve the MDGs at a cost of US$ 110 per capita per year on an accelerated timeline of five to ten years as a *proof-of-concept* project. Of the

12 MVP sites, this case study has been carried out in the first MVP site in Sauri, Kenya, where routinization of the interventions is known to have occurred with documented outcomes over a period of three years. While the emphasis is on the distinctive aspects of the rural development project based on implementation experiences in three mutually reinforcing sectors (i.e. health, agriculture and education), the case study reviews the local-level institutional and policy environment in which the MVP is executed. The primary objective is to obtain a clear understanding of the conditions necessary for the sustainability of project achievements within the MVP site and the scalability of the approach to other rural communities in the host country.

The Millennium Villages Project

The MVP targets the most vulnerable segment of the population, that is, subsistence farming communities living in remote rural areas with limited service provision. The MVP is operational in 12 sites in hunger hot-spot areas of 10 sub-Saharan African countries,[1] each site located in a different agro-ecological zone. The project benefits approximately 400 000 people living and working in rural areas (Figure 1).

The MVP delivers an integrated package of proven high-impact interventions, as identified by the UN Millennium Project. The overall objective of the project is to assist and empower rural communities to lift themselves out of poverty and achieve the MDGs in five to ten years (Sanchez et al., 2004). The underlying hypothesis is that simultaneous multisector interventions have the potential to overcome pervasive capacity constraints to livelihood development and help resource-poor communities escape the poverty trap by increasing productivity, with linkages from agriculture to non-agricultural income-generating activities (Sanchez et al., 2007).

The case study focuses on the first MVP site in Sauri with a total population of approximately 55 000, located in Yala Division, Siaya District, Nyanza Province. The Sauri MVP cluster contains 11 sublocations. The pilot phase of the project started with a town hall meeting in Bar Sauri sublocation (MV1 villages: 5519 people) in July 2004. This meeting brought together the villagers, MVP staff and district government officials to identify local needs, priorities and capabilities (Millennium Villages Project, 2005). In May 2006, the MVP transitioned into a scale-up phase to cover 10 adjacent sublocations (MV2 villages: 50 000 people) surrounding Bar Sauri sublocation.

In the initial MV1 villages, household surveys indicate that 79% of the population lives on less than US$ 1 per day, and agricultural activities constitute the main source of income for three-quarters of the households (Millennium Villages Project, 2007). Baseline assessments in each sector facilitated identification and design of the interventions in the areas of agriculture and environment, health and nutrition, education and community development, basic infrastructure and enterprise development.

Framework and objectives

The MVP postulates that increasing the *availability* of proven interventions across these three sectors (among others) can lead to significant synergies in terms of health and poverty reduction outcomes in targeted communities, and aims to achieve universal access to the interventions. An example is the strengthening of the health-care system by providing a health clinic for every 5000 people, equipped with health workers and essential medicines. Another example is the provision of quality agricultural inputs at subsidized rates to correct for market failures in rural areas.

A comprehensive approach to community development through capacity building and empowerment is a central feature of the MVP and is expected to improve the *acceptability* of interventions in the health and other sectors, leading to their wider and sustainable adoption by communities. A primary intervention in this area is training of villagers on technical issues (e.g. new farming techniques) and leadership skills to build adequate capacity for operation and management at the village level. Another intervention is community education to increase awareness on priority public health and gender issues.

Increasing the availability and acceptability of interventions is necessary, but is not sufficient to ensure increased and equitable access to interventions. The MVP focuses on removing financial, social and geographical barriers to accessing health, education and agricultural services and inputs, particularly by vulnerable and marginalized groups. Elimination of user fees at the health clinics is an exemplary intervention addressing the *accessibility* dimension. Another example is the provision of full agricultural input subsidies to the poorest and most

---

[1] During the preparation of the case study, two more MVP sites were launched in Toya, Mali, and Gumulira, Malawi.

Figure 1. The Millennium Village Project sites

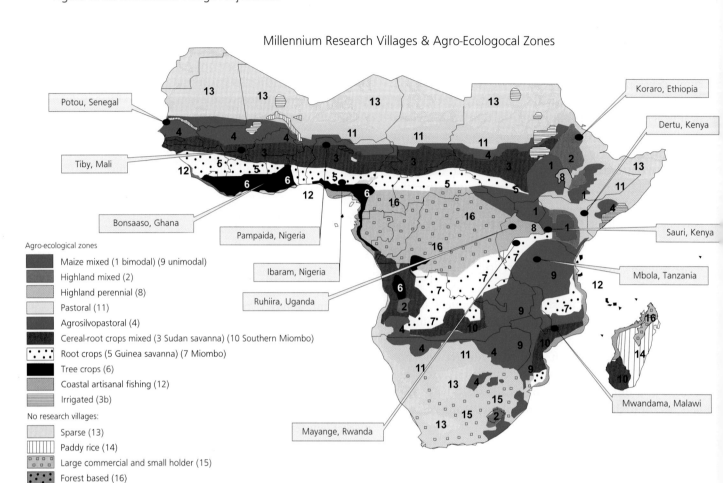

Millennium Research Villages & Agro-Ecologocal Zones

Agro-ecological zones

- Maize mixed (1 bimodal) (9 unimodal)
- Highland mixed (2)
- Highland perennial (8)
- Pastoral (11)
- Agrosilvopastoral (4)
- Cereal-root crops mixed (3 Sudan savanna) (10 Southern Miombo)
- Root crops (5 Guinea savanna) (7 Miombo)
- Tree crops (6)
- Coastal artisanal fishing (12)
- Irrigated (3b)

No research villages:

- Sparse (13)
- Paddy rice (14)
- Large commercial and small holder (15)
- Forest based (16)

Adapted from Dixon et al. 2001. Farming Systems and Poverty. FAO

marginalized households to support the accumulation of assets and increase their livelihood opportunities.

In sum, the MVP combines an integrated package of proven interventions in multiple sectors that target simultaneously the availability, acceptability and accessibility dimensions to achieve rapid progress towards the MDGs at the village level.

Project initiation and leadership structure

The MVP is designed by a team of scientists based at the Earth Institute at Columbia University and is implemented as a proof-of-concept project to galvanize support at the national and international levels for coordinated action and sustained investment within the 10-year time frame for the MDGs. Project implementation is overseen by the United Nations Development Programme (UNDP).

The intervention package is costed at US$ 110 per capita per year as per estimates of the UN Millennium Project

(Sanchez et al., 2004). Over the project term of five to ten years, on average, and depending on local needs and priorities, 40% of the funds is projected to be invested in health, 18% in agriculture and nutrition, 16% in water and environment, 14% in infrastructure, and 12% in education and community development (Millennium Promise).

The US$ 110 is financed from communities, governments and donors, i.e. US$ 10, US$ 30 and US$ 70 per person per year, respectively. The community share is mobilized by village sector committees and comprises in-kind contributions. The district government contribution is primarily towards basic infrastructure development, such as road and communication networks, as well as the provision of nurses, teachers and other essential government staff. The donor share is a sum of the contribution of the MVP through the Millennium Promise (US$ 50) and the contributions of local project partners, including nongovernmental organizations (NGOs), civil society organizations and the private sector

(US$ 20). This represents an increase in overall spending from pre-project levels. The level of increase is different in each MVP cluster, but it is estimated to be approximately US$ 50–70 per capita in view of the fact that some level of community, government and partner spending already exists in these communities.

While US$ 50 per capita per year is budgeted for baseline assessments and research activities in Sauri MV1 villages, the overhead costs of managing the project is US$ 10 per capita per year (Millennium Villages Project, 2007a), bringing the project budget to US$ 120 per capita per year. Fund-raising for the MVP is led by Millennium Promise, an NGO dedicated to supporting the MDGs. Private and governmental donors provide support to the MVP through Millennium Promise.

An underlying principle of the project is the building of a day-to-day decision-making capacity at the village level. This is mainly achieved through participation and empowerment of the villagers in the planning of project activities. The MVP initiated an implementation process in which villagers adopted a rural development approach and formed partnerships with the MVP, district government offices and other local NGOs. To facilitate this process, the villagers organized themselves into six different sector-specific village committees and a village executive committee, which monitors and evaluates if project activities meet community expectations. All committee members receive training on leadership and management skills in addition to technical issues. The village sector committees are responsible for developing community action plans in each sector, identifying existing community resources, and mobilizing villagers for active participation in project activities. The village sector committees meet every week and work closely with the project facilitators on the ground. The project facilitators are either hired by the MVP or seconded to the project as extension officers from the district government offices or other institutions.

8.2 Methods

This case study has been carried out in the Sauri MVP cluster where the routinization of interventions is known to have occurred with documented outcomes over the past three years. It aims to identify the distinctive aspects of project implementation and help in defining the conditions necessary for multisectoral action, sustainability and scalability of the approach.

Data collection and analysis

Two members of the case study team conducted in-depth interviews with 27 individuals who were identified as key informants, given their involvement with the MVP. The field work was completed in November/December 2007. The interview instrument used was designed and revised based on the results of cognitive interviews conducted in the initial phase of the study by the Principal Investigator. Cognitive interviews allowed for testing of interview length, flow and salience of the interview questions, as well as ease of response. The response format was open-ended; key informants used their own words to express their perspectives. The interview questions covered interventions and activities, achievements and implementation challenges.

The case study team further collected relevant project documentation from multiple sources to gather detailed information about programme context and content, and track the actual course of events to develop an understanding of the process of programme planning and implementation. The specific programme outcomes were substantiated by both in-depth interviews and documentary evidence.

Specifically, the case study data are from (1) primary sources: field interviews, direct observations during the site visit, participant observation at the project site through attending community meetings or social interaction with community members, and (2) secondary sources: project documents and programmatic data and records from multiple published sources. Documentary evidence was used to corroborate information obtained from in-depth interviews, and in-depth interviews were conducted with people in different status positions with potentially different perspectives and level of involvement with project activities (data triangulation). The case study focuses on current conditions, using past data to primarily substantiate the information gathered about the processes of programme planning and implementation.

The narrative and numerical evidence was compiled by the Principal Investigator and was critically reviewed by two senior MVP staff. The Principal Investigator contacted key informants with follow-up and clarification questions during the analysis phase, as needed. Preliminary findings of the case study were shared with a critical independent colleague and the draft report was revised accordingly (investigator triangulation).

8.3 Findings

Agriculture

Agricultural interventions are instituted to improve the nutritional, health and socioeconomic status of the population. Maize and beans are the staple food crops in this predominantly subsistence farming area, with an average plot size per household of 0.5 hectares for three-quarters of the households in MV1 villages (Millennium Villages Project, 2005). Most soils were depleted in essential nutrients as a result of continuous maize cropping, and maize production was insufficient to feed a household for an entire year. Fertilizer use was at a minimum, despite the severely depleted soils. For many households, small land holdings coupled with diminishing crop yields contribute to the problem of food insecurity.

Interventions and activities

Hybrid maize seeds, basal fertilizer and top-dressing fertilizer are distributed to all farmers at subsidized rates. To address the issue of project dependence, the agricultural input subsidy decreases each year over the term of the project. All farmers agreed to give 10% of their harvest surplus as a payback to the community in return for the agricultural inputs received. Therefore, the net input subsidy is 90% in year one, 45% in year two, 20% in year three, and 0% in years four and five (P. Mutuo, personal communication, 25 February 2008). Since the project's inception, a vast majority of farmers have received training in farming techniques from the agricultural extension officers seconded to the project from the district agriculture office (Millennium Villages Project, 2007b).

Since the end of 2006, farmers have started to diversify their crops for markets, including high-value vegetables, spices and fruits. Farmers have also engaged in non-farm income-generating activities through demonstration projects, such as livestock for dairy production, poultry and bee-keeping. Some start-up inputs (e.g. bee hives) were provided free of charge or through a flexible pay-back scheme in close partnership with local NGOs or private institutions. Producer groups are formed to promote these new activities.

Achievements

The interventions allowed households to achieve food security in a relatively short period of time, realizing and surpassing 0.6 tons of annual household maize demand, as shown in Figure 2. The interventions also allowed households to become market participants and increase their household income through the sale of harvest surplus, opening a pathway from subsistence to market-oriented farming.

Figure 2. Average annual maize production per household

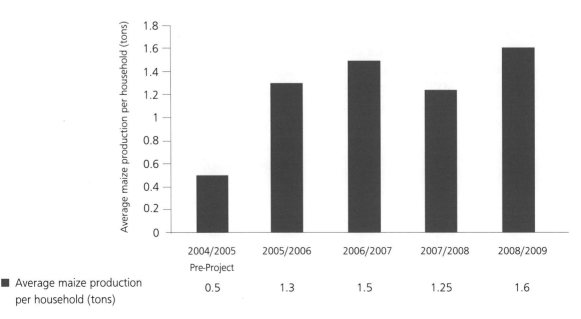

	2004/2005 Pre-Project	2005/2006	2006/2007	2007/2008	2008/2009
Average maize production per household (tons)	0.5	1.3	1.5	1.25	1.6

Interviews with the MVP staff, village committee members, and local government officers revealed the following effects of the agricultural interventions at the household level:

- Increased agricultural production was observed across all farming households and led to decreased short-term and inter-seasonal hunger.

- Increased agricultural production led to increased household income through the sale of harvest surplus.

- Increased agricultural productivity over the past three planting seasons availed land for production of high-value crops and diversification into non-agricultural income-generating activities.

- Increased household income allowed some farmers to purchase agricultural inputs to compensate for the reductions in input subsidies.

Implementation challenges

Interviews with the members of the various village committees revealed a conflict over the agriculture subsidy programme; most villagers expected full-input subsidy over the project term. This conflict was addressed by the MVP through discussions of the objectives of the subsidy programme with the community members at multiple meetings and was resolved by agreeing to provide full subsidy to the poorest and most vulnerable households, as identified by the Village Agriculture Committee, over the project term. The MVP organized information sessions to establish linkages between the farmers and local microfinance institutions. In 2007, few farmers applied for agricultural credit to make up for the reduction in input subsidies. The slow uptake of microfinance has been attributed to the recent introduction of the intervention and to the lingering discontent among farmers over the agriculture subsidy programme. The local MVP staff also noted that local microfinance institutions are risk averse towards agricultural lending.

Interviews with the local government officers at the district agriculture office revealed some early concerns about the agriculture subsidy programme. The MVP directly procured agricultural inputs from external providers and bypassed local agro-businesses in years one and two. In 2007, a voucher system for agricultural inputs was introduced to strengthen linkages between farmers and local agro-dealers, and training was provided to local agro-dealers. As a result, appropriate agricultural products became readily available in the local market.

The district agriculture office values the relationship formed between farmers and local agro-dealers as it is expected to survive beyond the project term.

The primary partnership between the project and the district government is the secondment of agricultural extension officers to the project, which provides necessary logistical resources to facilitate the work of extension officers in the communities, along with an additional stipend. The district agriculture office is unlikely to sustain these extension activities at this heightened level beyond the project unless there is an increase in the annual district budget for logistical expenses.

Health

Health sector interventions are implemented with the goal of improving the overall health and well-being of the population, while also promoting economic activities locally. Prior to project commencement in 2004, there was no health clinic in MV1 villages. Yala subdistrict hospital, with a catchment area of 96 000 people, borders the Bar Sauri sublocation; however, there was no medical doctor employed, and most villagers could not afford the services provided. The Sauri MVP population is a high-risk community for malaria with perennial transmission, and HIV/AIDS prevalence is estimated at 10–30% in this area (Millennium Villages Project, 2005). At project start-up, antiretroviral therapy (ART), HIV testing, and prevention of mother-to-child transmission (PMTCT) services were not available.

Interventions and activities

The MVP aims to provide a basic package of health-care services by operationalizing a health clinic for every 5000 people with health personnel, curative and diagnostic capability, reliable provision of essential medicines and periodic staff training. The MVP also introduced a cadre of community health workers (CHWs) to provide health outreach services. CHWs are trained in the prevention and treatment of common diseases, and remunerated and supervised. Drawn from the community, each CHW works with approximately 200 households.

In July 2005, the Sauri health clinic opened; it is staffed by one Registered Community Health Nurse, one Clinical Officer, two Enrolled Community Health Nurses, one Laboratory Technician, and six CHWs (Millennium Villages Project, 2006). MV1 Sauri residents receive free health-care services at the health clinic while nonresidents are charged a user fee equivalent to that charged at other government facilities. Starting in late 2006 and throughout 2007, similar clinics were established in MV2 villages.

The prevalence of intestinal parasites (*Ascaris lumbricoides, Trichuris trichiura,* or hookworm) in MV1 Sauri residents was 48% for children aged 2–4 years, 80% for children aged 9–10 years, and 75% for women aged 15–49 years (Millennium Villages Project, 2007). A school-based deworming programme was instituted in the three primary schools in MV1 villages in May 2005, and expanded to the 28 primary schools in MV2 villages in 2006.

The MVP distributed free long-lasting insecticide-treated nets (LLINs) to reduce malaria transmission and eventually malaria mortality rates. MVP Sauri residents have received 36 642 LLINs. The Village Health Committee, other community leaders and members were involved in informing and mobilizing the community about bednets (Millennium Villages Project, 2007c). Clearing of mosquito breeding sites around households is another ongoing intervention and recently, indoor residual spraying has been added to see if this cost-effective intervention would have an additional impact on malaria prevalence and incidence.

In collaboration with the Ministry of Health and the Centers for Disease Control and Prevention (CDC), HIV/AIDS services were strengthened. ART, HIV testing and PMTCT services commenced at Yala subdistrict hospital in 2005 (Millennium Villages Project, 2005). The MVP provided substantive budgetary support to the hospital for recruitment of additional health staff and infrastructure development. Over the course of 2007, HIV/AIDS services were decentralized to the health clinics and ART, HIV testing (both voluntary and diagnostic) and PMTCT services were made available at multiple health clinics (Millennium Villages Project, 2007c; Millennium Villages Project, 2007d).

Achievements

Since the opening of the Sauri health clinic in July 2005, MV1 Sauri residents are able to access health-care services closer to their place of residence and free of charge. Figure 3 shows a dramatic drop in utilization in July 2006, which marks the end of the long rainy season (and hence the cessation of malaria and other diseases related to rain), and stays at this low level during 2007.

Interviews with the members of the village sector committees highlighted that malaria has become less of a health problem. The MVP evaluated the impact of the intervention on malaria parasitaemia and anaemia through blood sampling. Initial blood sampling was conducted in March/April 2005 with a representative sample of MV1 Sauri residents, while repeat blood sampling was conducted in December 2006. The results showed that the prevalence of non-zero parasitaemia and high-density parasitaemia had decreased by 79% and 86%, respectively. Similarly, the prevalence of high-

Figure 3. Utilization of health-care services at Sauri Health Clinic – MV1 Sauri residents only

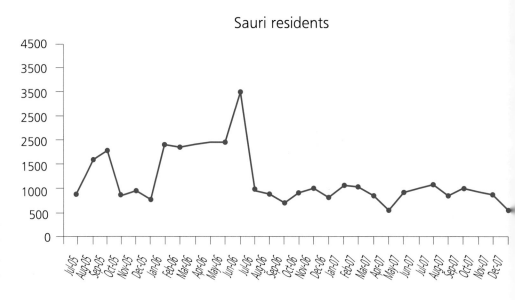

density malaria parasitaemia among children under three years of age had declined by approximately 92%.

Further analysis revealed that the impact of the interventions had significant benefits for the poor. The prevalence of malaria parasitaemia among those earning less than US$ 1 per day was 36% higher than among those earning US$ 1 per day or more at baseline. Following the interventions, the malaria prevalence decreased significantly in the poorer segment of the community and

Figure 4. Prevalence of non-zero malaria parasitaemia for an identical population during baseline (March/April 2005) and repeat blood sampling (December 2006), by income group

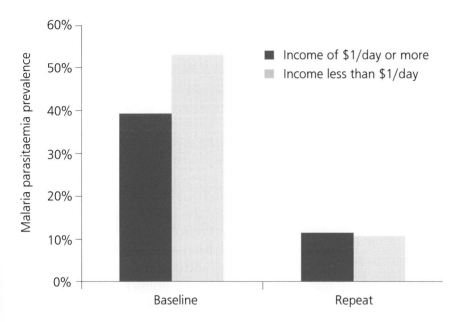

was lower than that of the wealthier segment (Figure 4). The MVP staff noted that the more significant outcomes among the poor are likely to be driven by the fact that, pre-project, fewer of those in poor households had access to bednets, basic health services and food.

Baseline assessments in MV1 villages indicated that 17% of children under the age of 2 years were underweight and 55% underheight (stunted) for their age. The findings of an anthropometric survey at year 3 showed reductions in the prevalence of underweight and stunting of 72% and 45%, respectively, for the same age group.

With support from Yala subdistrict hospital and CDC, HIV/AIDS services have been scaled up in all health facilities in the MVP cluster. This includes provision of testing services, ART and PMTCT. Antiretroviral (ARV) drugs are provided by CDC. By the end of March 2008, 660 people living with HIV/AIDS (PLWHA) in the MV1 villages were identified, of whom 103 are on ART. At Yala subdistrict hospital, 5342 PLWHA were identified of whom 2851 are receiving ARVs.

Implementation challenges

A number of significant challenges arose during project implementation. The MVP's commitment to working within government systems meant that interventions had to be agreed to by the district government office and sometimes by the national government, thus slowing decision-making in some situations. In particular, the recruitment of health personnel at the health clinics proved difficult as these new positions had to be approved by the Ministry of Health. The MVP provides salary top-ups to attract competent staff to the health clinics and Yala subdistrict hospital. This has led to some level of resentment between the government health workers and the new health staff employed through the MVP. While new recruits enjoy higher pay, their full integration into the health-care system as government employees is not guaranteed beyond the project. Overall, salary top-ups have been a contentious issue. Although the Government of Kenya has successfully introduced an allowance scheme for medical doctors, dentists and pharmacists, it currently is not considering the introduction of financial or non-financial incentives for nurses and other lower cadres due to fiscal constraints (Mathauer and Imhoff, 2006).

One of the core health interventions is the establishment or strengthening of a cadre of CHWs. Based on global best practice, the MVP aims to ensure a cadre of remunerated and trained community members who assist in the health facilities and visit households at least once a month to provide health education and awareness on priority health issues. The government recently announced its own CHW policy, which decided against remuneration. Finding literate, motivated community members to train as CHWs was a significant challenge for the project. In order for CHWs to be effective, they need to be readily available and make regular home visits to provide health outreach services. This proved difficult with a volunteer cadre, as proposed by the government. Volunteers often noted that they had to work in their fields for planting or harvesting, thus reducing the time available to undertake voluntary activities. Therefore, the MVP proposed to pilot a remuneration system for CHWs, which is not in line with the current national health sector policy.

The provision of sufficient amounts of essential medicines to health facilities was a significant hurdle. Forecasting increases in utilization as a result of improved health services, removal of user fees, and construction of additional facilities proved difficult, and sufficient medicines and consumables were not available in the government stores. Although the newly constructed Sauri health clinic was registered as a government facility in 2006, it has not received provisions from the Ministry of Health due to delays in regulatory processes. The MVP was often required to procure medicines from external sources, and it was difficult to estimate per capita costing of the health interventions in accordance with the MVP guidelines. There have also been reports of MV2 residents being inappropriately charged user fees in some of the health clinics.

Education

The education sector interventions aim to achieve universal primary school completion with a longer-term goal of transforming societies socially and politically. In Kenya, free primary education was instituted in 2003; however, the estimated primary school enrolment rate is only 76%. There are a number of reasons contributing to this low enrolment, including lack of schools and teachers, child labour and poverty. Although school fees have been abolished, parents are still being charged levies for maintenance and upkeep of school facilities, which affects school enrolment decisions at the household level.

In Sauri, the net enrolment rate in primary education is 84.6%. There are three primary schools in Bar Sauri sublocation. The schools were understaffed, and the classrooms overcrowded. Only one of the schools had a connection to the electricity grid. In the scale-up phase of the project, the total number of primary schools covered went up to 31.

Interventions and activities

The primary activities included renovation and construction of school facilities, removal of levies charged to parents and secondment of teachers. Most of these activities were spearheaded by the Village Education Committee in close collaboration with the head teachers, School Management Committees, local MVP staff and the wider community. The Village Education Committee mobilized the entire community for contributions instead of relying on only parents' efforts. For instance, farmers support the school meals programme with their harvest surplus under a payback scheme for agricultural subsidies received through the MVP. Pit latrines for improved hygiene and privacy in

schools were constructed with the participation and in-kind contribution of the community. The project initiated a sanitary napkin campaign to further increase school attendance of girls.

Achievements

The school meals programme aims at improving school performance and attendance of students. Prior to project commencement, most of the primary schools were committed to providing meals to students only in the higher grades. By the end of 2007, all 31 primary schools in the MVP cluster were equipped with new kitchens and cook stoves, providing nutritious lunch meals to 17 514 students (Millennium Villages Project, 2007b) at an estimated cost of US$ 32 per child per year (Millennium Villages Project, 2006). The local MVP staff and the two head teachers interviewed indicated that the enrolment rates have increased substantially following the interventions, and the primary schools are also attracting students living outside of the MVP cluster. The pupil–teacher ratio was 48:1 at baseline and is now 55:1. The need for more teachers to address this situation was brought to the attention of the district education office. The school attendance rate is currently about 93% in the three primary schools in Bar Sauri sublocation, which is partly attributed to the school meals programme.

Due to increased school attendance, coverage of the deworming programme has gradually expanded over the past three years. Deworming has become a routine intervention and is repeated as per WHO guidelines every four months in all primary schools in the MVP cluster, in close collaboration with the District Health Office.

Implementation challenges

The MVP covers approximately 60% of the costs of the school meals programme while farmers contribute to the programme by giving 10% of their harvest surplus. Parents cover one third of the costs through in-kind contributions, e.g. bags of maize and bean. Although all primary schools are provided with the necessary infrastructure, the sustainability of the school meals programme beyond the project period is questionable because of high recurrent costs. Interviews with the district government officials indicate that there are no plans to take over the school meals programme due to current budgetary constraints. Some of the schools that have land are setting up small farms to produce the necessary inputs.

The District Education Office is extremely underresourced, resulting in its inability to actively support project activities although they highly value the interventions, particularly the school meals programme. Area education officers regularly visit the primary schools in the MVP cluster, and project-related information is shared between head teachers and district education officers. However, understaffing and limited resources are districtwide issues in this sector.

Each primary school in Siaya district has a School Management Committee, comprising members of the community. This committee oversees the school operations and the allocation of resources disbursed by the district government. There was considerable conflict between the School Management Committee and the Village Education Committee, which was established under the MVP. These two committees had overlapping goals, and it proved difficult to establish a working relationship in the beginning. The conflict over the roles and responsibilities of the two committees was clarified by the area inspector of schools from the District Education Office and the local MVP staff.

8.4 Discussion

The MVP demonstrated that, under certain conditions, it is possible in a very short time to achieve the set development goals through a multipronged approach, setting the community at the centre, i.e. proof of concept. However, a number of issues arose during the implementation. These are discussed below under the three themes: managing multisectoral processes, ensuring sustainability and going to scale.

Managing multisectoral processes

The development challenges faced by the rural poor do not fall under specific sectors. Despite frequent commentary regarding the potential value of integrating interventions within the health sector (World Health Organization, 2007; Travis et al., 2004) and throughout the complex development process, implementation models and evidence of success in integrated projects has been limited.

The MVP experience is useful to the extent that it feeds into setting of policy priorities and allocation of resources at the local level. Many of the interventions are mutually reinforcing and collectively target systematic

disadvantages to which rural communities are subjected. For instance, the health status of children depends not only on the delivery of health-care services but also the availability of nutritious food and safe drinking water, and the education of mothers. Agricultural growth depends not only on improved farming techniques and quality agricultural inputs but also the health of farmers and reliable access to local markets. The emblematic example of the donation of a portion of the increased agricultural yield by farmers to the school meals programme, which then leads to increased school attendance and performance, which then contributes to the coverage and success of the deworming programme highlights the potential synergies if integrated activities are pursued. One condition for successful collaboration is the realization of complementarity and dependency of action to achieve sector-specific outcomes. This includes an understanding that action on availability, acceptability and accessibility to support achievements of sectoral outputs may need to be skilfully orchestrated in several other sectors. Integration across sectors is, however, difficult due to the vertical budgets of district government offices and staff shortages.

Communities understand and appreciate the linkages between interventions, and their initiatives and abilities do not adhere to the artificial verticality of government and donor programming. However, decision-making processes at the community level are often not effectively linked to priorities and resource allocations established by local governments and donors. The MVP makes a concerted effort to develop community capacity for collective action through establishment of village sector committees and producer groups, and aims to link communities with the local government and other actors involved with developmental activities in the area.

The role of district governments and decentralized district offices in service provision is generally locality specific, as is the extent to which NGOs and other local actors are involved with service delivery. The MVP stresses the importance of working within government systems and strengthening the capacity of district governments through strategic partnerships in the areas of training, infrastructure development and budgetary support. In establishing and coordinating such partnerships, it needs to be taken into account that different players might have different success criteria and constraints. One example found in the MVP was the hesitation of the microfinance institutions to increase their risks by providing loans in the agricultural sector. Another example was the extreme underresourcing of the District Education Office, which prevented this sector from participating to its full potential.

Poverty reduction strategies and pro-poor growth policies in rural areas should be informed by not only the local conditions but also the diversity of local development processes. There is much to be learned about the complementarities and trade-offs within and beyond the agriculture sector and the village level.

Ensuring sustainability

The MVP, with its emphasis on increased agricultural production, demonstrates the potential of pursuing agricultural input subsidies as a way of kick-starting agricultural growth. Subsidized provision of fertilizers and improved seeds allowed households to achieve food security in a relatively short period of time and increased household income through the sale of harvest surplus. However, small land-holding may limit the effectiveness of agricultural input subsidies and hence the extent to which increased crop yields may lead to improved livelihoods, particularly in the poorest households. The MVP also promotes diversification into non-agricultural income-generating activities, which can intensify household investment in agriculture as well as other crucial areas for human capital development, such as health and education.

The interventions in the agricultural sector have led to a pathway from subsistence to market-oriented farming, providing much-needed livelihood security to small-holder farming households in the MVP cluster, and underpin the need for reliable access to input and output markets, information and credit as part of a multisectoral development strategy in rural areas. An increase in agricultural productivity coupled with higher food prices may generate faster growth and can be an exit route out of poverty for those farmers who are net sellers.

It is understood that the communities will not pay for their own health and education services at the end of five years. External government and donor support to sustain the various achievements attained in the health, education and other social sectors will need to continue. While there is a strong sense of ownership of the interventions at the village level as a result of the project's efforts at community participation and empowerment, the communities will need district government support to pay for medicines, health workers, teachers and other core elements of the sectoral responses. Despite the reliance

on external funding for long-term sustainability of the social sectors, the project's efforts to build community capacity and engagement in their own development challenges will persist beyond project completion. The MVP further illustrates that, for agriculture to become a sustainable vehicle for rural economic and social growth, investments in physical and logistics infrastructure needs to come forward together with ensuring economically viable sizes of land plots.

The primary aim of the project is to prove that the MDGs can be achieved at a modest cost and in a relatively short period of time, and advocate for a more appropriate distribution of donor and government funds to support rural communities, in line with current financial commitments by the G8 and other donor countries. Sustainability should not be viewed from a narrow community, district or national perspective. Subsidies and external support from international sources will be needed to sustain production and workforce capacity for a long time to come.

Going to scale

Closely linked to sustainability is the question of scaling up the project's strategies and interventions to cover all the geographical areas in need. The diversity of sites and range of challenges highlight lessons of key barriers and facilitators, carrying implications for replication and scale up to other contexts. Scaling up will require at a national level additional resources and redistribution of current resources; changes of national policies, e.g. for salary top-ups, allowances for CHWs; as well as availability of sufficient technical, administrative and managerial capacity at central as well as district levels and beyond.

The MVP delivers a package of high-impact interventions in areas critical for increasing human, social and physical capital, and agricultural productivity, which can bring about immediate socioeconomic gains to rural communities in the short term and within a defined area. However, larger-scale public investment is necessary, for instance, in roads, telecommunications, and input and output marketing systems, to ensure that villagers stay on a self-sustaining path as they transition from subsistence agriculture to non-farm, off-farm and other commercial activities. There are cross-talks among the Government of Kenya, which is committed to meeting the MDGs by 2015, the MDG Center in Nairobi, and donor agencies to adopt the MVP approach and scale it up to the district level in eight different districts, indicating some level of ownership at the national level. The MVP stresses the need for higher-level policy-setting to be based upon insights gained at the local level; however, it is well understood that the project is not designed to provide insights on wider issues in scaling up such as facilitating an enabling political and institutional environment to promote pro-poor growth in rural areas. These are issues of considerable debate at the national and international levels, and pose difficulties in setting and implementing rural development policies.

Although the MVP relies heavily on donor investment, the project costs are informed by constraints established by the international agreements for ODA. The MVP provides not only a proof of concept, i.e. it can work in a tightly controlled, pilot project context – the MV1 villages; it also provides a first test of feasibility of scale up – the MV2 villages. The scaling up of the advocated rural development approach in rural parts of Kenya and other sub-Saharan countries will strictly depend on fulfilment of the ODA commitments. Distribution of the increased funding must be informed by demonstrated successful projects such as the MVP.

8.5 Conclusion

The MVP demonstrates that integrated interventions which target simultaneously the availability, acceptability and accessibility dimensions are feasible, and can lead to high-impact programmes in terms of health and poverty reduction outcomes at the village level.

Where integration faces its most significant challenges is the coordination of service provision, resource flows and technical assistance among local actors, particularly within the local government where existing vertical structures are heavily entrenched and where they need to get support from multiple ministries, each of whom work against separate deadlines, budgets and workplans. This makes integrated development work a challenge at the district level. On the other hand, the MVP experience shows that communities can organize themselves to work across programmatic silos with different development partners, if empowered to lead in their own development.

However, larger-scale public investment is necessary, for instance, in public sector staffing, roads, telecommunications, and input and output marketing systems, to ensure the sustainability of project achievements within the project area and the scalability

of the approach to other rural communities in Kenya.

Governments and donors need to become more flexible and establish internal mechanisms to facilitate intersectoral synergies and increase their responsiveness to community priorities. Given the trend towards decentralization in many countries, local governments are not only service providers and decision-makers but also serve as coordinators among local actors and advocates of local interests at the regional and national scale. What is not clear yet is whether or how the MVP experience will contribute to this process.

References

1. Ashley C and Maxwell S (2001). Rethinking rural development. *Development Policy Review*, 19:395–425.

2. Cabral L (2006). Poverty reduction strategies and the rural productive sectors: what have we learnt, what else do we need to ask? In: *Natural resource perspectives*. London, Overseas Development Institute. Available at: http://www.odi.org.uk/publications/nrp/nrp100_web.pdf (accessed on 2 March 2010).

3. Ellis F and Biggs S (2001). Evolving themes in rural development 1950s–2000s. *Development Policy Review*, 19:437–448.

4. Farrington J and Lomax J (2001). Rural development and the 'new architecture of aid': convergence and constraints. *Development Policy Review*, 19:533–544.

5. Mathauer I and Imhoff I (2006). Health worker motivation in Africa: the role of non-financial incentives and human resource management tools. *Human Resources for Health*, 4:24.

6. Millennium Promise. Available at: http://www.millenniumpromise.org/site/PageServer?pagename=mv_unlock (accessed on 2 March 2010).

7. Millennium Villages Project (2005). *Sauri annual report: July 2004–June 2005*. New York, Earth Institute, Columbia University.

8. Millennium Villages Project (2006). *Sauri annual report: July 2005–June 2006*. New York, Earth Institute, Columbia University.

9. Millennium Villages Project (2007). *Sauri baseline report*. New York, Earth Institute, Columbia University.

10. Millennium Villages Project. (2007a). FAQ on the Millennium Villages. Available at: http://www.millenniumvillages.org/resources/index.htm (accessed on 2 March 2010).

11. Millennium Villages Project (2007b). *End of year one report: July 2006–June 2007*. New York, Earth Institute/Millennium Promise/UNDP.

12. Millennium Villages Project (2007c). *Sauri 3rd quarter report: July–September 2007.* New York, Millennium Promise/Earth Institute, Columbia University.

13. Millennium Villages Project (2007d). *Sauri 4th quarter report: October–December 2007.* New York, Millennium Promise/ Earth Institute, Columbia University.

14. Sanchez P et al. (2004). *Millennium Villages: a prototype for scaling-up a package of science based development interventions at the village level based on the recommendations of the Millennium Project.* New York, The Earth Institute, Columbia University.

15. Sanchez P et al. (2007). The African Millennium Villages. *Proceedings of the National Academy of Sciences,* 104:16775– 16780.

16. Travis P et al. (2004). Overcoming health-systems constraints to achieve the Millennium Development Goals. *Lancet,* 364:900–906.

17. UN Millennium Project (2005). *Investing in development: a practical plan to achieve the MDGs.* London, Earthscan.

18. World Health Organization (2007). *Everybody's business: strengthening health systems to improve health outcomes – WHO's framework for action.* Geneva, World Health Organization.

Immunization programme in Anambra state, Nigeria

An analysis of policy development and implementation of the Reaching Every Ward strategy

9

Benjamin Uzochukwu,[1,*] Benjamin Onwughalu,[2] Erik Blas,[3]
Obinna Onwujekwe,[4] Daniel Umeh,[5] Uche Ezeoke[6]

---

[1] Department of Community Medicine, College of Medicine, University of Nigeria, Enugu-campus,
Nigeria & Health Policy Research Group, College of Medicine, University of Nigeria, Enugu-campus, Nigeria
[2] Ministry of Health, Awka, Anambra State, Nigeria
[3] World Health Organization, Geneva
[4] Department of Health Administration & Management, College of Medicine, University of Nigeria, Enugu-campus,
Nigeria & Health Policy Research Group, College of Medicine, University of Nigeria, Enugu-campus, Nigeria
[5] Ministry of Health, Awka, Anambra State, Nigeria
[6] Department of Community Medicine, College of Medicine, University of Nigeria, Enugu-campus, Nigeria
* Corresponding author: bscuzochukwu@yahoo.com

Abstract

Routine immunization coverage in Nigeria has remained low for over a decade, despite several efforts to increase it. There are significant variations in coverage between and within states. The "Reaching every ward" strategy has been in place since 2004 to scale up immunization activities and increase coverage. This would address aspects of the social determinants of child health linked to access to immunization services. However, there has been limited consideration of how the forces underlying the processes of designing and implementing these policies intended to promote equity (such as immunization) influence their achievements. This study explored the roles of stakeholders in the development and implementation of the Reaching every ward (REW) policy for delivering immunization services in Nigeria, and the factors influencing their roles. The exploration involved interviews with policy-makers and health-care providers using a two-case study design approach, with contrasting cases of implementation experience with the REW immunization programme. In addition, relevant documents were reviewed. The strategy got derailed by local and international interests and stakeholders at different levels due to weak management of the policy change and scaling-up processes. As a result, inequities between local government areas increased rather than decreased, which was the original objective. The study concludes that it is possible to drive specific average and equity targets, but short-cut driven approaches increase the risk of relapse and collapse. While involvement at the highest political level is necessary, local-level ownership is indispensable for improving and sustaining equity in immunization coverage.

9.1 Background

Routine immunization against childhood diseases is proven to be one of the most cost-effective interventions for reducing childhood illness and mortality. However, the 1990s experienced a decline in performance of the immunization system. This created a renewed interest in routine immunization (WHO, 2007). Nigeria's immunization coverage also remained low and this increased the burden of vaccine-preventable diseases in the country. There was evidence of low immunization uptake in virtually all parts of the country. The national immunization coverage survey of 2003 showed a national diphtheria, pertussis and tetanus third dose (DPT3) coverage of 24.8%, with widespread inequities in coverage, as children of parents in the lowest socioeconomic quintile were nearly 12 times less likely to be immunized than children of parents in the highest (National Population Commission [NPC] and ORC Macro, 2004). Further, very few states had immunization coverage above 40% (Figure 1).

Figure 1 displays clear differences in coverage between the north and the south as well as variations within the south. However, what is not shown by the mapping is that there are also considerable differences in coverage within each state between local government areas (LGAs) and within each LGA between wards. In order to increase the national and state immunization averages and, at the same time, reduce inequities within states, the Federal Ministry of Health with support from development partners adopted the "Reaching every ward" (REW) strategy in December 2004. This strategy builds on and is in line with the Reach every district (RED) strategy (WHO, 2006) and follows the recommendations made by the 12th Task Force on Immunization (TFI) meeting held the same year in Bamako, Mali.

The main tenet of the REW strategy was to focus particularly on and increase the immunization coverage in those LGAs and wards with a DPT3 coverage of less than 35%. The basic assumption was that low performance is a management issue and can be remedied by supporting and strengthening management. The five operational components of the strategy are: (1) improving access to immunization services through establishing or re-establishing fixed and outreach/mobile immunization sites; (2) supportive supervision of health workers; (3) linking the community with service delivery through the establishment of village and ward health committees; (4) regular monitoring and use of data for action; and (5) planning and management of human and financial resources. All these are aimed at providing accessible, regular, effective, quality and sustainable routine and supplemental immunization services in every ward. The idea was to roll out the REW to all states and, within

Figure 1. DPT3 immunization coverage by state

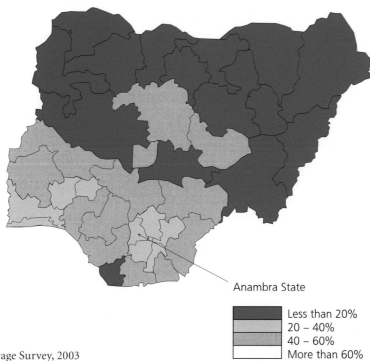

Anambra State

Less than 20%
20 – 40%
40 – 60%
More than 60%

Source: National Immunization Coverage Survey, 2003

each state, to roll out first to those LGAs with less than 35% coverage. As of December 2006, the REW strategy was being implemented in 446 of 774 (57.6%) LGAs in Nigeria, with planned coverage of the remaining LGAs by the end of 2007 (FMOH, 2006).

However, despite all the efforts made to increase immunization coverage, substantial variations persist not only between states but also within states, LGAs and wards. The slow progress threatens the realization of the fourth Millennium Development Goal (MDG) of reducing child mortality by two thirds by 2015.

Internationally, there has been only limited consideration of how the forces underlying the processes of designing and implementing such strategies and policies influence their achievements (Hill and Hupe, 2002), despite wide recognition of their importance for policy change. In most cases, the fact is ignored that implementation processes always involve contestation bargaining and negotiation among a range of actors, who either deliberately or accidentally make or fail to make the decisions that shape policy (Walt and Gilson, 1994).

This study set out to review the development and implementation process of the REW strategy in Nigeria. It explores the roles of stakeholders in implementing the scheme and the factors influencing the processes of

going to scale, managing policy change and ensuring sustainability.

9.2 Methods

The study was conducted in Anambra state, Nigeria. The state comprises 21 LGAs, 235 districts and 330 wards, with the capital at Awka. The 2006 census population of the state was 4 453 964 with 890 793 in the 0–59 months' age group and 2 093 363 in the 0–15 years' age group. There are 33 secondary health facilities, 382 primary health-care centres and one tertiary health institution in the state. Private health-care providers also offer services.

If the REW strategy had worked, the average DPT3 coverage in all LGAs would have increased and the gap between the highest- and the lowest-performing LGA would have narrowed. At the same time, the inequity between wards within each LGA would have decreased. From administrative reporting, it was anticipated that this would not necessarily be the case and, if not, the study would attempt to seek explanations. Based on initial explorations, five subunits of analysis were chosen for the study, i.e. DPT3 coverage, commitment and engagement, power and politics, resources, communication and community involvement.

The study was designed as an explanatory two-case inquiry (Yin, 2003) with contrasting implementation experiences of the REW immunization programme undertaken within Anambra state. Anambra state was chosen for this study for convenience of access and because it was one of the states in the federation with a relatively high, albeit still unsatisfactory, immunization coverage according to the 2003 National Immunization Coverage Survey (Figure 1). Two LGAs out of the 21 were selected for the study. The two LGAs were chosen to represent contrasting LGAs, a high performer (Ekwusigo) and a low performer (Orumba South) based on their reported DPT3 immunization coverage in 2006, i.e. 62% and 29%, respectively. In each LGA, one well-performing and one low-performing health centre were selected based on their immunization coverage. Both LGAs started REW implementation at the same time in all the wards. Thus, the criterion for success of the case study was for the poorest performing site to catch up.

Data collection involved in-depth interviews with key informants, including policy-makers at both the national and state levels, immunization managers and health workers at the state, LGA and facility levels. A total of 24 interviews were conducted, two at the national level, six at the state level, four at the LGA and 12 at the facility level. The key informants were interviewed separately and independently, using an interview guide, and each interview lasted for between 60 and 75 minutes.

All the interviews were tape-recorded except the one with the WHO acting State coordinator who did not agree to recording of the interview. Notes from all interviews were edited and transcribed verbatim immediately after the interview. The transcripts indicated the designation of the interviewee, date/time and duration of the interview only. Information identifying the name of the interviewee was omitted from the interview transcript but was left in the consent form. The interviews were transcribed and coded according to the subunits of analysis following the research questions and emerging issues. In addition to the interviews, relevant programme documents and reports were reviewed.

9.3 Findings

DPT3 coverage

Service data showed an increase in DPT3 immunization coverage in both Ekwusigo and Orumba South (Table 1). Coverage improved consistently during 2005, 2006 and 2007, and had more than doubled in Ekwugiso by 2007 compared with 2004. However, in Orumba South, the coverage declined in 2005 and 2006, although it picked up somewhat in 2007. While the coverage gap between the two LGAs in 2004 was 7 percentage points, this gap increased to 51 percentage points by 2007.

A focus at the ward level reveals different patterns across the two LGAs. In Ekwusigo, a systematic levelling up occurred from 2005 to 2007, when all but one of the wards had achieved a DPT3 coverage of more than 50% according to their service reporting (Figure 2A). In Orumba South, on the other hand, the situation worsened from 2004 to 2006, with one of the wards dropping from the 20–30% to the 10–20% range. Coverage in the highest performing ward also dropped. Only in 2007 did coverage in the wards start picking up (Figure 2B).

Over the time frame reviewed (2004–2007), the inequity in immunization between the two LGAs increased markedly, i.e. the gap in DPT3 coverage increased more than sevenfold. However, within Ekwusigo, the considerable inequities between wards in 2004 consistently reduced in the following years. In Orumba South, the picture is less clear – though the overall coverage increased in 2007, so did the variation in performance across wards.

Commitment and engagement

The drive to introduce the REW came from outside Nigeria. The initial evidence that the strategy could work came from experiences in other African countries. There was also a pressure to catch up with the polio eradication target since Nigeria had one of the last reservoirs in the world.

Table 1. DPT3 coverage, Orumba South and Ekwusigo LGAs, 2004–2007

LGA	DPT3 immunization coverage by year (%)			
	2004	2005	2006	2007
Ekwusigo	42	43	62	96
Orumba South	35	33	29	45

Source: Service data

Figure 2. Reported DPT3 coverage from 2004 to 2007 in the 14 wards of Ekwusigo and the 18 wards of Orumba South

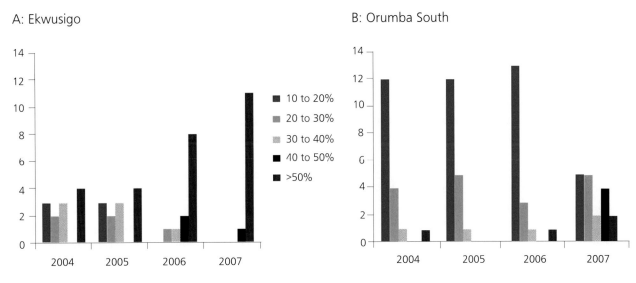

Source: Service data

"*The persistent low coverage of immunization in the country called for new approaches and there were success stories from other African countries. It was also informed by the fact that it was a regional [African] decision. REW is an outcome of an extensive consultative process with all key stakeholders, i.e. political, community, traditional, religious leaders as well as national and international public health experts*" (policy-maker, national).

From the interviews as well as document reviews, it was obvious that the Minister of Health played a key role in the introduction of the REW policy. This was not only due to his formal position as Minister but also because he had strong support from the President who was eager to eradicate polio in Nigeria to respond to the international demand. All REW activities are deployed within the framework of the Interagency Coordinating Committee (ICC), where government and partner agencies are represented. The major stakeholders in the ICC are: the Federal Ministry of Health; World Health Organization (WHO); United Nations Children's Fund (UNICEF); United States Agency for International Development (USAID); Rotary International; the European Union; Department for International Development (DFID); embassies of Canada, Japan and Norway; Christian Health Association of Nigeria; Medecins sans Frontieres (MSF); Red Cross; and Coca Cola.

This multiplicity of agencies was reflected in different ways at the different administrative levels. Although there were political and financial commitments at the

national level, this was not the case at the state and LGA levels. "*At both LGA and state level, REW is seen as a WHO and UNICEF affair. Hence, there is lack of political commitment and inadequate funding at the state level but not at the national level*" (policy-maker, national). According to the policy-makers interviewed at the state level, some important organizations were left out during the planning and implementation stages, including the Nigerian Medical Association, the Nigeria Midwifery and Nursing Association, and the Association of Local Governments of Nigeria (ALGON). Leaving out the latter was seen as a major problem. "*Leaving out ALGON was a big mistake. They are a very powerful group. This is why we have problems at the local government level. You know, this association is made up of all local government chairmen in the Federation and they decide what happens in their local governments. If they were carried along, we would not have had any problems in funding the REW at the LGA level*" (policy-maker, state).

The REW was marketed to the states as a blueprint to resolve their long-standing problems of achieving and sustaining high immunization coverage. Nevertheless, the REW strategy in Anambra state evolved into a Reaching every child (REC) strategy. When queried on why this was so, the explanation was that the state felt that the best way to increase immunization coverage was to go from house to house through supplemental immunization activities and thus focus on one of the components of the REW. This decision was taken by the state immunization team. "*You see, the only way to reach these children faster is to take* the services to their houses" (state programme manager). The shift or "drift", however, may also have come about due to the approach of one of the involved agencies, which was not fully in line with the REW strategy. "*It is not that reaching every ward is not realistic, but from the last meeting we had, the way the UNICEF consultant explained it we understood that it is more realistic reaching every child…*" (PHC Coordinator, Ekwusigo). Achieving a high instant coverage appeared to have taken precedence over building sustainable and equitable routine immunization services, as was envisaged in the REW strategy.

In Anambra state, some LGAs were designated UNICEF LGAs and at a point some were designated as Global Alliance for Vaccines and Immunizations (GAVI)-funded LGAs. "*Here in Ekwusigo, we are very lucky because we are a UNICEF-assisted LGA. So, they provide us with lots of resources*" (Immunization officer, Ekwusigo). In Orumba, which was not funded by UNICEF, the situation was different: "*We are not as lucky as the UNICEF LGAs which are bombarded with a lot of things. I believe the LGA has the resources to implement the REW. But the problem is that in Anambra state these resources are not controlled by the LGA. They are running what they call a 'central purse' and the LGA finds it very difficult to access these funds*" (PHC Coordinator, Orumba South).

Not being among the chosen few not only meant a shortage of or difficulties in accessing funds, it also meant a shortage of attention and guidance: "*Initially, nobody told us anything, they just said there is this new thing called REW and that we should start doing it. Suddenly they realized it was not working and now it is training from all quarters. Today it is UNICEF, tomorrow it is WHO, and so on and so on. The right thing should be done first and that is situation analysis and advocacy with both the community and health workers*" (Immunization officer, Orumba South). At the LGA level, the impetus for action appeared to rest with external agencies, as was also expressed by a manager from Orumba South. Independent local ownership, commitment and engagement, aside from a few health officials, appeared to be very limited at state and LGA levels.

Power and politics

Although implementation of the REW strategy was phased at the national level and supposed to start with those LGAs with less than 35% coverage within the states, Anambra state decided to start the REW strategy in all the LGAs at the same time. This was due

to political considerations. Although the decision was probably political, it was rationalized technically as put by a state policy-maker: "*There was no way we could have implemented the REW in some LGAs leaving the others out because generally routine immunization coverage is low in almost all the LGAs. So implementation was started in all the LGAs at the same time.*"

The process of implementation was delayed, as indicated by both the national- and state-level policy-makers interviewed, by an intraministerial struggle for the control of immunization between the National Programme on Immunization (NPI) and National Primary Health Care Development Agency (NPHCDA), which ended with the NPI ceasing to exist and its functions being subsumed by the NPHCDA. However, those interviewed at the national level did not believe this impacted on the implementation levels. In this process, a range of interventions were added to the original focus on routine immunization services, including: supplemental immunization activity (SIA), immunization plus days (IPD), insecticide-treated nets (ITN), antihelminthics, vitamin A supplementation, soap distribution, etc.

Further interviews revealed that power struggles and conflicts about control existed throughout the system. At the LGA level, "*Initially resources were controlled by the PHC coordinators, but due to mismanagement, it was moved to immunization officers who are administratively under the PHC coordinators. The coordinators felt overlooked. This is causing problems and may affect this new strategy*" (policy-maker, state). At the ward level, there was also conflict about who should control immunization. One of the cardinal changes brought about by the REW was the appointment of a ward focal person who was in charge of all immunization activities within the ward. The guidelines stipulated that this should be a qualified nurse/midwife or a community health officer. However, most of the nurses were newly employed and junior to the majority of the community health extension workers (CHEWs), who were predominantly found in the health centres and were also senior to the nurses by civil service rules. The CHEWs felt that the REW was challenging their competence to head the health centres. This created a lot of resentment and confusion as reported by one of the state policy-makers: "*The CHEWs protested against this arrangement and wrote a series of petitions even to the State Governor. In fact, they sabotaged the REW at some point until it was resolved.*" According to the same interviewee, there have always been such conflicts in the health sector which were merely being exposed by the

REW. He, however, did not offer any suggestion as to why this was so.

Political instability was also one of the concerns raised by policy-makers as negatively impacting implementation of the REW in the state. This was illustrated by one policy-maker who said: "*The state has witnessed a lot of political upheaval in the past with the abduction of the state governor at one point and his subsequent removal at another point.*" Sustainability at the state level is ensured through the State Social Mobilization Committee, chaired by the Commissioner for Health and in which all the major actors in the state are members, e.g. senior staff from the state immunization programme; the Ministries of Education, Information, Women's Affairs, and Planning; Local Government Service Commission; UNICEF; WHO; the National Orientation Agency; Rotary International; the House of Assembly Committee Chair of Health and Religious Institutions; etc. However, the functionality of the committee changes when the Commissioner changes. Anambra has in the recent past had Commissioners who were interested in moving the REW agenda as well as some who were not, thus affecting continuity and lowering the focus on immunization. The political instability also had direct operational implications for government funding: "*There was a time when we applied for funds, but at that time there was an impasse in the state and the governor was not there, so the funds could not be released. This has been happening on and off. Today one governor is in, next month it is another*" (policy-maker, state).

Resources

One of the issues raised by health workers was the inequitable distribution of resources and budgets. As mentioned above, in Anambra state, some LGAs were designated UNICEF LGAs and some GAVI-funded LGAs, while the rest had to rely on government funding. In particular, the UNICEF LGAs got more financial and material resources for the REW than the others, including, for example, solar-powered cold chain equipment. "*UNICEF sponsors our vaccine distribution. Every month they release money to us for collection and distribution of vaccines as well as for outreach. We have motorcycles. They also sponsor our monthly health workers' meetings and are planning to conduct training for outreach services for our health workers*" (Immunization officer, Ekwusigo).

Orumba South, being neither a UNICEF- nor a GAVI-funded LGA, did not benefit from such largesse but had to make do with slow, erratic and scant funding from the state and the LGA. This situation left the Orumba South programme not only with insufficient funding for implementing the REW strategy but also with a raised level of frustration among its managers. The PHC coordinator suggested that it should be the role of the government to even out resources across administrative areas.

The lack of resources in Orumba South affected performance in several ways – frequent and prolonged vaccine stock-outs, shortfall of resources and transportation for covering hard-to-reach populations – constraints that were not experienced by Ekwusigo. However, a deeper and more complex constraint related to human resources. "*We don't have enough staff to carry out REW activities. This LGA is at the extreme of the state. Most of the health workers when transferred to this place stay for a very short time, soon they all leave and vanish to other LGAs. So one thing I have to suggest in this matter is to have rural compensation from the state for those working in rural areas. That is the only way to keep them*" (Immunization officer, Orumba South).

It was not just the absolute shortage of staff that affected the performance of Orumba South. In addition to shortage of staff at the facility level, those interviewed indicated more absenteeism in Orumba South compared with Ekwusigo. As a result, the remaining staff was frequently charged with double and competing duties. "*We are short of staff and most of those we have don't come to work regularly. There is even a health facility head who is also the LGA Roll-back Malaria manager. How do you expect that one to be present at the facility when she is always busy going from one workshop to the other*" (Immunization officer, Orumba South). The shortage of qualified staff at the health facility level translated into concrete problems that directly affected implementation of the strategy: "*We don't have enough health workers to carry out the outreach services, and when we do, we have to close the health centre. Even when we have staff, they are mainly untrained or auxiliary workers. We are only two trained health workers. This is a rural area and the nurses especially don't like to work here*" (health worker, Orumba South). Together with vaccine stock-outs, this contributed to failure in adhering to set service schedules, postponement or cancellation of outreach activities, inability to provide services when mothers came to the centre, etc. According to those interviewed, mothers lost trust in the services and it was difficult to convince them to come back when they had been let down at times.

Communication and community involvement

Better integration of immunization services into community structures through involving the community in the planning and delivery of health services was one of the five operational components of the REW. However, this was found to be a major weakness by one of the state policy-makers interviewed. He said: *"One of the great challenges in ensuring the sustainability of the REW is how to get the community to own the programme. They see it as a government thing. Thus, there is poor community involvement and participation leading to a supply-driven approach …. Efforts are being made to strengthen the capacity of health workers to implement the REW, little is done to strengthen the capacity of the community to understand, use and benefit from the programme."* He found that the talk about community involvement *"started and ended at the state headquarters".*

According to the REW field guide, the community is supposed to be involved through the establishment of ward and village health committees consisting of community members and health-care providers in the catchment area. However, the programme manager shared the view of the policy-maker: *"The REW training so far has stopped at the level of the health facility and we have not yet moved down to the community."*

Although there seemed to be information-sharing about the policy from the state level during the implementation of the REW in the form of the monthly monitoring meetings of LGA immunization officers, disease surveillance and notification officers, and social mobilization officers, some health workers complained about the lack of consultation with them and the communities before implementing the REW. There was minimal training in Orumba South as this LGA was neither UNICEF- nor GAVI-supported.

When facility workers were asked if communities were involved in developing microplans, the responses indicated that community participation was more in Ekwusigo than in Orumba South. The differences in involvement were linked with broader issues of relationship between the community and the health facility. One of the health facility workers interviewed in Orumba South said: *"To be frank with you, I know my community very well, so I don't need the community members to help me in the microplan. Besides, they are always asking for money each time you invite them to the facility for one thing or the other."* Another health worker commented: *"I don't get*

them involved because there are a lot of political differences in the community. So who are you going to invite and leave out? You don't know who to follow." Health workers in Orumba South also mentioned during the interviews that they sometimes charged unofficial fees, i.e. payment for services that were supposed to be free. Their justification was that the government did not provide funding for running costs such as cotton wool, cleaning of the health facility and transportation to collect vaccines from the headquarters.

In Ekwusigo, the relationship with and attitudes towards the community were almost the opposite. *"We have committees that help us to make sure that our aim is being achieved……I have to involve the community…. at least involving the community will make them take the health centre as their own and they will help you to show you where you need to do advocacy ……. they know everybody in the community and all the things there. So I use them a lot to carry out my duties. I mean the health committee members"* (facility worker, Ekwusigo). The health workers interviewed in Ekwusigo saw community mobilization as one of their main functions and illustrated the point by explaining that communities at times contributed to the transportation costs of providing outreach services, complementing the resources received for this purpose from UNICEF. However, also in Ekwusigo, there were some initial problems with staff attitudes. The PHC Coordinator reported in the interview: *"There was a time when some of these health workers in charge of health facilities were not serious about this REW and I removed those that didn't change their attitude to work, demoted them and posted other people to take charge of their health centres. So others learnt their lessons and there was a great improvement."*

9.4 Discussion

The proof that the RED strategy could work had already been provided earlier and informed the decision to introduce the REW in Nigeria. A subsequent evaluation of the RED approach in the African Region has further shown that it works on a large scale across many countries (WHO, 2007). The doubling of DPT3 coverage in Ekwusigo and the fact that all but one ward in this LGA ended up in the best performing category shows that, under the right conditions, it is also possible in Nigeria to boost achievements dramatically within a very short time frame. However, it appears that the LGA which was already performing well benefited from additional support from external agencies, while the poor performer that was eligible under the original REW strategy for support had to rely on State funding only. Thus, the LGA that had more was given even more. The one that did not was left to sort things out on its own. As a result and contrary to the objective, the REW enhanced rather than reduced inequity during the time frame of review. The major process issues that might have contributed to this outcome are discussed below.

Going to scale

The key feature of the REW was to start with those LGA/wards with 35% or less coverage and to focus support on these for them to catch up. Instead, it was decided by the State team to do something in all the LGAs and wards, i.e. a significant digression from how the REW was conceived. Two arguments were given: first, that all LGAs were performing poorly, i.e. an operational reason; second, that there would be strong reactions from those that were not included, i.e. a political reason. A third argument, which was not brought up in the interviews, is the agency argument. Had the original idea been followed, then REW implementation would not have started in the UNICEF-supported Ekwusigo LGA before immunization and management improvements had taken hold in Orumba South.

REW scale-up issues were discussed primarily at the national level. There were limited consultations with politicians and policy-makers at the state and LGA levels, who appeared to see the REW as a WHO and UNICEF affair. Although the REW policy stressed the inclusion of political, community and religious leaders in planning and implementation, in practice they were not effectively involved. Lack of community involvement in planning and implementing immunization programmes in Nigeria has been noted as one of the reasons for the rebellion against the polio vaccine in Nigeria (Chen, 2004). Exclusion of community members and leaders translates to communities' lack of share in ownership of the programme. As noted by Rifkin (1996), "the community must be included in the conception, development, and implementation of the new immunization campaign and programme". The REW was "marketed" to the states based on output rather than process, as mentioned by one state policy-maker: "*They showed us the graph of their performance so we believed that if we bought the idea, we would also improve in our coverage.*" Selling an idea based on the desired results it could bring is probably an effective entry point to catch the attention of policy-

makers. However, unless the complexity of bringing about these results is understood and it is accepted that gains do not come without pain, implementation can result in the opposite of what was anticipated, i.e. increased inequity.

Improving equity in a situation where there are poor performers and very poor performers can be particularly challenging. Both groups need to be advanced; however, the poorest performer needs to be lifted the most. This requires differentiation in funding and attention. With respect to the latter, the focus also needs to be on the upstream determinants of the inequitable outcome of immunization between political and administrative areas. From the findings, it appears that, compared with Ekwusigo, Orumba South was not only different in that the former received UNICEF funding and the latter did not, but it also appeared to have faced a wider spectrum of adverse determinants and a stronger clustering of disadvantages including poor health staff availability and performance; poor relationship with the community, geographical remoteness, poor infrastructure, internal community tensions, etc. The PHC Coordinator expected the government to provide a continuum of services. The primary onus for such a continuum in the case of the REW would be at the State level with the secondary onus at the LGA level. The role of a continuum at these levels would not only be to level out differences in resources, for example, to counterbalance eventual additional external funding for some areas, but also to address the upstream determinants of the differential performance and outcome. While this cannot be the role of an immunization programme, there are broader health systems issues as well as issues that can be addressed only by the local government, planning, finance, and from both the political and civil service angles. The failure to effectively sell the "whole package" rather than just the shiny idea to those with the means to act possibly contributed to the increased inequity and certainly to the delays in progress in Orumba South.

What is the role of a case such as Ekwusigo in a large scale-up process? It is probably limited. It sets unattainable standards, contributes to frustration among those who do not benefit but are held accountable for not delivering equal results. It appears to provide evidence that money is the solution and thus diverts attention from the upstream determinants that must be addressed but are so much more difficult to handle. Similar effects on equity of choosing easy picks have also been demonstrated with respect to the Integrated Management of Childhood Illnesses (IMCI) (Victora et al., 2006).

Managing policy change

From the review of documents, it was obvious that the Minister of Health played a key role in policy development of the REW due to his formal position as the Minister as well as strong support from the President. Such high-level involvement and commitment undoubtedly had a determining role in the conception and launch of policy processes. Personal leadership and alliances of progressive actors often play critical roles, as a range of actors always influences policy change by bargaining, negotiating and contesting new policy ideas (Gilson et al., 2006).

However, from a simple vision of getting routine immunization services to those wards that had hitherto not been reached, the agenda quickly expanded and drifted. The core idea shifted from a base of equity and values to an opportunistic, utility base and the strategy became "a vehicle to ferry interventions, political and stakeholder interests". These were possibly all well intentioned as immunization services can potentially support, and be supported by, additional health interventions. However, taking forward an expanded agenda is much more challenging than taking forward a narrower one, as also noted by Gwatkin when comparing the roll-out of the oral rehydration therapy (ORT) and IMCI programmes (Gwatkin, 2006). The capacity to handle the additional complexity does not appear to have been present in this case.

The change from the REW to the REC strategy implies a shift in the level of the equity focus, i.e. from the political and administrative to the individual level. This might have been an appropriate adjustment to problems and realities encountered during programme implementation. However, it also means taking a short cut that might not provide an appropriate solution to the problems in the longer run. The REC agenda is less controversial than the REW agenda, as it puts the responsibility on the individual health worker and child (family) rather than the system – the ward and LGA. It does not challenge the structural determinants of the inequity situation. The "project" will deliver immediate results – but will those last? Probably not; the immunization history of the nineties is likely to repeat itself.

The pattern of change is usually shaped more by political imperatives and processes than rational planning (Reich, 1996). The decision to modify the strategy from the REW to the REC was taken at the state level, and seems at least in part informed by advice from UNICEF. The state-level interest would be to push the responsibility downwards to the LGA, wards and individual health facilities, rather than addressing the structural social determinants, which would have been a primary responsibility of the state. For UNICEF, a vested interest could be to report quick results to constituencies supported by it in the LGA, rather than being constrained by having to wait for others or redirect funds.

This illustrates some of the challenges that the Federal Ministry of Health (FMOH) has with respect to State Ministries of Health (SMOH) within a federal governance arrangement. For instance, the FMOH cannot compel the SMOH to implement policies and programmes. This makes stewardship of the health sector very challenging. The federal government and donor agencies established and disseminated the policy through the ICC. However, as warned by Gilson et al. (2006), national governments and international agencies cannot make health systems work better through exercising their own power. Instead, they need to develop managerial environments, understanding and skills that allow for the appropriate exercise of power throughout the health system. In the case of the REW, this would have meant at least four things. First, the parties of the ICC should have stayed faithful to the policy and not followed their own individual paths. Second, much more effort should have gone into explaining and making sectoral policy-makers at the state and LGA levels understand the core concepts and principles of the REW, and what it would imply in terms of input from and changes on their part, i.e. not selling the REW as a "miracle cure", but as requiring an active change of lifestyle. Third, targeted, possibly conditional, financing from a pooled source should have been accessible to remove bottlenecks and catalyse corrective action with respect to those LGAs below an established threshold, i.e. those with immunization coverage below 35%. Fourth, appropriate organizational and structural changes to support the strategy should have been instituted. This could include changes to programmes, such as those undertaken by merging the NPI and the NPHCDA, changes in functions as seen with respect to the NPI managers and PHC coordinators, and CHEWS and staff nurses/midwives. Such changes should ideally be the outcome of a planned process rather than a power struggle, which diverts energy and resources from the strategy. As noted by Gilson et al. (2006), power can be exercised by implementing actions, blocking actions or shaping other actors' understanding of the policy itself. Persuading public sector health workers and managers to support and accept new policies must begin by taking better account of their views and concerns. Their resistance to new policies is often a response to the perceived imposition of new policies without any form of consultation as well as wider workplace concerns (Kamuzora and Gilson, 2007).

Ensuring sustainability

Failure to sustain the immunization coverage achieved during the 1980s in the African Region triggered a renewed interest in routine immunization leading to formulation of the RED approach (WHO, 2007). The RED strategy encompasses two concepts of sustainability – of the outcome, i.e. immunization rates; and of the structure, i.e. routine immunization services, concluding that the first depends on the second. However, the RED Guidance Note (WHO, 2006) also realizes that viability of routine immunization services depends on sustainability of financial resources. In Ekwusigo, such resources were available at least for the period reviewed due to support from UNICEF. In Orumba South, such resources were neither available in the community nor in the health services. Strengthening and sustaining routine immunization structures in Orumba South would require substantial resources and not the modest additional amount suggested in the RED Guidance Note. Significant resource shortfalls led to an inability to attract and retain an adequate, qualified and motivated workforce; acquire, maintain and operate adequate facilities and equipment; and meet other operating expenses, such as allowances for outreach, supplies, etc. Further, while recommending that community members should be involved in both the development and implementation of the REW, consideration should be given to remunerating them, since there are personal opportunity costs of these community-level activities which, particularly in low-income communities, may be substantial (Uzochukwu et al., 2004).

Without buy-in from and ownership by the political powers and administration, including financial commitment, it is difficult for health programmes to be sustained. Although there was strong political will at the national level supported by donor influence and international pressure, this was not so at the state and LGA levels. At these levels, the REW was seen largely as "a WHO and UNICEF affair". Overlooking the ALGON during the planning stages was a missed opportunity to get the local governments on board, institutionalize the equity component of and sustain routine immunization services in general. The local governments not only set priorities across sectors but also hold the "purse" within sectors for their respective local areas.

The importance of involving the administrative aspect of the local governments in addition to the political aspect was further accentuated by the political instability experienced in Anambra during implementation of the REW. Even during stable periods, politicians come and go and so does the political focus. While political will and support can be critically important when introducing new policies, sustainability of immunization services is probably best ensured by tying them closer to the administrative rather than the political agenda. There was no indication that the local administrative and political ownership and integration in Ekwusigo were any greater than in Orumba South.

Immunization is considered a public good, which is the reason why it is provided free almost everywhere. This implies that financing of immunization is a national and international public concern. Financial sustainability of immunization and the REW strategy therefore has two aspects: ensuring a sufficient and continuous flow of resources, regardless of whether the source is national or international; and ensuring effective allocation. The latter includes reallocation in situations where there is a particular donor focus and influx of funds to a certain area. This did not happen in Anambra. Allocation and reallocation is a task of governance and the importance of governance is increasingly referred to by implementation theorists (Hill and Hupe, 2002).

Limitation of the study

The results of this study should be interpreted with some caution because Anambra state is just one of the 36 states of the Federation and some of these findings may not be representative of the country as a whole. However, as the information from the different sources converge into a general picture, it is reasonable to assume that the same factors could be at play across Nigeria as well as elsewhere.

9.5 Conclusion

Nigeria is among the countries that have benefited from financial and technical support from partner agencies for implementation of the REW policy. However, the REW got derailed by local and international interests at different levels due to weak management of the policy change and scaling-up processes. As a result, inequities between LGAs increased rather than decreased, which was the original objective of the REW. It can be said that the strong leadership required to achieve greater equity was missing. Equity is about taking on powers and redistributing resources; if not, existing powers and structures will prevail and deepen inequities, which is exactly what happened in the two cases discussed.

It is possible to drive specific average and equity targets but short-cut driven approaches increase the risk of relapse and collapse. While involvement of the highest political level is necessary, local-level ownership is indispensable. Thus, steering from the top must be combined with a demand from below. It is therefore important to involve all key stakeholders in the planning, implementation and monitoring of the programme. This study shows that the concrete problems in implementation that exist on the ground can hamper or even block implementation of the best intentioned programmes.

Acknowledgements

The authors are grateful to the Consortium for Research on Equitable Health Systems for their input to the design of the study.

References

1. Chen C (2004). Rebellion against the polio vaccine in Nigeria: implications for humanitarian policy. *African Health Sciences*, 4:206–208.

2. FMOH (2006). *11th Meeting of the Expert Review Committee (ERC) on Polio eradication in Nigeria*. Abuja, Nigeria, 7–8 December 2006.

3. Gilson L et al. (2006). *Applying policy analysis in tackling health equity-related implementation gaps*. EQUINET Discussion Paper Number 28.

4. Gwatkin D (2006). IMCI: what can we learn from an innovation that didn't reach the poor? *Bulletin of the World Health Organization*, 84:768.

5. Hill M and Hupe P (2002). *Implementing public policy*. London, Sage Publications.

6. Kamuzora P and Gilson L (2007). Factors influencing implementation of the community health fund in Tanzania. *Health Policy and Planning*, 22:95–102.

7. National Population Commission (NPC) and ORC Macro (2004). *Nigeria Demographic and Health Survey 2003*. Abuja and Calverton, Maryland, NPC and ORC Macro.

8. Reich M (1996). The politics of health reform in developing countries: three cases of pharmaceutical policy. In: Berman P (ed.). *Health sector reform in developing countries*. Cambridge, Harvard University Press.

9. Rifkin SB (1996). Paradigms lost: toward a new understanding of community participation in health programmes. *Acta Tropica*, 61:79–92.

10. Uzochukwu BSC, Akpala CO, Onwujekwe OE (2004). How do health workers and community members perceive and practice community participation in the Bamako initiative programme in Nigeria? A case study of Oji River local government area. *Social Science and Medicine*, 59:157–162.

11. Victora CG et al. (2006). Are health interventions implemented where they are most needed? District uptake of the Integrated Management of Childhood Illness strategy in Brazil, Peru, and the United Republic of Tanzania. *Bulletin of the World Health Organization*, 84:792–801.

12. Walt G and Gilson L (1994). Reforming the health sector: the central role of policy analysis. *Health Policy and Planning*, 9:353–370.

13. WHO (2006). *The reaching every district strategy*. Available at: http://www.who.int/immunization_delivery/systems_policy/RED-FactSheet.pdf (accessed on 07 March 2010).

14. WHO (2007). *In-depth evaluation of the Reaching Every District approach in the African Region*. Brazzaville, World Health Organization. Available at: http://www.comminit.com/en/node/297864/292 (accessed on 07 March 2010).

15. Yin RK (2003). *Case study research – design and methods*. Thousand Oaks, California, Sage Publications Inc.

Women's empowerment and its challenges

Review of a multi-partner national project to reduce malnutrition in rural girls in Pakistan

10

Kausar S Khan,[1,]* Agha Ajmal[2]

[1,2] Community Health Sciences, Aga Khan University, Karachi. Pakistan
* Corresponding author: kausar.skhan@aku.edu

Abstract

Over the past years, malnutrition figures for children below the age of 5 years have been stagnant in Pakistan. Substantive inequities in health, and low female literacy, low school enrolment and high drop-out rates for girls in primary schools have remained a challenge. The Tawana project addressed these issues. Initiated by the Federal Ministry of Women and Development, it was a national project launched in 29 districts. It focused on empowering local women by giving them the opportunity to plan and manage a feeding programme, and demonstrate how malnutrition could be reduced. Following this, enrolment and retention of girls in government primary schools increased. This central role played by women was supported by multilevel collaboration between the Aga Khan University (AKU), eleven local nongovernmental organizations (NGOs), district governments, Pakistan Baitul Maal (PBM) and the Federal Ministry. The project provided freshly prepared meals in 4035 government primary girls' schools over a two-year period and reduced the acute form of malnutrition (wasting) by 45% and increased enrolment by 40%. However, the biggest challenge for Tawana came from its sociopolitical context and from some of the collaborators. Despite the success, the government replaced the project and substituted fresh food with packaged milk and cookies. This case study seeks explanations as to why things evolved as they did and draws lessons by looking into three themes: going to scale, managing multisectoral processes and ensuring sustainability.

10.1 Background

Poverty has increased and food insecurity has become more acute in Pakistan over the past years. "*Soaring food prices and shortages of staples mean about 77 million people of Pakistan's 160 million population are food insecure, a 28 percent increase over the past year, according to U.N. World Food Programme (WFP) estimates. The term food insecure means people are unable to get sufficient nutritious food to meet dietary needs. While there have not been serious food protests in Pakistan, analysts say there is a danger anger could explode in a society that has already fallen prey to Islamist militants bent on bringing down the government*" (Aftab Borka http://uk.reuters.com/article/idUKISL2696320080711?sp=true). When the Tawana[1] project was initiated in 2002, the situation was not as grim. The political situation too has altered considerably since the inception of the project. General elections have taken place and a new government is in power, but a political impasse prevails around the issue of the judiciary and the rising cost of living.

Pakistan is a federation consisting of four provinces – Punjab, Sindh, North West Frontier Province (NWFP) and Balochistan. In addition, there are the federally administered tribal areas (FATA), the federally administered northern areas (FANA) and Azad Kashmir (AJK) with their own political and administrative systems. The Pakistani society has two parallel systems of governance – the formal, legal system, and the non-formal system governed by customs and traditions. Instead of the formal system influencing the non-formal one, it is the latter which prevails, especially in the rural sector as the elite (tribal and feudal chiefs in an area) carry greater power than those in the formal sector. Furthermore, when the State is weak or indifferent to maintaining security for all, and politics are played out more for self-gain than for public good, poverty and health inequalities are bound to flourish.

Health indicators in Pakistan are monitored through averages and rates, and inequities are thus not highlighted. Urban–rural differences are found in health data, but inequities within the urban and rural populations are not monitored systematically. Similarly, differences in mortality on the basis of gender are highlighted, but differences on the basis of class and other stratifiers of equity are not used to unpack the averages of the health data. The Health Management Information System (HMIS) provides information on morbidities in a

[1] The word means robust and healthy in Urdu.

district, but inequities cannot be assessed because of the way it is organized. However, available data show marked differentials in health-care use and outcomes. The proportion of births attended by skilled health personnel for mothers in the lowest education quintile is nearly one third that of those in the highest quintile. Among their offspring, measles coverage is about 40% lower and under-five morality about 60% higher (Table 1).

There is a visible association between health-care use and outcomes and level of the mother's education (Table 2). However, adding to inequities is the fact that education is also unevenly distributed. There are large differences between males and females, between urban and rural areas, and within the rural areas between provinces. While 79% of the urban male population is literate, this is the case for only 13% of the females in Balochistan (Table 2).

It is in this context that Tawana was launched. In its three years of existence (2005–2008), the project demonstrated a reduction in the rates of malnutrition, e.g. in underweight by 22% and stunting by 45% (Badruddin et al., 2008), an increase in enrolment in primary schools (Table 3), and rural women's ability to manage funds and a feeding programme. It was a step towards establishing a tradition of collective action by women, and thereby forming a foundation for grass-roots democracy.

In the 1990s, the School Nutrition Project (SNP) had demonstrated that, given the opportunity, women and men of rural Sindh, together with NGOs and the private Aga Khan University (AKU) in Karachi, could implement a community-based programme within the purview of a government department, which positively impacted both school enrolment and the nutritional status of girls. About three years after the closure of the SNP, the Federal Minister of the Ministry of Women's

Table 1. Key maternal and child health indicators by education level of the mother – lowest and highest quintile (WHO, 2009)

	Education level of mother	
	Lowest	Highest
Birth attended by skilled health personnel	27%	74%
Measles immunization coverage	51%	81%
Under-five mortality rate (per 1000 live births)	102	62

Table 2. Key education indicators by geographical area and sex

	Male (%)	Female (%)
Overall primary school enrolment 2000–2007 (a)	73	57
Urban literacy rate in 10+ population 2005–2006 (b)	79	64
Rural literacy rate in 10+ population 2005–2006 (b)	57	31
Punjab	58	37
Sindh	54	17
NWFP	62	27
Balochistan	46	13

Sources of data: (a) WHO, 2009; (b) Pakistan Social and Living Standards Measurement Survey quoted in UNESCO, 2008

Table 3. Increase in primary school enrolment in Tawana project areas during the three years of the project's existence (Badruddin et al., 2008)

	Punjab	Sindh	NWFP	Balochistan	AJK	FATA
Increase (%)	52	37	26	12	29	33

Development (MoWD) called AKU to assist in developing a project to address the twin problems of malnutrition and low enrolment and attendance in rural government girls' schools. Planning began in November 2001 and by September 2002, Tawana was introduced in 29 districts and operational in about 4000 government girls' primary schools, supported by AKU and 11 NGO partners.

Field work continued till June 2005, during which period daily meals were served to over 410 000 girls. Comprehensive training in participatory approaches, nutrition and anthropometric measurements, and the importance of girls' education were imparted to 663 field workers (FWs), young women from within the 29 districts of Tawana. Four thousand three hundred eighty-three School Committees (STCs) were formed after the village women were introduced to the purpose and method of the project. The STC would identify a woman from among themselves to become the community organizer (CO). She was responsible for facilitating the STC to manage the feeding programme. The CO and at least one schoolteacher were trained in nutrition, record-keeping, management and team-building. Thus, about 4400 COs and schoolteachers were trained; over 95 000 village women were also trained through a structured continuing education programme, and received information about malnutrition and its impact, what constituted a balanced diet, the importance of education for girls and its benefits.

The feeding programme, the hub of Tawana, required the village women to plan and deliver a balanced meal each day under the aegis of the STC. Funds for the programme were provided by the government and included an additional Rupees 1000 a month (about US$ 20) to address any need related to the school. For managing the funds, STC had to open a bank account, and since in many remote areas of Pakistan banks are not available, post office accounts were opened. For most women of the STC, this was their first experience of opening and operating a bank account. For the banks and post offices too, it was their first experience of serving rural women.

After three years of operation, Tawana in the form described above was closed down, despite the availability of government funding for at least another two years of operation. The project was replaced by one that contracted with the commercial sector to provide milk and biscuits to the schools instead of the food freshly prepared by the village women. This case study aims to seek explanations as to why things evolved as they did and draws lessons by looking into three of the Priority

Public Health Conditions (PPHC) (http://www.who.int/social_determinants/resources/pphc_scoping_paper.pdf) themes: going to scale, managing multisectoral processes and ensuring sustainability.

10.2 Methods

The study used a single-case explanatory design (Yin 1993) and was launched from the initial theoretical proposition that while participatory approaches worked well and had an impact at the community level, there were too many implementing parties with unclear terms of reference who were unable to understand each others' points of view and had diverging interests. Together with weak and underdeployed oversight structures, this caused closure of the original Tawana and replacement by a milk-and-cookie programme. This proposition led to the choice of four subunits of analysis: process and effect of the participatory approach; implementing parties and their respective roles; divergence of ideas; and oversight mechanisms.

As a first step in data collection, published and unpublished project documents and reports were reviewed. These included 14 quarterly, three monitoring, and five bi-annual reports. The news items published about Tawana from November 2002 till December 2006 were also studied. On the basis of these reviews, a guide for in-depth interviews and focus group discussions (FGDs) was developed.

Interviews were conducted with government officials in the education and concerned ministries of four project districts in Sindh province, as well as their counterparts at the provincial and federal levels. Managers of AKU and NGOs, field staff of implementing partners, and members of the STC were also interviewed. A total of 25 interviews and 11 FGDs were conducted.

The interviews and FGDs were tape-recorded and transcribed into Roman Urdu. The transcripts were then saved in Rich Text Format and imported into the QSR NVIVO 2.0 program for analysis.

The analysis was conducted as a participatory exercise wherein all team members gave their inputs on the validity of the text coded against each subunit of analysis. The coding report on each subunit was generated for each stakeholder.

10.3 Findings

Process and effect of participatory approach

The key tenet of the Tawana approach was empowerment of village women to take decisions and control resources. At the district level, NGOs had salaried FWs – young local women who introduced Tawana to the village women, then trained, mentored and monitored the implementation. With support from their district supervisor, they systematically introduced Tawana in the schools through the following steps:

1. Formation of a School Tawana Committee (STC)

2. Identification of a CO by the STC, i.e. a woman from within the STC who would get a monthly stipend of Rs 1500.00 (about US$ 30.00)

3. STC to open a bank account or post office account (where a bank was not available) with two signatories, i.e. a member of the STC and the schoolteacher

4. Information on the bank account and the two signatures would be forwarded to the District School Nutrition Committee, so that funds could be released.

The feeding programme would start once the above steps were completed. AKU's information system tracked the progress of the steps and delays were pursued at district, provincial and federal levels.

In addition to the tangible and documented impact on girls' anthropometric measurements and their school enrolment, as mentioned in the introduction, Tawana had effects on social determinants such as household knowledge and practices, status of women in the community, participation in the workforce, and began to touch upon the norms regarding women's role in the society.

The women interviewed in the villages could mention the three food groups, knew about the importance of a balanced diet and of hand-washing before preparing food and eating. "*Women started thinking that if they are having daal (lentils) and if they add vegetables in it, the food would be more balanced*" (FW, NGO). At least some of this new knowledge and new practices remained beyond the programme: "*The feeding programme has gone, but what we learnt is with us*" (village woman, member of STC). Reportedly, it was also understood by the villagers why girls' health and education are so important.

However, according to those interviewed, the biggest change introduced by Tawana was that it brought women out of their homes. Women got involved in decision-making and started taking things in their own hands. Reference was made in the interviews to STCs of two schools which had demonstrated in front of the District Education Office because of non-release of funds. Tawana was seen as giving young women a confidence that is now part of their life. "*The project worked for women and among women, not only for a dominant group….it built participation on a voluntary basis*" (CEO, NGO). "*The community liked the programme as everything was in their hands. They made all the decisions*" (CEO, NGO). Such observations were also made by the village women themselves. "*We got the opportunity to learn about a balanced diet, keeping records, keeping accounts. For the first time, women went to open an account in a bank. To have an account was a great thing (apna account hona bari baat hai)*" (village woman).

Young women who had never thought that they would be able to visit any place alone became salary-earning members of their families. "*Women became more confident due to Tawana …If I talk about myself, I used to be a frightened girl. When Tawana started I joined as a CO, before I could not even go into the house next to mine. But in Tawana I sat on a bus alone and went 15 kilometers away from my house at 7:00 in the evening. I felt so much improvement in myself that my household members were astonished*" (a young village woman who is now working as an FW for an NGO). Being involved in the STCs, and in particular as a CO, was for several of the women a first step to a salaried job. *Tawana produced a skilled human resource for the market* (PBM, District). In the first instance, they found employment with the NGOs. "*About 70% of the women who participated in the project are still working and among them 60% are with us*" (DS, NGO). However, some went further into the wider labour market using the qualifications and skills they had acquired. "*When they hear that we have worked in Tawana, they not only accept us but give us preference*" (a female FW).

In addition to empowering individual women, empowerment also occurred at the community level. According to information provided during the interviews, some of the STCs were converted into community-based organizations and continued organizing the villages around women's and girls' issues. However, the empowerment of village women released forces and, when demanding space and rights, this frequently created friction in their contact with the government services, in particular, the district authorities and civil service. *"The community, which is difficult to organize, was linked by the design of the Project with a power that was more powerful. This was a mismatch and we faced problems in this connection"* (DS, NGO).

Implementing partners and their respective roles

Tawana was a multi-party project, and thus had many stakeholders at four levels – village, district, province and federal. Some of them were vertically linked, notably government ministries and agencies. The NGOs had their own hierarchies. Within the districts, there were the elected representatives as well as the staff of the local government. Then, at the village level, there was the STC composed of village women who implemented the core of Tawana – the feeding programme. Finally, there was AKU spearheading the entire project.

At the federal level, the partners were the MoWD that had initiated the project, the Ministry of Social Welfare and Special Education that took over when the original ministry was split into two after elections brought a new government into power. The Federal Ministry worked on Tawana through two units within it: the National Implementation Unit (NIU), established especially for the Project; and the Pakistan Baitul Maal (PBM). AKU had a formal agreement with the MoWD to implement the programme at the district level.

In each province, the Minister and Secretary of Education were taken into confidence and meant to provide support by monitoring the district-level education departments through the District Education Officers, who would thus provide a link between the district and the province. However, the social mobilizer of PBM, who had a key role at the district level, reported to the Provincial Chief Secretary. The Provincial Coordinator of PBM was also included in the provincial-level deliberations and meetings of Tawana. However, the Province played a secondary role, receiving updates of the programme, and helping to resolve problems as they were encountered. PBM was primarily responsible for disbursement of funds to the districts and had representatives placed at the district level. The provincial NIU had a team that visited the districts for monitoring purposes.

At the district level, the Department of Education, the PBM Coordinator, the Senior District Administrator, and the seniormost elected representative played key roles. AKU was responsible for implementation through its 11 NGO partners. At the individual school level, there were three main actors; the schoolteachers, the School Management Committee of the Education Department, and the STC. Funds for the feeding programme were released by the Federal MoWD and deposited in a special account opened in the name of District School Nutrition Committee (DSNC). From here it was sent to the STC account; the Executive Director of the District Education Department was required to sign the cheques for depositing the money.

Tawana was launched at a time when the devolution plan of the federal government was introduced. The plan required government departments to report to the elected council of the district. It was a time of considerable confusion as the new roles of the elected representatives and the government service providers and civil servants were not clear. The first changes in roles came within the first year of implementation. PBM at the federal level decided to change the role of their district-level workers from helping the funds to reach the school accounts and collect the data from the school level. Instead, they were to monitor feeding activities and the use of funds at the school level. As they were all men, their entry into girls' schools and villages was restricted because of the male–female segregation practised in rural areas.

The many different partners and their shifting roles created challenges for implementation, particularly when problems arose. *"In some districts (Lodhran, Pakpattan) the DCO[2] had a positive stance in resolving problems. When we started in Kotli it [Tawana] was run wonderfully. It was also run well in the northern areas, a few districts in Peshawar and also in Kohistan. It depended much on the NGO partner, if that was strong, it was an easier run"* (PBM, Federal). The many partners created many interfaces that were frequently difficult to deal with, in particular when, as reported by those interviewed, every second or third month they were informed of operational changes. *"We were actually working in schools that belonged to the government not to us, not to communities and not to AKU. But government is a power that is not in anybody's control and they do not have consistent views and thoughts on various issues. In such conditions it was*

---

[2] DCO is the coordinating head of the District Administration. He/she has the authority to review and assess the performance of the groups of offices, i.e. health, education and works, etc. and give directions for taking action to improve efficiency.

difficult to work" (CEO, NGO). Over time, as far as the NGOs were concerned, they found ways of operating. "*Initially we had difficulties but later we understood that we had to implement this project through a learning-by-doing strategy*" (another CEO, NGO).

One of the challenges most frequently mentioned by the NGO managers was the de-link between those controlling the funds and the implementers. "*You empower those at the lower level, and give the control to a higher level – that's a recipe for conflict*" (DS, NGO).

The burden of the complex overhead structure was also felt directly at the field level: "*If a woman is at a cooking stove, and ten women try to guide her, then problems are bound to arise… something like this happened in Tawana*" (FW).

Divergence of ideas

The three partners AKU, PBM and NIU were meant to work as a team, but differences in interpretation quickly became the source of misunderstanding and conflict. Conflicts were augmented by the political situation, which resulted first in the Minister who had initiated the project leaving after a change in government. Then, the Ministry was split into two and a new Minister took charge. With her came a new Secretary and the head of the NIU was replaced. During its three years, the Project saw three Secretaries, all were critical of Tawana, questioned the role of AKU and the terms of the agreement it had signed with the Ministry.

Tawana was conceived based on a holistic idea of simultaneous actions to reduce inequities with respect to three determinants of health, i.e. nutrition, education and gender. The SNP had provided a proof of concept with the main drivers: money from the government to prepare food locally; a participatory approach that gave decision-making power to village women; and support and guidance from FWs. However, these core ideas were not understood by all. "*It was an excellent project but unfortunately people did not understand the spirit of it*" (PBM, Province). The CEO of an NGO was of the view that although the SNP had provided the learning base, it had been limited to AKU. He suggested that the learning should have been shared in the strategic planning meetings with the government and NGOs. Others suggested an intermediary phase between the SNP and full scale-up. "*It should have been implemented in one district from each province and then gradually up-scaled*"

(PBM, Federal). According to the documents reviewed and the interviews, the divergence in understanding widened as the challenges of implementation grew.

The PBM decided after three months that only girls enrolled in school would be allowed to access the daily feeding in order to facilitate record-keeping. This argument was contested by AKU and the NGOs, but the decision prevailed. A further change was in the signatory for the STC bank account. It had begun with the STC identifying a woman from among them to be the signatory along with the schoolteacher. This was changed to the CO, i.e. the woman who received a monthly stipend. Here, the reason was that a volunteer should not be a signatory to the bank account. This created additional paperwork and caused awkwardness when an external decision was imposed on village women while the participatory approach had placed women at the centre of decision-making. Despite protests, this change was also enforced. Several interviewees argued that boys' schools should have been included. Their argument was that malnutrition was also prevalent in boys. Further, a CEO of an NGO found that the feeding programme had diverted the attention of teachers to feeding rather than educating the children, and that the programme in general had received too much attention.

However, despite these differences, the work at the district level proceeded with its own local dynamics. Feeding took place, but with frequent hiccups in resource flow due to differences in concepts of control. While funds moved smoothly to the district accounts, there were delays in funds reaching the school accounts. These delays were caused by the reluctance of government officers to sign the checks for the schools as they were not accepting of a nongovernment person providing the verification and the district PBM had been specifically instructed from the federal level not to verify the accounts. "*The project suffered because of the bureaucratic hassles that are inherent in the government system such as having to tender everything. There should have been some flexibility in the government rules and regulations as these things slow the processes*" (PBM, Federal).

Some interviewees felt that the difference in understanding was deepened by the programme design omitting a critical actor. "*There was disconnection between implementation – through project partners and financial disbursements – through the district government which was not a project partner. This ruined the project. It caused discontinuation of feeding and broke the momentum*" (CEO, NGO). The lack of a shared understanding, according to some, resulted in a mistrust that affected implementation. "*Throughout the project we were afraid of AKU and AKU was afraid of us. This caused huge problems in the project*" (PBM, District).

The lukewarm buy-in from the district bureaucracy was, according to those interviewed, accentuated by the frequent transfers of DCOs and Executive District Officers (health, education, agriculture, works and services, etc.), requiring dedicated action on part of the NGOs to overcome the problems. "*A few assumptions were not aligned with the ground realities, for instance, the assumption that the DCO and EDO (Education) would sign cheques smoothly was a flaw….we made them work for the project on the basis of personal relationships*" (DS, NGO).

When the new Tawana was launched by the government, it was significantly changed. The new programme was managed entirely by the government. This meant that "*instead of women preparing fresh meals, contracts were given for supply of milk, juice and biscuits*" (AKU person). Contracting followed a normal government business model, facilitated tendering and adherence to standard accountability measures.

However, several interviewees from both the government and NGOs suggested that there might have been other reasons for the new look of Tawana. "*Some officials in our district supported milk and cookies because they knew they would get their share*" (District Administrator). Similar sentiments were expressed by the NGOs. "*The concept of milk and cookies is an old one and an easy way out. It is also linked to commissions – perks and money – that people get from the branded juice companies* (CEO, NGO). Among the FWs and communities there was dissatisfaction and a sense that the changes were introduced to benefit government officials and the industry. "*We do not want synthetic juices. We want fresh food for our children. They are sick with juices and cookies in just two months. They have sore throats. We want Tawana with fresh food again*" (woman of STC). In some districts, this dissatisfaction resulted in protests that stopped the new programme – however, the "old" was not brought back.

Oversight mechanisms

The National Steering Committee chaired by the Minister only met once during the brief tenure of the first Minister and then never met again during the entire life of the project.

"*The PBM played quite a different role, compared with how the people who wrote the proposal had conceived it. Instead of a partner they [PBM] became the monitor* (Manager TPP, AKU). The PBM, administratively part of the Ministry and hence with easy access to the Secretary, was most critical of Tawana and submitted the criticism in writing. He (Managing Director, PBM) criticized AKU for not submitting reports on time; expressed that the NIU had no role; and that there were no clear control and command structures. The NIU, having been created specially by the Minister, was marginalized. The Secretary called for an audit and filed a reference with the National Accountability Bureau (NAB), the federal government department investigating severe cases of corruption in the government sector. This created great anxiety and suspicion of the entire project, putting the reputation of the partners at stake. "*The Ministry failed to provide leadership, and people down the ladder did not take interest. ….The project struggled because the leadership that conceived the project was not part of it at the time of implementation. The new Secretary actually himself sent the project files to the NAB and asked them to audit them. The district government used to say that if the funding Ministry does not accept its own child, why would we participate in it? We will also be audited if we release funds for this programme*" (NIU).

The growing disagreements between the three partners, PBM, NIU and AKU, led to the formation of a special committee. The decision was taken at a meeting in the Planning Commission of Pakistan. The committee had the approval of the newly appointed Minister to investigate the working of Tawana and was headed by the Chief Economist of the Planning Commission. However, the report and recommendations of the committee were never shared with the partners.

The district governments were not considered implementing partners but were required to only release the funds. In the early part of the project, there was confusion over who would call the district meetings. The PBM representative was understood to be calling the meetings, but would not and eventually an NGO had to shoulder this responsibility. This, according to some, contributed to the district governments' reluctance to release the funds and be held accountable. There were several suggestions offered by those interviewed on how to make the district government an implementing partner, including: "*There should have been a separate Project Management Unit of the project at district level*" (CEO, NGO) and "*The project should be under the Education Department*" (CEO, NGO). However, those interviewed from the NGO sector pointed to the leadership vacuum created by the change of government, as expressed by one of their CEOs: "*The then government, which wrote the project, was very strong, and therefore they thought that their baby would easily be adopted. But they could not stay in power for even six months and that changed the scenario.*"

In the Tawana planning document, the target was to reach 26 districts, 5000 girls' primary schools and 500 000 girls. However, later the federal government added three more districts with 300 schools, expanding the scope to 530 000 girls. Once the implementation of Tawana began, it became clear that the given targets would not be met. The number of schools stipulated did not exist and thus, the number of girls to be covered could also not be met. "*The expected 5300 schools were not there to initiate projects either because of non-availability of teachers or the schools were there on paper but did not exist in reality* (AKU, Tawana Project Manager). This became a source of contention between the federal ministry and the implementers. The three consecutive secretaries of the ministry over the three-year period persistently pointed out this discrepancy as a failure of the project.

Throughout the history of the programme, data quality remained a concern. "*Maintaining data integrity was the key issue. AKU focused on that a lot but found it really difficult to train NGOs to put rigour into data collection*" (AKU, Tawana Project Senior manager). This was suggested to have contributed to mistrust and overemphasis on monitoring. "*There were so many monitors in the project. PBM had its own and NIU had its own. Then other government departments were also monitoring things*" (CEO, NGO).

A communication strategy was developed under the responsibility of the NIU. However, the approval to launch the strategy had to come from the Secretary of the ministry but was never given. This created an information gap, and rumours and speculations flourished.

10.4 Discussion

Going to scale

Going to large scale means moving into a real world where there are several external factors at play, most of which cannot easily be foreseen or controlled, and where management is passed over from the hands of those who

initiated the "project" to various actors, either existing or created for the project.

Tawana was the successor of the SNP which had been implemented in Sindh province by AKU. The AKU also had the contract with the MoWD to implement Tawana at the district level during the scale-up process. AKU considered the SNP as the pilot for Tawana. However, the SNP had been implemented in one province only and with AKU in direct control in each district. The SNP had proven the concept that empowerment and feeding at the community level would lead to improved school attendance and nutritional status of girls. What the SNP had not tested were the managerial structures and systems to support a large-scale implementation of these concepts.

Very soon after the launch of Tawana, there was confusion about the extent of the scale, including the operational and conceptual boundaries of the programme. The number of districts and schools to be covered was increased; in some instances, beyond reality. This became a source of contention when things went sour. On the one hand, the parent ministry used the confusion to argue that the targets were not met. On the other hand, the implementers, i.e. AKU and the NGOs, argued that the targets were not based on reality, but none of the parties had a clear picture of what this reality was. Another change with respect to the magnitude of the scale-up was the decision to limit the feeding to girls in schools, i.e. not to include out-of-school girls in the same age group, which was a part of the original blueprint. This was not only a matter of numbers but also an issue related to which objective was the most important – improving nutrition or improving school attendance. However, the deepest-rooted dispute about the boundaries of the programme was in relation to the empowerment objective and the intrinsically related questions of accountability and autonomy in decision-making. By nature, the empowerment objective would blur the boundaries of the programme and make it less centrally controllable.

Tawana was a complex government programme implemented by the nongovernment sector. In the original plan, the programme was envisaged to be led directly by the Minister of Women and Development, supported centrally by two bodies set up specifically to oversee programme roll-out – the Tawana Steering Committee and the NIU. As the initiating minister left the Ministry, the Steering Committee effectively ceased to exist and in the leadership vacuum created, the NIU was sidelined. The loss of central oversight and leadership function early in the scale-up process left the programme unable to correct two critical flaws of the original design – the lack of formal anchoring of the programme at the district level and a weak monitoring system. This left room for rivalry, creation of parallel systems and disputes about what was actually happening in the programme.

The combination of unclear boundaries, loss of central leadership, and inadequate management structures and systems proved fatal to the survival of Tawana, despite the documented achievement of outcomes for all three objectives of the programme.

Managing intersectoral processes

In Pakistan, a sector is a defined domain within the government system. Each sector has its hierarchy of managers and service providers at district, provincial and federal levels. Separate from but interacting with the government sectors at all levels in Tawana was the nongovernment sector, i.e. AKU, NGOs and communities. Although a concerted effort of the actors was crucial for implementation, they tended to work vertically.

For the NGOs, the participatory approach was of intrinsic value, as it encompassed the concepts of democracy and empowerment. This view was clearly not shared by the government sectors' civil servants, whose work values were based on command and control. The participatory approach worked well at the village level but became difficult to pursue as unilateral decisions were taken by the ministry. AKU and its implementing partners protested because they found that this compromised the project and caused loss of credibility vis-à-vis the village women.

More differences with respect to ways of working soon came to the fore. Apart from the participatory approach, getting things done was more important for the NGOs than following the correct procedures or adhering to defined roles. For example, when it was unclear as to who should call the district meetings, the NGOs took on that role. When things were not working or the processes became too heavy, the NGOs made use of personal contacts to cut short the red tape. This was good as it made things happen and produced immediate results. However, it kept the programme as an NGO project and prevented integration.

A particularly delicate interface between the civil service and Tawana was with respect to the handling of money. On the one hand, the civil service did not understand what it required to work with the community. On the other hand, AKU and the NGOs did not understand how the government works and what it requires, for example, in terms of audit trails. This interface was the Achilles heel that eventually brought Tawana down. The programme relied on the regular flow of government money to keep the feeding activities running. However, by releasing the money without proper documentation and due processes, the individual civil servant would run a personal risk of being accused of improper administration and thus exposed to audit investigation. A district civil servant who was not prepared to run such a risk could turn off the flow to the individual STC. However, the Secretary who found the risk too uncomfortable had only the choice of filing a reference with the NAB. While it cannot be ruled out that corruption, as suggested by several of those interviewed, was a factor influencing the decision to change, the main reason was possibly that tendering for supply of items which can be weighed and counted fitted into the standard way of doing business. Giving money to village women to buy and do something that could never be entered into government ledgers did not fit in with any format that the civil servants were used to.

There were indications of problems from the start, and AKU and the NGOs should have acknowledged and put more effort into developing the interface with the government structures. Implementing a programme such as Tawana requires a participatory approach to involving both the community and the civil services. It requires a change in the way that civil servants think and work, and an appreciation by the nongovernmental partners of the limits of such change. One potential solution could have been for the NGO in each district to act as an intermediary with respect to handling of funds, i.e. to provide the government with what is required in terms of accountability and "countability", while maintaining flexibility on the community side where the accounting standards and options are different. However, changing the way that the bureaucracy works might not be only a procedural matter. Improving equity, including gender equity, and empowering village women is about changing social norms and some of the very premises that the society is built on – bureaucracies by definition are conservative.

The three interlinked determinants – nutrition, education and gender – could all be seen as falling within the mandate of the initiating MoWD. However, when it came to implementation, additional sectors and line-ministries became concerned. For example, the key venue of operation – schools – is in the education sector, general nutritional status in the health sector, etc. While there was common ground, each sector had its own objectives, measures and targets. Sometimes, these were conflicting and compromises needed to be worked out. There are several examples in Tawana of this. Including only girls attending schools in the feeding programme makes sense from the exclusive viewpoint of increasing enrolment, while from a health perspective, it does not make any difference whether the undernourished girl is in school or not. From an equity perspective, the girl out of school is likely to be more vulnerable than the one at school. Another example is the question of inclusion of boys in the programme. While the equity objective would call for a focus on levelling the gap between boys and girls, pure "average" health and education objectives would not necessarily differentiate between them. Clear choices were made in the original programme design. However, when it came to implementation, there was no forum to articulate and explain these choices, and to integrate the interests of the different sectors, whether at district, province or federal level. Leaving out the district government was a serious oversight, particularly as decentralization took place in parallel with the roll-out of Tawana.

Ensuring sustainability

Sustainability in the case of Tawana can be discussed from at least two perspectives: the perspective of what was sustained after Tawana ended; and how the programme could have been sustained in the longer run, instead of being closed despite the availability of government resources.

Over its short lifetime of three years, Tawana had built over 4000 women's groups in 29 districts, supported by their husbands and NGOs at the micro level and, in many instances, also by officials at the district level. The women gained skills, confidence and acceptance not only to provide better nutrition to girls and their families in general, but also to start addressing and influencing the social norms that underlie gender inequity in much of rural Pakistan. There was ample indication from the interviews with both officials and women that the seeds provided by Tawana had germinated and were beginning to take root. Had the programme continued, it could have built a self-sustaining social base for greater participation of women to better the conditions of the poor and the disadvantaged. From Tawana's experience,

a large human resource was developed and its importance lies in the fact that Pakistan does not have adequate and effective human resources for social improvement.

The upstream social determinants addressed by Tawana were the social norms that shape downstream determinants of what women can or cannot do and how girls are regarded, educated and fed. Changing such norms on a large scale requires a combination of a dedicated political leadership and building of an impetus from below. As discussed above, a momentum was forming at the grass-roots level to support such change processes. However, due to political turbulence, the original central political leadership, the MoWD, lost office and subsequently the ministry was split into two. With the devolution of power to the districts, challenges as well as opportunities emerged for the programme to establish the required political commitment to sustain efforts. However, in most but not all cases, these opportunities were missed and the challenges not appropriately dealt with, such as through adjusting the programme design.

One of the most important threats to the sustainability of Tawana was probably that the programme never came to grips with whether it was an NGO project implemented with government money or a government programme implemented by NGOs. Instead of addressing the implementation and thereby institutionalization and sustainability challenges head on, instant short-cuts were pursued, creating friction and distrust between the civil servants and NGO implementers. The focus shifted from outcome to process and in that the rural village women lost out.

10.5 Conclusion

Tawana demonstrated on a large scale that malnutrition can be reduced and school enrolment for girls increased through a community based-programme that actively involves rural women in decision-making roles. Turning the Tawana model into a national project is a decision a government can take. The issue is of political will and government courage, which can be influenced and supported from the grass-roots level and through advocacy by NGOs and other civil society groups.

Several lessons can be drawn from the Tawana experience regarding where more emphasis could have been put or where things should have been done differently. First, implementing a complex programme addressing social norms requires the involvement of many actors. Effectively managing the interfaces between these are critical to the mission. Differences in cultures, values and modes of operation must be identified and dealt with appropriately. As a starting point, all those involved have to accept and understand their own and others' roles, constraints and need for change. Only then can the necessary mutually supportive learning and action commence. Second, moving from small-scale pilots to large-scale operations covering vast geographical, cultural, political and administrative areas requires a phased roll-out to test processes and management mechanisms and tools, as the lines of immediate control get longer and thinner. Third, sustaining a large-scale and nationwide programme addressing social norms will require government buy-in and complementary action by government and nongovernment actors. NGOs have a critical role in challenging and educating both the civil services and the public in this respect.

Finally, without a proper forum, such as a national steering committee, and a mechanism for continuous monitoring, learning and adjustment of design and approaches, even the most promising programme will soon lose momentum in a complex and ever-changing real world. Tawana fell short of such a forum and mechanism almost from the start.

Acknowledgements

First and foremost, we would like to thank all the stakeholders who gave their valuable time for the interviews. Their patience and readiness are greatly appreciated. They shared their thoughts frankly and without any hesitation, especially the women who once were members of the STC, and the schoolteachers of the schools where Tawana was implemented. The staff of the NGOs, even those who were no longer employed by the NGO, willingly took part in the review of Tawana. The CEOs of the NGOs deserve special thanks as they accommodated the interviewers in their busy schedule. Special mention must be made of the respondents of the PBM and NIU, who gave interviews over the phone, and ensured that the interviews were not interrupted. We would also like to acknowledge the work of our field team, and the support provided by the administration of the Community Health Sciences department of AKU. Last, but not the least, we would like to thank WHO for the opportunity to write this case study, and especially Dr Blas for valuable guidance on understanding case study as a research approach, and in organizing the paper.

References

1   Badruddin SH et al. (2008). Tawana project—school nutrition program in Pakistan—its success, bottlenecks and lessons learned. *Asia Pacific Journal of Clinical Nutrition*, 17 (S1):357–360.

2   UNESCO (2008). *Needs assessment report on literacy initiative for empowerment – Pakistan.* Government of Pakistan, Islamabad, Project Wing, Ministry of Education.

3   Yin RK (1994). *Case study research: design and methods* (2nd ed.). Thousand Oaks, CA, Sage.

4   WHO (2009). *World health statistics 2009.* Geneva, World Health Organization.

Local Health Administration Committees (CLAS)

Opportunity and empowerment for equity in health in Perú

11

Laura C. Altobelli,[1,]* Carlos Acosta-Saal[2]

[1] School of Public Health and Administration, Universidad Peruana Cayetanto Heredia, Lima Peru and Peru Country Director, Future Generations
[2] General Directorate of People´s Health, Ministry of Health, Lima, Peru
* Corresponding author: laura@future.org

Abstract

Local Health Administration Communities (CLAS) in Peru are private, non-profit civil associations that enter into agreements with the government and receive public funds to administer primary health-care (PHC) services applying private sector law for contracting and purchasing. CLAS is an example of a strategy that effectively addresses the social determinants of health (SDH), which refers to the social, cultural and economic barriers at the local level that keep people from effectively utilizing health-care services. Initially, this started as a small-scale initiative backed by a Supreme Decree, and now there is a national law on CLAS. The Peruvian government provides a structure for more flexible financial management with social participation, which gives citizens direct control of the transparent management of PHC services. Evidence is presented comparing CLAS to PHC services administered through the traditional public system, which still operates in 70% of the Ministry of Health PHC system. This shows a positive equity effect of CLAS and greater efficiency in the use of resources. However, the process to get the CLAS to where it is now was both long and difficult, and required political trade-offs that went right to the core of the programme idea.

11.1 Background

Health and inequities

Between 1990 and 2007, Peru's gross national income per capita doubled from 1270 to 2570 (PPP Int. $) and, from 2000 to 2006, the per capita total expenditure on health rose by 36%, i.e. from 232 to 316 (PPP Int. $). During the same period, the government's share of the total expenditure for health increased from 53.0% to 58.3%.

Over the past two decades, Peru has experienced a marked reduction of more than 70% in mortality rates for infants and children below the age of 5 years, and more than 20% reduction for adults. Males have consistently higher mortality rates compared to females (Table 1).

There are considerable inequities in the health indicators according to place of residence, wealth and education (Table 2). The largest inequities are with respect to "birth attended by skilled health personnel", where the ratios range from 2.0 for place of residence to 4.8 for wealth. For all three health indicators, the largest inequities are in the indicator for wealth. The least variation across health indicators is found for "place of residence".

The CLAS programme

Peru delivers health care through a mix of providers. The Social Security Institute (EsSalud) provides obligatory employee health insurance with payroll deduction, serving approximately 20–24% of the population with formal employment. The Armed Forces has its own system of care for military families, which comprise 3% of the population. The wealthiest 5% utilizes private services and the private health insurance industry. The poorest 65–70% of the population is covered by the Ministry of Health (MOH) network of primary health-care (PHC) services and hospitals. Of this group, we estimate that 45% have access to health-care services and 20% remain excluded due to geographical, social, cultural and economic barriers.

Peru is among the few countries in the world which has a government health programme with legalized, regulated and institutionalized community participation. At present, the Shared Administration Programme (Spanish acronym PAC), formalized in April 1994 by Supreme Decree 01-94-SA, gives responsibility and decision-making power over the management of public resources for the administration of 31% of the MOH–PHC system. Participation is formalized through a contract signed between the Regional Health Department and a non-profit entity – the Local Health Administration Community (Spanish acronym CLAS) based on a local health plan. The CLAS is obligated to manage and ensure implementation, and the MOH to finance the plan.

Of 6871 MOH–PHC facilities, 2133 (31%) are administered by 783 CLAS. Individual CLAS administer one facility, and aggregate CLAS can administer two or more PHC facilities (Figure 1). CLAS comprise 42%

and 52% of large health centres in rural and urban areas, respectively, and 43% of larger rural health posts. Among small health posts in rural and urban areas, CLAS administer only 26% and 27% of them, respectively. Of the larger health posts in urban areas, 33% are administered by CLAS (Altobelli, 2007). When the CLAS programme was initiated in 1994, the early CLAS tended to be small health posts with one doctor. These have developed over time into larger facilities with more personnel, infrastructure and equipment.

A CLAS is organized as a non-profit civil association under rules of the Peruvian Civil Code. Its General Assembly is composed of two elected representatives from each community in the jurisdiction of the CLAS, one representative from each community-based social organization, and one representative each from the health facility(ies), the micronetwork centre, the municipality and the regional government.[1] Members of the General Assembly have a four-year term and, among themselves, elect seven members to form the Board of

Table 1: Mortality rates in Peru from 1990 to 2007 (WHO, 2009)

	1990	2000	2007	Reduction
Infant mortality rate (MGD 4)				
Male	62	35	18	71.0%
Female	54	30	16	70.4%
Under-five mortality rate (MDG4)				
Male	82	42	21	74.4%
Female	73	37	19	74.0%
Adult (15–60 years) mortality rate				
Male	164	163	124	24.4%
Female	123	120	98	20.3%

Table 2: Key indicators of health inequity in Peru, 2006–2007 (WHO, 2009)

		MDG 5	MDG 4	
		Births attended by skilled personnel (%)	Measles immunization coverage among 1-year-olds (%)	Under-five mortality (death per 1000 live births)
Place of residence	Rural	30	56	100
	Urban	60	69	78
	Ratio urban–rural	2.0	1.2	1.3
Wealth quintile	Lowest	16	36	121
	Highest	77	76	60
	Ratio highest–lowest	4.8	2.1	2.0
Education level of mother	Lowest	27	51	102
	Highest	74	81	62
	Ratio highest–lowest	2.8	1.6	1.6

[1] The original structure of CLAS included only six elected community members who among themselves chose the three-member Board of Directors. This was changed with the 2007 law.

Directors with a President, Secretary and Treasurer, who have two-year terms. The health facility Medical Chief is the CLAS Manager. The relationship between CLAS, the local municipality and the government through the Regional Health Directorate (Spanish acronym DIRESA) is formalized with a Co-Management Agreement, with responsibilities on all three sides specified in detail. An annual operational plan and budget called the Local Health Plan (Spanish acronym PSL) is a key instrument for co-management beyond standard clinical services and includes specific community-identified needs.

CLAS-run health services depend primarily on government funding through: (1) direct cash transfers from the public treasury, (2) cash reimbursements from the government health insurance programme (SIS) for the poor, and (3) in-kind receipt of medicines and other supplies purchased in bulk by the DIRESA. All of the above, plus fees collected from patients for non-covered health services, are transferred into a commercial private bank account controlled by each CLAS as opposed to non-CLAS health services which do not control funds. CLAS are also able to directly receive and administer third-party donations. All funds are publicly owned and CLAS provides monthly financial reports to the DIRESA. Expenditures of public funds for acquisitions

and infrastructure are faster and simpler under the CLAS system and CLAS are not required to return unspent funds to the central government at the end of each fiscal year. The success of CLAS has been attributed to their agility in financial management, with more efficient spending on priority and community-identified needs for better quality of health care. For example, a CLAS can purchase laboratory equipment or contract services to third parties, renovate the health facility, hire more personnel, purchase security equipment and services to prevent thefts, and make other improvements that enhance the quality of care.

Social control over finance and health personnel is exercised by CLAS and the community is empowered to feel ownership of the health services and demand accountability by health personnel. Personnel are hired and fired by CLAS under private labour contracts that provide for health insurance, a one-month vacation, twice-yearly bonuses and severance pay. On the other hand, the labour regimen of the government's payroll personnel provides permanent job security, a six-hour work day and a public pension.

"Peru's CLAS programme is one of the world's best demonstrations of rapid expansion with decentralization

Figure 1: Growth in the number of primary health-care facilities administered by CLAS and the number of CLAS from inception in 1994 to 2007

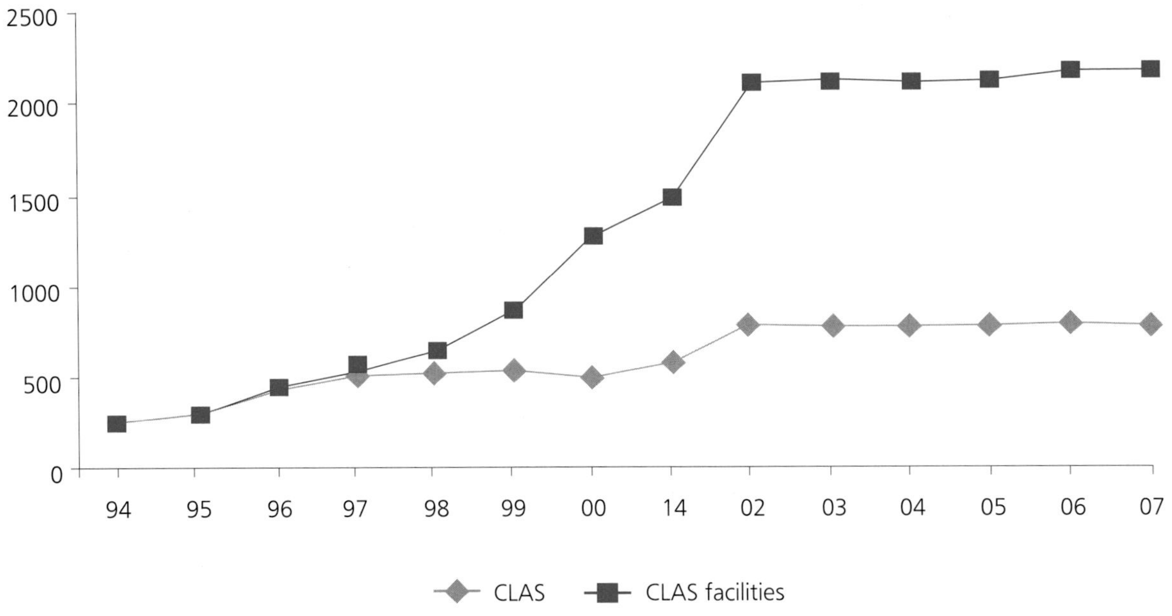

Source: Ministry of Health, 2007

of the Alma-Ata model of community-based primary health care" (Mahler et al., 2001). Further, studies comparing CLAS and non-CLAS facilities by and large show positive effects of CLAS in the areas of equity, quality and coverage of health services (Altobelli, 1998a, 1998b; Cortez, 1998, 1999; Vicuña et al., 2000; Altobelli and Pancorvo, 2000; Altobelli and Sovero, 2004).

Most Peruvian communities have strong traditions of internal organization, though their relationship with the government has swung between dependence, independence and mistrust. The development of CLAS has been influenced by government and health sector politics as well as physicians' and health workers' unions. The almost two decades since the CLAS programme was initiated has gone through periods of strength and growth as well as periods of near extinction. This case study reviews what has shaped the CLAS to become what it is today by drawing lessons with respect to the following broad themes: going to scale, managing policy change, adjusting design and ensuring sustainability.

11.2 Methods

This case study focuses on the process of implementation of CLAS, with four types of implementation processes of particular interest: (1) *going to scale* – the challenges faced in moving from a small pilot programme to a widespread intervention; (2) *managing policy change* – in terms of formulating policies to benefit the poor and vulnerable, influencing the political environment, the role of individuals as policy champions and managing opposing views; (3) *adjusting design* – adjustments made to the original programme design during implementation; and (4) *ensuring sustainability* – issues in securing ongoing financial viability and promoting institutional integration.

The case study enquiry was made along two tracks: (1) achievements in promoting equity; and (2) the life history of CLAS.

Data collection combined several methods. Qualitative data were collected through semi-structured interviews with a range of stakeholders on the retrospective and current knowledge and perspectives. These stakeholders had played key roles in the development and implementation of CLAS (Table 3). Interviews were tape-recorded, if permitted by the respondent, and transcribed. Three regions were selected for interviews of CLAS presidents and managers on the basis of geographical distribution (coast, mountains, high jungle) and the level of regional support to CLAS (high, low, medium). In each region, three "good" CLAS and three "poor" CLAS were selected utilizing the MOH classification based on management criteria.

Documents reviewed included government legislation, regulations, administrative directives, etc. Published and unpublished reports and evaluations on the Shared Administration Programme were also reviewed, including quantitative analyses of programme performance comparing CLAS and non-CLAS PHC facilities.

Table 3: Persons interviewed during the data collection

Persons interviewed	Number
Present member of Congress	1
Past Health Minister	1
Past and present national coordinators of the PAC	5
Past and present general and executive directors in the Ministry of Health	4
Past programme coordinators and government advisors	6
Past and present leaders of the physicians' union and association	2
Past and present international consultants and advisors	2
CLAS association presidents	18
CLAS managers	18

Figure 2: Average number of physicians per health post and health centre whether CLAS or non-CLAS, rural or urban, 2006

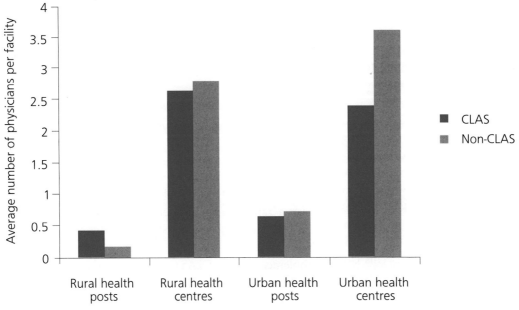

Source: prepared by author based on data from the *National inventory of infrastructures, equipment, and human resources*. Lima, Peru, Ministry of Health, 2006

Figure 3: Percentage of patients in the three lowest income quintiles with full or partial fee exemption by CLAS and non-CLAS rural health facility

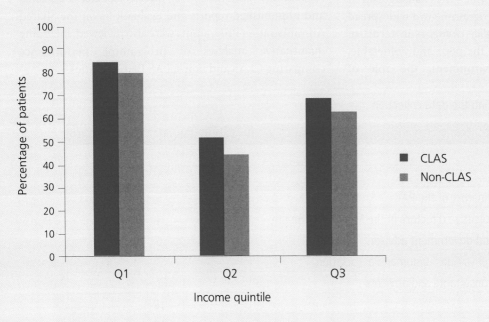

Source: Altobelli L. *Health reform, community participation and social inclusion: the Shared Administration Programme*. Lima, Peru, UNICEF, 1998. Data are from the 1997 National Living Standards Survey in Peru.

Figure 4: Percentage of sick rural children below the age of five years taken for health care by residence within the catchment area of, respectively, CLAS and non-CLAS health facilities (1996–2000)

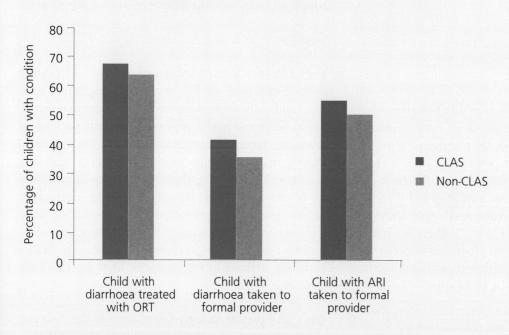

Source: Altobelli L (2006). *Comparative analysis of health impact and health services utilization in CLAS and non-CLAS primary health care services in Peru, Lima.* Lima, Future Generations. www.future.org (Data are from the Peru Demographic and Health Survey IV, 2000.)

Figure 5: Percentage of rural children below five years of age with chronic malnutrition by education of mother and by residence in a catchment area of, respectively, a CLAS and non-CLAS health facility (1996–2000)

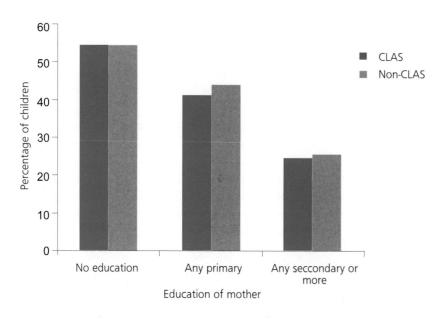

Source: Altobelli L (2006). *Comparative analysis of health impact and health services utilization in CLAS and non-CLAS primary health care services in Peru.* Lima, Peru, Future Generations. (Data are from the Peru Demographic and Health Survey IV, 2000.)

11.3 Findings

Achievements

Availability of physicians

Rural CLAS health posts have more than twice the average number of physicians compared to rural non-CLAS posts, 0.41 versus 0.16, while the number of physicians is similar for urban health posts, i.e. CLAS, 0.63 and non-CLAS, 0.74. Urban non-CLAS health centres have significantly more doctors on average (3.62) than both rural non-CLAS (2.8) and rural and urban CLAS, i.e. 2.63 and 2.40, respectively (Figure 2). There is a marked difference in the availability of physicians between rural and urban CLAS for both health posts and health centres than is the case for the non-CLAS facilities.

Access

The Peru Demographic and Health Survey (DHS) data show that CLAS catchment populations in rural areas were on average poorer than rural non-CLAS populations (Altobelli, 2006). Furthermore, CLAS facilities were also consistently more likely to grant fee exemptions than non-CLAS facilities (Figure 3). Nearly all CLAS reported having a sliding scale of fees-for-services to increase access for the poor.

Health-care utilization

Records from 2002 of all the 675 health facilities (200 CLAS and 475 non-CLAS) in the Cusco, Huánuco and La Libertad regions show almost double the average number of annual clinic visits for children below five years in the catchment areas of rural CLAS versus non-CLAS (2.32 versus 1.22). For urban areas, the number was 2.94 for CLAS versus 1.73 for non-CLAS (Altobelli and Sovero, 2004).

For specific conditions, i.e. diarrhoea and acute respiratory infections (ARI), data show a consistently higher use of health-care services in CLAS as compared to non-CLAS facilities in the catchment areas (Figure 4).

Outcome

Figure 5 shows that, among rural children whose mothers had any primary schooling, the rate of chronic malnutrition was 40.8% for those living in CLAS catchment areas and 44% for those living in non-CLAS

areas. This difference is significant ($P<0.01$). For the other education categories, the difference was not significant.

Quality of care

The CLAS presidents and managers who were interviewed defined quality of care as shorter waiting times, non-discrimination, no mistreatment, longer opening hours, having sufficient health personnel, particularly medical specialists, having enough medicines, etc. They reported making management decisions: (1) to motivate health personnel by increasing wages, (2) to orient expenditures to improvements in infrastructure and equipment, (3) to present proposals to the regional or local government for financing of infrastructure and other projects, and (4) to improve their own capabilities by taking training in management, legal aspects of the PAC, etc.

The CLAS presidents interviewed were of the view that relationships with health personnel have improved since they became accountable to health personnel. Requests by the community for changes or improvements in health services are generally channelled through the CLAS association members. In case a patient is mistreated, the line of decision-making is not standard, but nearly always involves a collaborative decision between CLAS members and the CLAS manager, and sometimes referred to the DIRESA for a solution and final action.

Building social capital

The CLAS presidents interviewed considered their CLAS membership to be an honour; they found that they were highly respected by the community, and were seen as having the power to change what needed changing to improve health services and the health of the community. In all the CLAS interviewed, the number of female members of the General Assembly has increased over time. One third of CLAS interviewed had a majority of women members; four or more of the seven members were women.

Life history of CLAS

Primary health care (PHC) was placed on the health policy agenda for the first time in 1985 by the then Health Minister Dr David Tejada, a former Deputy Director General of WHO under Dr Halfdan Mahler. Though many were enthused by the PHC approach, there was little support for the strategy either technically, administratively or financially in the centralist and hospital-oriented health sector. As a result, the initial enthusiasm for PHC faded within a couple of years. Hyperinflation, the Shining Path terrorist activity, and government estrangement from international financing had eroded public health services by 1990. With the change of government in 1990, budgetary deficiencies and terrorist activity continued in rural areas. Also, the cholera epidemic of 1991 diverted health sector attention. Following capture of the Shining Path leader in September 1992, Peru began to move rapidly towards a new economic model that slowed inflation and stimulated greater international investment and donor financing. The Ministry of Economy and Finance (MEF) initiated the "Peruvian Government Reform Project" and within that the "Health Sector Reform". The MEF commissioned the development of legal norms to modernize the health sector, applying concepts of social-oriented market economics and democracy (Vera, 1994).

There was a new orientation to poverty reduction and growing political commitment to decentralization as part of the regional trend in Latin America. Jaime Freundt took over as Minister of Health in mid-1993 with the intention of strengthening PHC services: only 300 health posts were operational in rural areas, out of a total 4318 health centres and posts in the country (Ministry of Health, 1992). Innovative solutions were required. A new major programme financed by the public treasury and administered through a special quasi-public programme, the Basic Health for All Programme (Spanish acronym PSBPT) had the goal to rapidly increase PHC coverage to the neediest populations. By 1996, over 2000 PHC facilities were reactivated with human and material resources with the greatest proportional increase in the poorest areas (Valdivia, 2002).

Dr Freundt saw the need for an alternative form of administration for PHC, which would begin to solve the problems of lack of resources and poor quality of services. Privatization was becoming acceptable and the idea was to design a programme that would involve community participation, recognizing that the State could not manage everything, that "things work when those who are most interested in having it work well are involved" (personal communication, Freundt 2007).

Dr Freundt sought advice from an international expert on community participation, Carl E. Taylor,[2] who was

in the process of developing an evidence-based theory of community change, which incorporated new roles for empowered communities, the government and outside change agents (Taylor and Taylor, 1995 and 2002). In January 1994, Carl Taylor and two Peruvian experts, Juan Jose Vera and Patricia Paredes, visited mountain communities where the Shining Path was active to find out why villages did not want to reopen MOH services. Villagers told them that doctors were uncaring and treated them as though they were ignorant, and mainly wanted to return to the city. The villagers wanted to have medical care on their own terms and have a say in it.

The programme was initiated with minimal publicity to avoid the fate of a similar, widely publicized community-controlled programme in the education sector in 1993, which was seen as a threat to teacher autonomy, and was quickly brought down by the powerful teachers' union (Ortiz de Zevallos et al., 1999).

The legal framework provided by the Peruvian Civil Code and its articles for creation of civil associations was seen as the ideal model for building community-based health administration committees. The most relevant prior experience was the Programme for Revitalization of Peripheral Health Services, a UNICEF-supported project that had applied the principles of the Bamako Initiative to a community-administered revolving drug fund.

From January to April 1994, the legal and institutional framework of the new programme was drafted and a Supreme Decree Nº 01-SA-94 was signed by the President on 5 May 1994. This created the Shared Administration Programme (PAC) with the formation of CLAS, and the Shared Administration Programme for Pharmaceuticals (PACFARM). PAC was set up as a sub-programme of the PSBPT. Dr Freundt was so convinced of the need to go forward with CLAS that he bypassed two signatures in the MOH before sending the original Supreme Decree on CLAS to the President.

A highly qualified technical team with multidisciplinary membership and committed to the idea of community participation was assembled and remained for the first four programme years even with changing health ministers and national politics. Later national coordinators of the PAC were physicians who had previous experience as CLAS managers and could provide operational guidance to other physicians around the country who were managing

[2] Founding Chair and late Professor Emeritus of the International Health Department at The Johns Hopkins University School of Hygiene and Public Health (now Bloomberg School of Public Health)

CLAS on the ground. The PAC technical team began the identification, formation and training of regional health staff, PHC facility personnel and communities.

The first pilots of CLAS were inaugurated in July 1994 with thirteen PHC facilities in Ayacucho, home of the Shining Path, and coastal Ica. By the end of the first year, 250 health facilities were incorporated into the programme, each with a CLAS association. Two evaluations of CLAS conducted in 1995 and early 1996 had very positive findings on the progress and value of CLAS (O'Brien and Barnechea, 1996; Taylor, 1996). By mid-1997, 10% of all MOH PHC facilities in Peru were administered by CLAS: 558 CLAS administered 611 health facilities (out of about 6000 total facilities) in 26 out of the 33 health regions.

An important reform that contributed to decentralization and improved equity was the development of two government health insurance programmes that were eventually combined into the Integrated Health Insurance programme (Spanish acronym SIS). The Free School Insurance programme (Spanish acronym SEG) was created in 1996 to fulfil President Fujimori's 1995 re-election campaign promise to provide public school children with free medical and dental care. Health facilities became quickly overwhelmed since they had received no resources for hiring additional personnel to meet the increased demand for health services by schoolchildren. The second public insurance scheme began in 1997 with a pilot for the Maternal–Child Insurance programme (Spanish acronym SMI), which focused on reducing financial barriers to preventive services and childbirth. The pilot took place in three areas where CLAS were already well established.[3] As a CLAS was able to directly receive insurance reimbursements, it could immediately respond to the increased demand by hiring more personnel and enhancing services. Non-CLAS facilities were not considered in the SMI pilots and the role of the CLAS in the success of the SMI pilots was not widely known or understood at the time.

By the end of 1997, resistance to CLAS was building from various sides. Groups of regional-level health administrators criticized the CLAS, physicians' unions and health workers' unions called for a boycott of CLAS, and groups of officials and technical advisors in the central ministry belittled the value of CLAS. Health reform teams working on the design of health management "networks and micro-networks" refused to incorporate

CLAS into their proposals. Under pressure to close CLAS, the new Minister of Health decided to freeze CLAS expansion and commissioned an internal programme evaluation (Vicuña et al., 1999). At that point, over 150 additional CLAS had been organized and were waiting to be recognized. Another 200 were at various stages of formation. By not considering that a decentralized model was functioning through CLAS, consultants charged with designing a decentralized model omitted CLAS from their design frameworks. Instead, they preferred the idea of handing PHC services over to management by local municipalities, even though that idea was widely seen as questionable due to incipient capabilities in most municipalities. As a compromise, the new law on CLAS incorporates the local municipal government as one of three signatories on the co-management agreement, thereby satisfying the goal to articulate PHC services with the local government, while maintaining a share of community control.

The health reform teams designed a model called the "health management network" in which PHC facilities were regrouped into networks and smaller micro-networks related by geographical accessibility that centralize health information and channel referrals between facilities of increasing resolutive capacity. The larger network management centres manage funds, including SIS insurance reimbursements, health budgets for goods and services, and for results-based budgeting. This heterogeneous framework was superimposed on CLAS, creating a competing organizational model.

Management of CLAS in its early stages was placed in the DIRESA Community Participation Units, staffed with sociologists and anthropologists who were experts in community participation but had difficulty in comprehending the decentralized financial and human resource management aspects of CLAS, and were therefore ineffective in correctly representing the programme to the rest of the MOH. These officers were sometimes a source of criticism for CLAS, particularly in the first years of CLAS when power struggles occurred between communities and the government, as both learned new roles and ways to share power in decision-making and control over resources.

The World Bank took an interest in CLAS as a strategy for modernizing the public sector, improving transparency and ensuring social control of public

---

[3] SMI was piloted in CLAS-administered networks in the regions of Tacna and Arequipa, and the Moyobamba province in the region of San Martin.

expenditures. Other agencies also became interested and commissioned papers on the programme, including the Inter-American Development Bank (IDB) (Altobelli, 1998a), International Development Research Centre/ IDB (Cortez, 1998), and UNICEF (Altobelli, 1998b). All these papers found that, compared with non-CLAS, the performance of CLAS was better with respect to health-care coverage and equity.

In January 1999, the CLAS programme was reinstated. A new strategy was prepared for rapid expansion, incorporating additional health facilities into existing CLAS. These were referred to as "aggregate CLAS", whereby one CLAS administered more than one health facility; some administered as many as 40 facilities. The pros and cons of the aggregate CLAS model were addressed in a case management paper, which suggested that community involvement declined with aggregate CLAS, though efficiency could increase (Altobelli and Pancorvo, 2000). Thereafter, it was decided to divide larger aggregate CLAS into smaller ones.

Scaling up of the SMI programme also began in 1999. At this time, non-CLAS were included in SMI, but they could not receive the insurance reimbursements directly. In CLAS, however, SMI reimbursements were received directly into their co-managed bank accounts and provided the base to improve staffing, infrastructure and equipment, allowing CLAS to enter an upward spiral of improved supply and demand. Within three years, CLAS went from covering 10% to more than 30% of the primary-level facilities. The decision to rapidly scale up both CLAS and SMI in 1999 was a result of the World Bank Programmatic Social Reform Loan to Peru using a new mechanism in which policy decisions and benchmarks were agreed upon with government social sectors (health, education, food assistance, justice) as conditionalities for loan disbursements.

Funding for SMI expansion was part of a proposed 1999 funding package of US$ 264 million from the World Bank, IDB, and a consortium of bilateral funders (Britain, Canada, Japan and others). The package was intended to subsidize all recurrent costs of the SMI for three years, after which it was expected that the Government of Peru would begin to take over the costs. The MEF put pressure on the MOH to comply with the agreed policy changes. These included expanding CLAS by a specified percentage each year for three years between 1999 and 2002, as one

of the conditionalities for loan disbursement to the MEF.

However, the transitional government in 2000–2001[4] wanted to put the SMI expansion loan package on hold until the next elected government was in place. The delay resulted in donor withdrawal. Without these loans, the SMI insurance reimbursements were left to the responsibility of the public treasury. The lack of secure financing for SMI adversely affected the ability of CLAS to improve the quality of services. Further, there was no technical support for CLAS from the World Bank-funded technical assistance project, PARSalud, due to perceived wavering of political commitment to CLAS. However, the dedicated national technical team of Shared Administration was a constant that provided the underpinning technical support to keep CLAS alive during this time.

The dramatic increase in CLAS during 2001–2002 (Figure 1) can be attributed to the World Bank Programmatic Social Reform Loan (PSRL) conditionalities, in addition to the committed advocacy of the National Coordinator of Shared Administration, Victor Baccini, who was able to convince the Minister to not delay CLAS expansion. This was a major achievement in spite of the conservative orientation of the then Health Minister who, together with his Vice Minister, reversed gains in women's access to health services (Coe, 2004). When the Vice Minister became Minister in 2002, he took overt action to delay CLAS expansion.

Most nongovernmental organizations (NGOs) worked on projects funded by donors and, by and large, played only a small role in supporting CLAS. Eventually, Pathfinder and CARE Peru incorporated some support to CLAS as part of their larger projects on reproductive health and health rights programmes. Future Generations was the only NGO that provided technical support to CLAS throughout the life of the programme and, beginning in late 2002, developed a "model CLAS" in the poor urban settlement of Las Moras in Huánuco Region on the eastern slope of the Andes. The model works with a methodology of community empowerment for strengthening social control and transparency of health management, with capacity building of all actors to strengthen social capital and local ownership of the development process (Díaz et al., 2006). Las Moras has been awarded several prizes and recognition in national competitions on quality improvement, and serves now as

---

[4] The transitional government was installed as a result of a fraud detected in the 2000 Presidential elections.

a model site and a self-help centre for action learning to help scale up the model, and help politicians and health officials see the value of CLAS.

The MOH in 2002 commissioned an evaluation of CLAS with the call to propose "other models of co-management". The evaluation reports provided a positive assessment of CLAS with useful recommendations (Sobrevilla et al., 2002; Velarde and Sobrevilla, 2002; Puntriano, 2002). Ignoring these papers, the MOH went ahead towards closure of CLAS through a series of Ministerial Resolutions[5] in late 2002. The only bilateral donor agencies at that time with a technical interest in CLAS were the Department for International Development (DFID) and United States Agency for International Development (USAID), though they provided little financial support.

When Dr Halfdan Mahler, former Director General of WHO, visited Peru in 2001, he made site visits to several CLAS, and spoke highly in favour of CLAS to dignitaries of the medical profession and the MOH. A health advocacy group, ForoSalud representing civil society, comprising health professionals and health-related NGOs, was established in 2003 and included civil society groups involved in health at the regional level. In general, ForoSalud was supportive of CLAS.

There were no major adjustments made in the laws and regulations guiding CLAS from 1994 till 2007, given that ten Ministerial Resolutions were passed during that period, which modified only minor details of the programme. However, three Ministerial Resolutions in late 2002 reduced the autonomy of CLAS, delineating how the MOH could close down a CLAS, and creating a commission to revise its legal framework. This stimulated Future Generations in January 2003 to initiate advocacy with the Health Commission of Congress on developing a new law decree to provide legal stability to CLAS and protect it from the fluctuating levels of support provided by changing leadership teams in the MOH. By the end of that year, a consortium of development agencies and NGOs, public health experts, and MOH officials[6] was assembled by Congressman Dr Daniel Robles, President of the Health Commission. A "Sub-Commission for the Study of CLAS" was formed and an initial draft of the law was discussed in a series of three macro-regional meetings in December 2003 and January 2004. Numerous subsequent drafts were produced during 2004 through

October 2005, but work on the law was put on hold as the 2006 Presidential election campaigns drew near and the political climate became uncertain as to how the new government would want to deal with CLAS (Future Generations, 2008).

Work on the CLAS law proposal in the Health Commission of the Congress stimulated a parallel effort within the MOH, which felt that it was their role to prepare the law proposal. For a time, there were two parallel and competing CLAS law proposals in process.

Despite the rapid expansion, increasing community demand and success of CLAS in delivering health care, resistance grew from the medical profession, regional DIRESAs and health worker unions. The Medical Federation claimed CLAS to be a move toward privatization of health, thus jeopardizing their goal to have all physicians on the public payroll. Physicians have long sought what they consider their lawful right to be hired as permanent public payroll employees for public sector jobs.

Strong resistance also came from the administrative staff in DIRESAs who lost control over resources as a result of the CLAS system that transfers funds directly to CLAS bank accounts. In addition, the use of low-cost, short-term, no-benefit contracts by CLAS generated resistance from the non-physician health workers' union FENUTSA,[7] despite the fact that the same type of contract was also widely used in non-CLAS PHC facilities.

Overt resistance to CLAS was building particularly from the Medical Federation, which feared the permanence of a potential CLAS law that they believed was contrary to their main goal of public payroll employment for physicians in government health services. A national physicians' strike led by the Medical Federation in late 2003 to early 2004 included as two of 10 demands the derogation of CLAS as well as public payroll employment of all physicians. By that time, MOH leadership had passed to a Minister who was a supporter of the physician unions, and under whom the physicians' strike began. It fell, however, on his successor to resolve the strike, which she did by agreeing in April 2004 to public employment of physicians with gradual incorporation over time. One expert interviewed described this as "the most regressive policy decision in public health to occur in the last ten or fifteen years", damaging the health system and the

---

[5] R.M. N° 895, R.M. N° 1743, and R.M. N° 1793
[6] Federación Nacional Único de Trabajadores de Salud (FENUTSA)

health reform process. Many feared that CLAS would be debilitated by the loss of social control over physician performance.

CLAS had survived the physicians' strike, but PAC was progressively dismantled as funding was cut and the PAC technical team was reduced from 35 persons to five over a period of two to three years. In December 2005, the remaining PAC team was transferred from the Programme for Administration of Management Agreements (an outgrowth of PSBPT) to the Executive Office of Health Services Management in the MOH, with final transition of CLAS financial management to the MOH General Accounting Office. While it was widely feared that PAC could suffer in administrative efficiency and lose technical guidance from this move, it was also seen as a positive action toward mainstreaming PAC into the general work of the MOH. On the down side, regional DIRESAs remained without a specific office in charge of regional CLAS management. Responsibility for CLAS continued to be assigned in an ad-hoc manner in each region.

In his inaugural speech on 28 July 2006, the President Alan Garcia stated that he would extend the experience of CLAS during his presidency to the education sector. Finally, in October 2007, the Peruvian Congress approved a new "Law on Co-Management and Citizen Participation in Health Facilities at the Primary Level of Care of the Ministry of Health and the Regions," bringing to an end five years of advocacy on CLAS from within the MOH and from outside change agents.

Despite the new law, the renewed expansion of CLAS has not yet occurred. Two explanations were given by those interviewed. First, MOH attention has been focused on the development of a new law on Universal Health Insurance, which does not contemplate the role of CLAS and evidence that public insurance for the poor depends on CLAS for its effectiveness. Second, major resistance comes from regional and network administrative units that struggle to not lose control over resources that should be devolved to CLAS. It is generally noted that these units make large procurements of equipment and supplies that are not always essential, based on suspected supplier "incentives".

As for the physicians and other health staff who have moved to public employment status, which requires permanent assignment to a specific health facility, the result has been their massive exodus from rural to urban

health services (Altobelli, 2007). Many of these physicians seek the new options for public-funded specialty training, after which they never return to their non-transferable PHC post assignments, which remain forever abandoned since budgeting for the post moves with the person.

11.4 Discussion

Contribution to improving equity

There are a number of indications that CLAS has made important contributions to improving health equity in Peru. The marked difference in the availability of physicians between CLAS and non-CLAS health facilities (Figure 1) suggests that CLAS made progress in addressing both the rural–urban divide in the distribution of physicians and the relative overstaffing of the urban health facilities with respect to this category of staff. Nearly one in two of the rural CLAS health posts is staffed by a physician, while this is the case for less than one in four of the non-CLAS health posts. With respect to urban health centres, CLAS has on average about one third fewer physicians compared to non-CLAS centres. These differences could be explained by the staffing of CLAS facilities, which is determined by the demand of the community, the means and the ability to set conditions of service, e.g. to attract physicians to serve in rural areas. For the non-CLAS facilities, the surplus of physicians in urban health centres might to a large extent be determined by the supply, i.e. the preference of physicians to serve at a particular location. However, the difference observed in the 2006 data between CLAS and non-CLAS centres could already have changed as a result of reverting to government employment instead of private sector contracts, and the tendency to abandon rural posts by public payroll staff from both CLAS and non-CLAS facilities.

CLAS could have a doubly positive effect on equity. First, it covers populations that tend to be poorer than the catchment populations of the non-CLAS facilities. Second, CLAS facilities appear consistently more willing to provide full or partial fee exemptions compared to the non-CLAS facilities, and thus lower the financial barriers to access for poor individuals. One of the results could be the observation that the health-care utilization of mothers with sick children is consistently higher in CLAS compared with non-CLAS populations.

The picture might be more complex with regard to the effect on malnutrition rate. Data on malnutrition in under-five children by education level of the mother show that there is a significant difference in CLAS versus non-CLAS populations only in the group "any primary education". There could be a number of explanations for this: malnutrition is influenced by other social determinants that have a stronger influence than access to and use of health-care services. While fee exemptions and outreach increase access to and use of curative services, the effective use of health promotion services could also be restricted by messages and communication methods not appropriate to the target clients. Further, the CLAS concept of community participation and control could by its very design be more appealing to groups with mid-level education, which could influence how promotion services are provided.

Going to scale

The CLAS programme was established during a period fraught with economical and political problems, and mistrust between communities and the government. As a result, only 300 out of 3800 health centres and posts were operational. One year after the start of CLAS in July 1994, 250 health facilities were incorporated into the programme, each with a CLAS association. By mid-1997, 558 CLAS associations administered 611 facilities and, from 2002, about 780 CLAS associations administered more than 2100 facilities. The key facilitators for this rapid scale-up are likely to have been the approach to piloting, the demand-driven nature of the scale-up, and the capacity of the CLAS model to absorb resources, among others.

The sites for the first 13 pilot CLAS/PHC facilities were in those areas where the government had previously been faced with the most opposition and distrust, and where public facilities had been the most dilapidated during the long period of economic and political turbulence. This meant that if the pilots could be made to work in these areas, the chance of them working in other areas would be greater than if the pilot experiences and learning had been done in "easy" areas and with a subsequent adaptation to more "difficult" areas.

Once the initial group of 13 CLAS was functioning, they served as demonstration sites, encouraging other communities to choose to enter the programme, thus maintaining the self-selection process that was an important feature of successful implementation. Self-selection and active community involvement from the start probably contributed to increasing the chances of successful implementation in each case. "Things work well when those who are most interested in having it work well are involved" (personal communication, Freundt, 2007). Further, community pressure possibly also played a political role in keeping up the momentum of scale-up, as in 1997 when resistance to CLAS was building, 150 CLAS were awaiting recognition and another 200 were in various stages of formation.

However, probably the single most important factor in the scale-up process was that the CLAS concept and model was actually "scalable". Compared with the non-CLAS model, the CLAS model matched perfectly with the injection of resources by the World Bank and bilateral donors through the demand side, i.e. the SMI and later SIS insurance schemes, as the CLAS could absorb resources and easily adjust capacity. Further, the conditionalities of the World Bank Programmatic Social Reform Loan that committed the government to a specific yearly percentage expansion of the CLAS prevented, at least for a while, bureaucratic and political obstacles to slow the expansion.

Managing policy change

The introduction and implementation of CLAS involved three key policy changes: (1) decentralization, i.e. devolution of power and control from the civil service to the community and moving the responsibility for provision of certain health services from the government to the nongovernmental sector; (2) deprofessionalization of governance, meaning that CLAS managers, i.e. medical doctors and sometimes nurses, were answerable for performance to lay people elected by the community rather than through professional hierarchies, e.g. in the MOH; and (3) the resource flows were reversed from being supply-driven to becoming demand-driven i.e. financial resources were provided through insurance and user payments directly to the individual health unit and human resources were employed according to the need and ability to pay. These changes were profound, both conceptually and politically, and it is remarkable that the whole programme did not collapse during its implementation. There can be several possible explanations for this.

The introduction of CLAS took place in a political and economic situation in Peru which left no doubt that reform and change were critically necessary. The general trend in Latin America as well as elsewhere in the early 1990s was privatization, decentralization and a reduced role of the State in service provision. Peru's new economic model based on these principles rapidly showed results in terms of slowing inflation and attracting foreign investments and donor support. At the same time, Taylor and Taylor were developing an evidence-based theory and approach to community change that matched well with the new model for development. Together, these factors created a conducive opportunity for the President, in May 1994, to sign the Supreme Decree that provided the legal and institutional framework for launching the CLAS.

Reorganization of power relations should be expected when incorporating community partners in the management of public services (Morgan, 2001), and it was anticipated from the conception that the new programme would trigger resistance, particularly from the medical profession. In order for the new programme to take root before facing the anticipated resistance, it was launched without being widely publicized. There were three main sources of resistance: the physicians' and health workers' unions, the regional health administration, and groups within the central MOH. For the first source of resistance, the main issue was the implication that CLAS meant shifting from government to private sector employment contracts and conditions. Eventually, the physicians' union got its way and physicians, later joined by non-physician health staff, are gradually converting to public employment even when working in a CLAS. For the two other sources of resistance, i.e. the regional health administration and certain groups of central MOH officials, the issue was the perceived loss of power, mainly of financial control, by the devolved control of resources and decision-making to the CLAS associations. Many misunderstandings still remain but these have not changed the tenet of the policy.

It is remarkable that the leadership function for the policy change was provided not by an individual or the same group of persons. Rather, leadership was provided by a series of individuals and groups over the period of 14 years, each making their particular leadership contribution at critical points in time. This included Dr Freundt, Minister of Health, who conceived and launched the idea in 1993, the National Coordinator of the PAC, the former Director General of WHO, a private non-profit organization, and Congressman Daniel Robles who as President of the Health Commission finalized and got the law passed in 2007.

The absence of a central leadership probably prolonged the process of finalizing the policy and being integrated in the overall health sector policies. It actually took longer to get the policy change in place than it took to scale up the programme. At times, the leadership vacuum gave rise to parallel processes that probably contributed directly to one of the most critical compromises to the original idea that health facility staff were to be contracted directly by the CLAS. The absence of a long-term leadership figure probably led managers to put greater emphasis on incremental achievements with respect to policy change and legalities, thus depersonalizing the programme and ensuring greater long-term sustainability. Loan-givers and donors did not take a direct role in the policy formulation process. However, they played an important role in managing policy change by setting and enforcing conditionalities and, through the MEF, by providing pressure and reducing the risk of reversal. However, the expansion stopped once this pressure disappeared (Figure 1).

CLAS has been the subject of numerous evaluations and studies, some of which served as an integral part of the scale-up process in the early phases of implementation. The early evaluations provided evidence of the efficacy of the approach. Later comparative studies of CLAS and non-CLAS facilities supported by the World Bank, Inter American Development Bank, International Development Research Centre/IDB and UNICEF showed a better performance of CLAS than non-CLAS with respect to health-care coverage and equity. A further study in 2002 of the CLAS model was undertaken by the MOH with the aim of proposing "other models for co-management". However, the results of this study also were in favour of CLAS.

Over its lifespan, CLAS has been involved with three pilots and demonstration projects. The first, in 1994 with the original 13 pilot facilities, showed that the approach could work, even under difficult circumstances. The second round of pilots in 1997 did not focus on CLAS but the SMI insurance programme. However, the contribution of CLAS to the working of the SMI was not recognized at the time. The last, started in 2002, was to demonstrate how model CLAS facilities could work to strengthen PHC services generally. Pilots, demonstration models and evaluations can be important components of managing policy change. The positive outcome of the various studies certainly provided the evidence to loan-givers and donors who needed to justify their support and conditionalities. However, for some politicians and other interested parties, the positive outcome of these studies was not sufficient to convince them as their success criteria were not necessarily health-care coverage and equity.

Adjusting design

Throughout the history of CLAS, it was a constant battle to maintain and keep the key components of the concept intact. There were a number of important adjustments made to the design during implementation. First, grouping of PHC facilities into "health management networks" was superimposed on the CLAS, creating a competing organizational structure. This led to the concept of aggregate CLAS (1999), where one CLAS could administer as many as 40 individual facilities. However, after a case management paper showed declining community involvement (Altobelli and Pancorvo, 2000), it was later decided to split up the larger aggregate CLAS. Second, the inclusion of local municipal governments as one of three signatories on the co-management agreement (2007) was a compromise as resistance grew from designers of government decentralization and "municipalization". The incorporation of this local "third party" into MOH-PHC services may potentially complicate decision-making and politicize management of PHC. The long-term effects of this design change that was imposed during the final debate prior to Congressional approval of the new law may be revealed in future.

The most substantial adjustment to the CLAS design happened in 2004 when, as a response to prolonged and fierce opposition by physicians' unions, the government took a U-turn and agreed to government employment of, eventually, all physicians. This was seen by many as ending the social control of this critical staff group, which could potentially reverse the achievements of CLAS and lead to loss of community faith and interest in the model. However, the new 2007 law requires public payroll employees in CLAS to adhere to CLAS control mechanisms. The real damage has occurred from allowing increasing numbers of public employees to move their budgeted positions to urban facilities, thereby, in effect, reducing public budgets previously designated for rural health facilities, whether CLAS or non-CLAS.

Ensuring sustainability

One outstanding feature of CLAS throughout the almost two decades of its existence is that implementation has not depended on a single person or group. This idea prevailed even through dramatic political changes. The following may have been the major contributing factors to this: right from the very beginning, CLAS was anchored in legal instruments, which have gradually been widened and deepened; and that the CLAS model provided a very efficient mechanism for financing the health sector through the demand side, i.e. through social insurance schemes.

11.5 Conclusion

This case study describes the positive effect of the CLAS programme on equity in availability, access and utilization of quality PHC services in Peru. It analyses the life history of the programme from 1993 to 2007, focusing primarily on the scaling-up and policy change processes.

It cannot be ignored that CLAS was initiated at a time that was conducive to the approach both locally, following the political, economic and government service collapse, and internationally, when the general public sector reform mode was a move towards a lesser role of the State and greater role of the private sector. However, there were some elements that made the CLAS approach unique and thus provided a learning experience for others. First, the initial roll-out of the CLAS programme was demand driven. It started with those most in need and created a momentum both managerially and politically, in that it became important enough to not be ignored. Second, the programme was scalable, i.e. it could absorb and put to work large sums of additional money by smoothly adjusting capacity while maintaining quality through a combination of social control and injection of resources through the demand rather than the supply side and third-party donations. Third, from the very beginning, CLAS followed the route of institutionalization and incrementally worked on establishing the formal and legal base for sustaining the programme.

A weakness has been that, aside from the initial phases, the programme has lacked continuing political leadership, resulting in two major compromises to the original idea – health staff converting to government employee status, contrary to the original blue-print where most staff were to be hired by the CLAS associations on private sector contracts; and reverting a portion of the resources previously managed by CLAS under the control of network management units. The possible impact of these compromises on equity in availability, access, utilization and quality, as well as the long-term viability of the programme will depend on health sector leadership, which only the future will tell. Contracted health personnel in the field express a general desire to convert to CLAS, seeing its positive effect on the quality of care and the advantages of private labour contracts. Thus, CLAS could eventually expand on its own merits, but perhaps not before the authorities demand accountability throughout the public administration system and create more effective policies regarding public sector employment.

Acknowledgements

This paper is dedicated to the late Carl E. Taylor who passed away in February 2010 at the age of 93. Many thanks go to Erik Blas and Sara Bennett of WHO for overseeing the development of this paper; to Luis Espejo, José Cabrejos and Alejandro Vargas who participated through Future Generations in Model CLAS and CLAS law development; to Julio Puntriano and Victor Baccini for assistance with field work for this paper; and to the many persons interviewed who generously shared their experiences with CLAS. This paper received funding support from the World Health Organization Alliance for Health Policy and Systems Research.

References

1. Altobelli LC (1998a). *Comparative analysis of primary health care facilities with civil society participation in Venezuela and Peru.* Prepared for the seminar *Social Programs, Poverty, and Citizen Participation,* 12–13 March 1998. Cartagena, Colombia, Inter-American Development Bank. Available at: http://www.future.org/publications/comparative-analysis-primary-health-care-facilities-with-participation-civil-society-ve (accessed on 8 September 2010).

2. Altobelli LC (1998b). *Health reform, community participation, and social inclusion: the Shared Administration Program.* Paper prepared for the Mid-term Evaluation of the UNICEF-Peru Cooperation. UNICEF Peru, August 1998. Available at: http://www.future.org/publications/health-reform-community-participation-and-social-inclusion-shared-administration-progra (accessed on 8 September 2010).

3. Altobelli LC and Pancorvo J (2000). *The Shared Administration Program and the Local Health Administration Committees: case study of Peru.* Case study prepared for the III Forum for Europe and the Americas on Health Sector Reform. San José, Costa Rica, World Bank. Available at: http://www.future.org/publications/shared-administration-program-and-local-health-administration-associations-clas-peru (accessed on 8

September 2010).

4. Altobelli LC and Sovero J (2004). *Cost-efficiency of CLAS associations.* Lima, Future Generations, Mulago Foundation, DFID. Available at: http://www.future.org/publications/cost-efficiency-clas-associations-primary-health-care-peru (accessed on 8 September 2010).

5. Altobelli LC (2006). *Comparative analysis of health impact and health services utilization in CLAS and non-CLAS primary health care services in Peru.* Lima, Future Generations Peru.

6. Altobelli LC (2007). *CLAS: retrospective and prospective.* Lima, Future Generations. (Invited presentation at the Institute of Peru – University San Martin de Porras. Data from the National Inventory of Infrastructure, Equipment, and Human Resources, Ministry of Health of Peru, 2006).

7. Coe AB (2004). From anti-natalist to ultraconservative: restricting reproductive choice in Peru. *Reproductive Health Matters,* 12:56–69.

8. Cortez R (1998). *Equidad y calidad de los servicios de salud: el caso de los CLAS.* Lima, Research Center of the Universidad del Pacífico [Working Documento N° 33].

9. Cortez R and Phumpiu P (1999). *La Entrega de Servicios de Salud en los Centros de Administración Compartida (CLAS): el caso del Perú.* Lima, Universidad del Pacífico, International Development Research Center (IDRC/CIDA), Inter-American Development Bank (IDB).

10. Díaz J et al. (2006). *Pilot project SCALE-Squared Training Center, CLAS Las Moras – Huánuco: mid-term evaluation 2003–2005.* Lima, Future Generations, Mulago Foundation, Duane Stranahan Charitable Trust.

11. Future Generations (2008). *Development of the "Law That Establishes Co-management and Citizen Participation in Primary Health Care Facilities of the Ministry of Health and the Regions": a documented chronology 2003 to 2007.* Prepared to commemorate the approval by the Peruvian Congress on 5 October 2007 and the promulgation by the President on 30 October 2007 of Law N° 29124. 15 January 2008.

12. Mahler H et al. (2001). *Memorandum on findings and recommendations for Peru's national system of community co-managed primary health care.* Franklin, WV, Future Generations. Available at: http://www.future.org/publications/memorandum-findings-and-recommendations-perus-national-system-community-co-managed-prim (accessed on 8 September 2010).

13. Ministry of Health (2007). *Health services management annual report.* Lima, Ministry of Health.

14. Ministry of Health (1992). *National inventory of health infrastructure.* Lima, Ministry of Health.

15. Morgan L (2001). Community participation in health: perpetual allure, persistent challenge. *Health Policy and Planning,* 16:221–230.

16. O'Brien E and Barnachea M (1996). *Informe Final: Evaluación*

del Programa de Focalización de Gasto Social Básico: Sub Programa Administración Compartida. Lima, Ministry of Health and Program for Analysis, Planning, and Implementation (PAPI)-USAID.

17. Ortiz de Zevallos G et al. (1999). *The political economy of institutional reforms in Peru: the cases of education, health, and pensions.* Lima, Instituto Apoyo, Inter-American Development Bank [Working Document R-348].

18. Puntriano J (2002). *Análisis del Modelo de Co-Gestión Vigente: análisis critica de la normatividad nacional que regula o incide en el diseño y el funcionamiento del Modelo de Cogestión CLAS.* Lima, Ministry of Health.

19. Sobrevilla A (2002). *Proposals for improvement of co-management of public health services.* Lima, Ministry of Health.

20. Taylor C (1996). *Evaluation and report on strengthening a national co-managed system of primary health: report to the Honorable Minister of Health.* Lima, Pan American Health Organization. Available at: http://www.future.org/publications/evaluation-and-report-strengthening-national-system-community-co-managed-primary-health (accessed on 8 September 2010).

21. Taylor-Ide D and Taylor CE (1995). *Community-based sustainable human development: a proposal for going to scale with self-reliant social development.* New York, UNICEF Environment Section. Available at: http://www.future. org/publications/community-based-sustainable-human-development (accessed on 8 September 2010).

22. Taylor-Ide D and Taylor CE (2002). *Just and lasting change: when communities own their future.* Baltimore, The Johns Hopkins University Press in collaboration with Future Generations. Available at: http://www.future.org/publications/just-and-lasting-change (accessed on 8 September 2010).

23. Valdivia M (2002). Public health infrastructure and equity in the utilization of outpatient health care services in Peru. *Health Policy and Planning*, 17(Suppl.):12–19.

24. Velarde N and Sobrevilla A (2002). *Proposals for adjustments to the CLAS Model and for the development of other experiences of co-management in health.* Lima, Ministry of Health.

25. Vera JC (1994). Modernization and opening of health services to participation of the private sector. In: *The privatization of health on the road to modernity.* Lima, Institute for Free Market Economy.

26. Vicuña M, Ampuero S, Murillo J (2000). *Analysis of effective demand and its relation to the management model in primary health care facilities: evaluation of the Shared Administration Program.* Lima, Peru, Ministry of Health-PAAG-SBPT-AC.

27. WHO (2009). *World health statistics – 2009.* Geneva, World Health Organization.

What happens after a trial? Replicating a cross-sectoral intervention addressing the social determinants of health

The case of the Intervention with Microfinance for AIDS and Gender Equity (IMAGE) in South Africa

12

James Hargreaves,[1,2,*] Abigail Hatcher,[1,2] Joanna Busza,[1]
Vicki Strange,[3] Godfrey Phetla,[2] Julia Kim,[1,2] Charlotte Watts,[1]
Linda Morison,[1] John Porter,[1] Paul Pronyk,[1,2] Chris Bonell[1]

[1] London School of Hygiene and Tropical Medicine, Keppel Street, London WC1E 7HT
[2] School of Public Health, University of the Witwatersrand, PO Box 2, Acornhoek 1360, South Africa
[3] Social Science Research Unit, Institute of Education, 18 Woburn Square, London, WC1H 0NR
* james.hargreaves@lshtm.ac.uk

Abstract

The evaluation and implementation of cross-sectoral interventions that aim to improve health outcomes by targeting their social determinants is complex. The Intervention with Microfinance for AIDS and Gender Equity (IMAGE) was an explicit attempt to design, implement and evaluate such an intervention in rural South Africa. The intervention combined an established microfinance programme with gender and HIV/AIDS training, and activities to support community mobilization. A cluster randomized trial found mixed outcomes while a process evaluation confirmed that the intervention had been largely delivered as intended during the trial. In this chapter, we draw on data from the six-year process evaluation and additionally from interviews with experts in the microfinance and HIV/AIDS communities. We describe the chronology of IMAGE delivery and management in South Africa, and the views of stakeholders with an interest in future deployment of the intervention. We highlight key lessons from our experiences in developing an intersectoral collaboration, expanding the scale of intervention delivery following a trial and exploring models for long-term sustainable delivery. The IMAGE experience underscores the potential of intersectoral collaboration in targeting the social determinants of health. It offers lessons for taking interventions to scale within partner organizations and highlights the complexity of engaging with multiple sectors, particularly since issues such as sustainability are judged rather differently by actors in different sectors.

12.1 Background

Sub-Saharan Africa is home to high levels of HIV/AIDS and intimate-partner violence (IPV). Over 60% of the world's HIV infections take place in the region, (UNAIDS, 2006) and 36–71% of African women report having been in a violent relationship (WHO, 2005). There is growing recognition that IPV can put women at increased risk for HIV infection, either directly through rape and sexual violence (Garcia-Moreno and Watts, 2000) or indirectly because of its downstream influence on other mediating variables such as risk behaviours (Andersson et al., 2004; Dunkle et al., 2006; Wong et al., 2008).

A common set of circumstances shape vulnerability to both HIV and IPV. Key social determinants such as poverty, underdevelopment and entrenched gender inequalities combine to fuel high levels of both (Rhodes and Simic, 2005; Mane et al., 1994; Gupta, 2002; Parker et al., 2000; Fenton, 2004; Garcia-Moreno and Watts, 2000; UNAIDS, 2002). Yet in both fields, there is limited experience in designing and implementing interventions that engage these social determinants. Where programmes do exist, it remains to be seen whether these can be taken beyond intensively managed pilot and research progammes to a regional and national scale. Expanding the coverage of an intervention poses real challenges, yet little research has focused on consistent implementation across settings (Gandelman and Rietmeijer, 2004; Glasgow et al., 2003)

or within new communities (Blankenship et al., 2006). Intervention trials should therefore be accompanied by process evaluations that examine the potential to maintain fidelity and acceptability as interventions are taken to scale (Rapkin and Trickett, 2005; Oakley et al., 2006). It is these latter issues that form the focus of this chapter.

This chapter discusses the Intervention with Microfinance for AIDS and Gender Equity (IMAGE), which combines group-based microfinance with gender and HIV training, and activities to support community mobilization (Pronyk et al., 2006). IMAGE was an explicit attempt to address poverty and gender inequalities in rural South Africa with the goal of reducing the rates of HIV and IPV. IMAGE was evaluated in a controlled trial and demonstrated mixed success in terms of measured health outcomes. Nevertheless, the implementing partners chose to scale-up intervention delivery following the trial. Throughout the trial and subsequent scale-up, there was significant interest in examining process and policy considerations for delivering this type of cross-sectoral intervention. This case study describes a process evaluation of the incremental scale-up of IMAGE over a period of six years in South Africa. It also describes the views of stakeholders from the fields of HIV/AIDS, gender-based violence, microfinance and development on the potential for further replicating IMAGE in other settings. Our discussion highlights opportunities, constraints and wider lessons for cross-sectoral programmes attempting to address the social determinants of health in sub-Saharan Africa.

The Intervention with Microfinance for AIDS and Gender Equity (IMAGE)

IMAGE was initiated in rural South Africa in 2001. The project brought together partners in the health and development sectors: the Rural AIDS & Development Action Research Programme (RADAR) represented a joint initiative of the School of Public Health at the University of Witwatersrand and the London School of Hygiene and Tropical Medicine, while the Small Enterprise Foundation (SEF) is a widely respected South African non-profit microfinance provider.

This research partnership emerged to assess how microfinance might serve as a vehicle for delivering an intervention to address the social determinants of health (Anderson et al., 2002). Working with women from the poorest households in target communities, IMAGE attempted to foster social and economic empowerment in ways that might reduce their vulnerability to HIV and IPV. The researchers drew on ecological theories of disease causation, and adopted the constructs of social capital, social networks and community mobilization (Babalola et al., 2001; Manandhar et al., 2004; Szreter and Woolcock, 2004). The approach was also influenced by Paulo Freire's transformative approach to adult education and the notion of critical consciousness (Freire, 1968). The intervention sought to strengthen individual and collective capacities to understand and address priority concerns in their communities, as this has been shown to be effective among a range of disempowered and marginalized populations (Parker, 1996).

The intervention that emerged had three components that were delivered to clients by different staff from the two specialist organizations: RADAR and SEF.

— *Microfinance (delivered by SEF):*

The poorest households in villages were identified through participatory wealth ranking (Hargreaves et al., 2007). Adult women from these households were eligible to join a programme of group-based micro-lending to support the start-up and expansion of small businesses. Approximately 40 women met fortnightly at loan centre meetings managed by fellow borrowers and supported by SEF staff.

— *Gender and HIV training (facilitated by RADAR staff):*

A compulsory 12–15-month training curriculum for SEF clients called "Sisters-for-Life" (SFL) took place during loan centre meetings. SFL comprised ten one-hour training sessions. Based upon participatory learning and action principles and techniques (Cornwall and Jewkes, 1995; Pretty et al., 1995; Freire, 1968), SFL covered topics that included gender roles, cultural beliefs, relationships, communication, IPV and HIV. SFL aimed to strengthen communication skills, critical thinking and leadership.

— *Activities to support community mobilization (facilitated by the same RADAR staff as SFL):*

This phase expanded the intervention to reach out into the community. Key women were selected by their centres for a further week of leadership training. Following this, they worked with centres to develop locally appropriate responses to priority issues including HIV and IPV. Community mobilization was an attempt to generate wider intervention effects among vulnerable groups in the households and communities where IMAGE was offered.

IMAGE trial results

From 2001 to 2004, a cluster randomized trial was conducted which compared women enrolled in the intervention with similar women from matched control villages. The study examined the direct effects among these female participants in the programme, while also assessing the indirect effects on HIV risk among 14–35-year-olds living in households and communities where the programme was offered. This was supplemented by complementary qualitative assessments which took place over the duration of the study (Kim et al., 2007; Pronyk et al., 2006; Pronyk et al., 2008; Phetla et al., 2007).

Over the three-year study period, the study provided:

- Good evidence of reduced levels of reported IPV among direct intervention participants compared with the control group;

- Good evidence that intervention participants reported changes in locally derived measures of gender empowerment, effects that were echoed by narratives in the qualitative data;

- Some evidence of reduced HIV vulnerability among the subgroup of intervention participants who were less than 35 years old at baseline, with this group reporting increased uptake of voluntary counselling and testing (VCT) and less unprotected sex compared with controls;

- Some evidence of improvements in indicators of economic well-being in the households of intervention participants;

- Some evidence of increased communication about sex and sexuality in the households of intervention participants;

- No evidence of an effect on HIV incidence or the rate of unprotected sex among indirectly exposed young people living in the households or communities of intervention participants.

Thus, the primary outcome results of the IMAGE trial were mixed and continue to be discussed both within the research team and beyond. Since data collection for the trial was completed in late 2004 but the results of analysis only began to be available many months later, it was primarily the positive experiences of staff and clients on the ground that drove the decision to undertake an initial scale-up of IMAGE beyond the trial site.

12.2 Methods: the IMAGE scale-up case study

Our process evaluation tracked the scale-up of IMAGE during and after the trial. We examined considerations for delivering the intervention, institutional partnership models, and policy opportunities to transfer cross-sectoral interventions such as IMAGE to new settings.

A six-year, mixed-method process evaluation was conducted, the detailed methods and results of which are reported elsewhere (Hargreaves et al., 2010). In brief, we collected quantitative data in the form of attendance registers, client questionnaires and financial records. During the IMAGE trial, we conducted 374 hours of participant observation, semi-structured interviews ($N=34$) and focus group discussions ($N=16$) with programme clients. During the IMAGE scale-up, we conducted semi-structured interviews with programme clients, staff and management ($N=98$).

The experiences with IMAGE in the field also led to an interest in whether IMAGE could be replicated in other settings. To investigate the potential for this, we conducted an external stakeholder analysis. We identified informants from three "policy networks" and used a purposive "snowball" sampling methodology to identify stakeholders ($N=31$, plus 10 focus group discussion participants) that would both be supportive and skeptical of transfer of IMAGE to new settings. We conducted semi-structured interviews and one focus group discussion to explore the barriers and facilitators associated with the potential transfer of IMAGE to new settings.

Many informants were aware of the IMAGE study prior to being interviewed, but all were provided with further information about the intervention and research in the form of an information sheet, and the IMAGE study paper from *The Lancet* (Pronyk et al., 2006). All gave written informed consent for their involvement. We provide below brief descriptive details of the informants who took part and the networks they represented.

HIV/AIDS researchers ($N=12$) included researchers from Europe, the United States and South Africa who have been influential in studies of social approaches to HIV prevention.

Microfinance practitioners ($N=11$, plus 10 focus group discussion participants): Those in the microfinance community with the greatest policy influence were consultants and employees of large, international microfinance initiatives (MFIs).

Donors and policy experts ($N=8$) included decision-makers from donor institutions as well as policy experts from health and development organizations.

12.3 Findings

Managing an intersectoral partnership

At the beginning of the trial, RADAR initiated the partnership with SEF and led the design of the training and community mobilization components of the intervention. During the trial, RADAR was responsible for implementing the training curriculum with new SEF clients, as well as managing the recruitment, training and performance of SFL staff. RADAR was also responsible for raising most of the programme's external funding. SEF contributed a well-respected model for delivering microfinance to the poor and was known within the microfinance community for having achieved demonstrable poverty alleviation among clients. Despite a previous reluctance to allow outside agencies to work with their clients, SEF joined the IMAGE partnership. As SEF's microfinance programme was reaching operational financial sustainability, it was a timely opportunity to initiate new activities. In addition, RADAR's enthusiasm for fund-raising, managing the intervention and maintaining SEF's operational model were key in getting the project off the ground (Panel 1).

However, the partnership also highlighted institutional differences between the implementing partners. These created both challenges and opportunities that demanded sensitivity to different organizational cultures. In some cases, the differences created tensions among field staff requiring action by managers. For example, two different types of staff (RADAR's health staff and SEF's microfinance providers) worked together with the same clients, so it became important to standardize working conditions and performance management expectations where possible.

As efforts began to move the intervention to scale after completion of the trial in 2004, the partners wished to explore the possibility of more fully integrating the management of the training and community mobilization within core microfinance activities. This was regarded as a potentially more sustainable strategy for delivering the model to large numbers of SEF clients. However, this was approached with some caution as managing a health programme lay outside SEF's core mission. Furthermore, the need to be seen as financially sustainable (with interest from loan repayments covering all operating costs) remained critical for SEF. Taking on additional programmatic inputs potentially conflicted with this mandate as health trainings would carry costs that might not provide financial benefits.

Panel 1: Project initiation and management, 2001–2004

Several institutions have approached [SEF] in the past, to use our institutional framework, our centre meetings, our people, the poverty level of them, to use the systems we had created, and we had always said no. Always. And this once we said yes. I think the fact is [RADAR] sold it as empowerment, as giving people knowledge and information, and that might spill out over into a better loan repayment.

SEF Manager

The cost was a big issue. That was the main issue. And we realised that it would not add any cost to our program that all the people that will be involved [SEF and SFL staff] would be fully paid from [RADAR].

SEF Manager

We did not want to disrupt SEF's core activities – microfinance is a tough business so we didn't want to disturb what they were doing and we just wanted to make sure that our relationship with them was smooth.

RADAR Researcher

These factors resulted in SEF being unwilling to house donor funds for the programme or become the legal employer for the health training team. As such, the IMAGE scale-up remained funded primarily through grants to RADAR rather than SEF. A complex, partially integrated management structure emerged which created operational challenges during the scaling-up process. These challenges included the following:

- *Programme management:* In the interests of cost efficiency, there was less investment in senior management staff for the training programme during scale-up. This occasionally led to compromises in the quality of the intervention, low field staff morale, and stretched monitoring and evaluation systems. This was compounded by a lack of depth in management capacity, with staff absence and illness resulting in further strain.

- *Ownership by the microfinance partner:* Not housing financial and administrative resources directly within the implementing body created complex lines of accountability and some lack of clarity around roles and responsibilties. This made it challenging to solve problems in a timely fashion.

Delivery models for moving to scale: IMAGE in rural South Africa

During the IMAGE trial (2001–2004), the combined intervention was delivered to 430 clients. Following the trial's completion, there was support for expanding programme activities. A scaled-up delivery of the intervention (2005–2007) reached over 3000 households in more than 100 villages.

Panel 2: Changes in views of the optimal delivery model for IMAGE, 2005–2007

2005

Now we're over the course of the scale-up, looking much more towards how to successfully mainstream and integrate (SFL into SEF).

RADAR researcher

2006

For me one of the things is that we have got to see if we can get the productivity of the training up, if we are going to have the integration thing then we have got to have the organizational cultures be close, and I worry that they are not.

SEF Manager

2007

So we have made the decision that ideally Sisters for Life should go into a separate NGO ... We would like to carry on in very much the same way we were doing in the trial where RADAR was a separate body who asked to bring in trainers and then coordination happened at the field-worker level.

SEF Manager

Over the course of 2001–2004, the intervention reached the target audience as planned. Programme attendance levels were high, and the finanical performance of the microfinance programme remained excellent. Loan repayment rates were measured as 99.7% and drop-outs were nearly half the institutional average during the early stages (Hargreaves et al., 2010).

By mid-2007, some 3000 clients had received the SFL training as the scale-up drew to a close. Clients still valued the high-quality training they had received, while both SEF and RADAR managers remained enthusiastic about partnering microfinance and health training for clients. These successes supported a continuation of the intervention beyond 2007.

However, the scale-up was not without problems. By 2007, both organizations felt that a new model for the partnership was necessary (Panel 2). As of 2008, the approach being developed had the gender and HIV training being delivered alongside SEF's microfinance operations but by a team based within a separate nongovernmental organization (NGO) that was itself responsible for acquiring external funding, and setting productivity and quality targets. This new institutional structure had set a new target of reaching 15 000 households by 2011 over a 4000 km² area.

Potential sustainable replication of IMAGE in other settings

By 2007, there was wide support for the idea of combining economic and health interventions among opinion leaders from the fields of microfinance, HIV/AIDS and gender beyond the IMAGE study teams. Microfinance practitioners felt that the IMAGE model aligned with their broader goals of women's empowerment:

It's opening up women's eyes to a lot of things, their own power is the main aspect, but the link between their kind of personal power and economic power is so intimate that I can see [IMAGE] working in a lot of other contexts.

Microfinance practitioner

HIV researchers felt the IMAGE study contributed usefully to the debate around addressing gender inequalities and poverty as underpinnings of the HIV epidemic by using rigorous research methods. There was also an increase in awareness of microfinance when the

Nobel Peace Prize was awarded in 2006 to Muhammed Yunus, the founder of the Grameen Bank, Bangladesh. Forging interdisciplinary partnerships also supported the aims of policy experts within international NGOs, which perceived IMAGE as having successfully operationalized a rights-based approach to HIV prevention, linking gender equity and livelihood entitlements to health promotion.

The IMAGE approach resonated with development NGOs that had been moving away from direct service provision toward providing communities with the skills to analyse their own situations and advocate for improvements through citizen action:

It kind of takes you back to the whole gender debate around practical and strategic gender needs. And in fact that is what poor people want, that is what women want. They do not live strategically one day, practically on another day, you know people live their life holistically. For me IMAGE is a good and quite solid approach in terms of supporting women to solve their problems.

Donor /Policy expert

However, opinion leaders from the various disciplines differed in how they envisioned further developments for the intersection of microfinance with health promotion for preventing IPV and HIV. Those with experience in delivering and evaluating HIV/AIDS programmes emphasized the need for greater research on outcomes:

You could present [IMAGE] as trying out a new approach or present it as refinements on an already proven approach, depending on what [donors] are looking for … this is my researcher bias in thinking there's always more important questions to investigate.

HIV researcher

HIV researchers argued that while there may be data supporting IMAGE as an intervention for the prevention of IPV – a worthwhile aim in its own right – the lack of impact on HIV documented in the trial meant that more evidence would be required on its potential contribution to HIV prevention before advocating the approach.

The results of the IMAGE trial were of much less importance to respondents from the microfinance sector. This group felt that the IMAGE study confirmed a pre-existing body of evidence that microfinance could alleviate poverty, empower women and have a role in reducing

IPV. Some felt that despite the results of the trial, impacts on HIV might also be expected in the future. They viewed the evidence base as sufficient to convince practitioners of the worth of the approach to women's lives, but needed more details on feasible operational models before they would consider committing their own organizations to implementing an IMAGE-style project.

I don't think the impact is disputed but it's operationalizing it that is the real issue, part of the research isn't just the impact – you won't have any problem in convincing microfinance people about impact. And you don't have to have a heavy duty empirical study to do that for microfinance people. But when you are coming to operational things, IMAGE does not have the model to show people how this works.

Microfinance practitioner

This group emphasized the existence of increased pressure on MFIs to be financially sustainable, ensure client repayment, and expand with minimal donor support, which would make it difficult for IMAGE to be delivered through a traditional MFI. This echoed SEF managers' concerns when seeking a feasible model for delivery of IMAGE.

In a microfinance institution aiming for sustainability, we account for every cent we spend... I think there are sufficient funders interested in the issue internationally to fund this. I really think [IMAGE] should always be externally funded.

SEF Manager

To the microfinance audience, SEF was seen as a particularly strong organization. Some felt this was beneficial since SEF could be expected to provide leadership in the area; others emphasized that even though SEF was able to implement such a project, others may not be able to. For example, the South African microfinance sector was seen as weak and it was felt that few MFIs would be able to support additional projects beyond their primary goal of disbursing loans.

Because if you talk about linking with microfinance institutions in South Africa, it's impossible, because the sector is so weak. They're struggling so much that they almost can't even think of doing it [an IMAGE-like programme]. And you wouldn't hear them speaking in kind of a mission-driven way either.

Microfinance practitioner

There was a consensus among microfinance practitioners that while the IMAGE model seemed promising, it should be the HIV community, not microfinance practitioners, who should take the model further.

Putting those kinds of interventions – education interventions together with microfinance – I think that can be a powerful sell. But my sense is that the audience that's going to be most receptive are people trying to say there are better solutions to problems like HIV infection rates, rather than people from the microfinance side.

Microfinance practitioner

Stakeholders from all informant groups noted that sectoral differences in funding and research agendas would make integration of the microfinance and gender training components of IMAGE difficult within any single given institution.

I guess in terms of the general policy environment, the first thing I would see as a challenge is the fact that these two worlds don't talk to each other at the policy level...You've got people with different backgrounds, different technical skills, a different view on the world.

Microfinance practitioner

Many opinion leaders therefore suggested that institutional partnership would be the most effective way to transfer the IMAGE model, a position that mirrored the experience of IMAGE partners through the scale-up.

12.4 Discussion

We have presented a chronology of IMAGE over a six-year period and documented the views of influential external stakeholders on the potential for IMAGE to be replicated in other settings in the future. Our experiences and interviews have generated lessons which may inform other cross-sectoral initiatives engaging the social determinants of health.

Intersectoral collaboration

IMAGE highlights the promise of partnerships between specialist organizations where there are mutual interests and common benefits. At the level of programme management, shared vision and ownership of IMAGE was critical. Meeting clients' basic needs provided an important incentive for participation and a strategic entry point for engaging wider health priorities. Our experience also suggests that the high quality of each component of the intervention was an important pre-requisite for integration, and that the presentation of a compulsory unified package to clients facilitated its acceptance.

Our evaluation also highlighted differences between the sectors involved in the intervention. Different sectors may have different value bases, success criteria and management cultures. Multisectoral interventions may fall outside the conventional priority-setting process in public health, which often demands well-packaged and sector-specific interventions with standardized protocols designed to produce measurable results. Interventions that work between sectors challenge the way government departments, academic institutions, international organizations and donor agencies are structured. In addition, the time required to see programme effects may be longer than usually provided. Such challenges were encountered early with regard to planning and resource mobilization for the study. Strong management, respect for each partner's strengths and a willingness to learn were essential in delivering IMAGE.

IMAGE highlights the potential for synergy in cross-sectoral interventions – where an integrated model may produce greater benefits than either component on its own. The addition of health training may have strengthened solidarity and group dynamics in participating loan centres, something that microfinance alone is less likely to do (Kim et al., 2009). Similarly, the microfinance platform facilitated the health training by contributing to high attendance rates, providing a forum for discussion, and attracting a client base that was rural and extremely poor. Traditionally, poor rural clients in South Africa are underserved by health interventions, and long-term health interventions with marginalized populations face challenges around consistent attendance.

Microfinance may not be the only entry point for linking economic, health and development gains. For example, research on South Africa's old-age pension system demonstrates that children in the home of grantees grow taller than their otherwise similar peers (Anderson et al., 2001). "Incentive-based welfare" in Mexico where poor households are given cash grants provided children attend school, go to clinics, and participate in health and nutrition education interventions has led to increased health service utilization, food expenditure and reductions in stunting (IFPRI, 2002). In Nicaragua and Honduras, programmes linking economic incentives to health interventions have led to increases in childhood vaccination coverage (Maluccio et al., 2000), levels of antenatal care and well-child check-ups (Morris et al., 2004). Despite these encouraging results and early success stories, the conceptualization of such models remains at an early stage. There is great potential for cross-sectoral programmes to engage the key social determinants of health, but the success of these approaches will require further innovation and ongoing operational research.

Taking integrated health programmes to scale

Core elements of IMAGE were implemented with strong fidelity to the original intervention. Despite the growing interest in structural programmes, few health interventions have been shown to be consistently implemented after a trial (Miller and Shinn, 2005). A process evaluation that demonstrates strong intervention fidelity is therefore an important finding.

However, adaptations to the delivery model were necessary to take IMAGE to scale and there were challenges as the scale-up progressed. The need for adaptations such as these align with a growing field of work around intervention transfer, which suggests that flexibility and ongoing quality improvement are needed when taking projects to scale after a trial (Baumann, 2004; Gandelman and Rietmeijer, 2004; Rapkin and Trickett, 2005).

For example, over time, the delivery of IMAGE shifted from a "linked" model (with integration at the point of delivery with clients) towards a partial "parallel" model during scale-up (where attempts were made to harmonize at a senior management level) and then an eventual return to the former option (Hargreaves et al., 2010; Dunford, 2002). Challenges were encountered in bridging institutional cultures, limiting the willingness of partners to house both components of the intervention within one organization.

The existing literature suggests that scaled-up interventions generally require greater management capacity to cope with delivery over wider areas, and more complex sets of inter-manager and manager–staff relationships (Binswanger, 2000). Lessons learned from the IMAGE partnership are of potential relevance to the scale-up of other cross-sectoral interventions. These include: the need to define roles and responsibilities of the various actors, including finance and staff management; the importance of each partner playing to their skills;

Panel 3: Facilitators, barriers and conditions for replicating cross-sectoral programmes like IMAGE

Facilitators	**Microfinance as growth industry:** more donors are showing an interest in the approach, burgeoned by the 2006 Nobel Peace Prize endorsement.
	Rights-based approaches: community mobilization phase fits well with the current emphasis on activism and building grass-roots advocacy.
	Cross-disciplinary focus: donor and policy-setting institutions promote efforts that take a multipronged approach to complex issues.
Barriers	**Vertical systems:** HIV and microfinance exist within different sectors that do not interact at policy, funding or operational levels.
	Unclear mechanism of action: results of the evaluation leave uncertainty regarding which components of the programme were most effective and why.
	Unproven impact on HIV: it is difficult to channel HIV funding and human resources into an intervention for which limited evidence of impact is available.
Conditions for change	**Additional information:** guidance is required on operationalizing the model, including the relative effect of different components.
	Resolution of internal debates: the microfinance field needs to maintain support for social development as the central mandate.
	Advocacy for IMAGE: outcome evaluation and academic language are not adequate to assist all constituencies in making informed choices.

sensitizing staff to the perspectives of new partners; harmonizing working conditions for staff between sectors; developing and implementing monitoring and evaluation systems; ensuring excess capacity exists to fill management gaps in the event of illness or absence; and that well-functioning microfinance is a pre-requisite for the introduction of additional training components.

Finally, challenges and opportunities within IMAGE relating to "scope" were also important. Many health sector interventions are passive, with clients accessing services at the point of care within well-defined geographical catchment areas. However, economic interventions such as microfinance expand rapidly to cover wider geographical areas. Our health programmes faced challenges in developing systems adaptable enough to quickly respond to shifting needs while maintaining the broader integrity of the interventions. In the case of IMAGE, the microfinance partner began to appreciate the added benefits of high-quality, gender-focused training for its clients. The health partner similarly gained a better understanding of the management, field systems and monitoring that is required in addressing the needs of large numbers of clients. This balance between scope and quality has proven critical to maximizing and extending the reach of other cross-sectoral programmes (Rotherham-Borus et al., 2000).

Sustainability of interventions

Finally, concerns regarding the sustainabilty of cross-sectoral interventions such as IMAGE are often raised. Panel 3 synthesizes the facilitators and barriers, and recommends ways forward for transfer and uptake of IMAGE which were identified by most or all of the stakeholder groups we interviewed. Many of the challenges and opportunities identified in Panel 3 are relevant to other cross-sectoral interventions as well.

Although the policy networks that could be involved in replicating IMAGE have distinct interests, priorities and key stakeholders, several themes emerged that demonstrated broad agreement on enabling IMAGE uptake and transfer. The multidisciplinary focus of the IMAGE model aligns with the current discourse within HIV and development circles which views health, gender and poverty as being inextricably linked. Opinion leaders across policy networks felt that IMAGE was taking place within an enabling policy context where donors and institutions were supportive of notions such as microfinance, institutional partnerships and rights-based approaches to development. Certainly, the increased interest over the past decade in structural approaches to HIV/AIDS (Latkin et al., 2005; Parker et al., 2000) may have created a supportive policy environment for transferring IMAGE to new settings.

However, respondents also cautioned that individual policy networks tend to approach programmes from "different worlds", drawing from distinct vocabulary, ideology and modes of communicating new ideas. Indeed, the concept of sustainability is different in the two sectors involved. Within the microfinance sector, there is a drive for organizations to achieve financial sustainability and reduce reliance on donor funds. In such a context, innovations such as health-related add-ons may be difficult to introduce. Opinion leaders reaffirmed this and suggested that funding for non-financial innovations will probably have to come from elsewhere. Conversely, in the public health sector, virtually all interventions require some form of subsidy or external support. Standardized interventions are developed and cost-effectiveness analyses allow decision-makers to weigh their value for money amid a spectrum of competing interventions.

While these differences might provide strength by offering a multidisciplinary response, they may also pose obstacles in the form of rigid policy, funding and organizational structures that are resistant to abandoning the specific aims of their respective constituencies. In a sense, the very strength of the IMAGE partnership, with its structural approach to poverty and health, fuels debates about its applicability to the specific aims of both microfinance and HIV prevention. Additional information – either specific to the logistics of planning, establishing and implementing an IMAGE-style programme, or more definitive data on its effects on HIV vulnerability – might alleviate some of the expressed qualms.

Finally, the broader policy and funding environment may need to shift from its current approach of championing single issues towards a more multidisciplinary approach. There are distinct examples of donors making strides towards the successful partnering of interrelated issues such as poverty and HIV but, on the whole, the development world continues to be characterized by policy "silos". Even as experts call for institutional partnerships, few organizations actually have the capacity or impetus to, for example, encourage dialogue between their distinct HIV/AIDS and poverty departments. In a funding environment where donors and organizations are rewarded for concrete deliverables on specific issues, it would be a rare institution that would be in a position to fully take on the IMAGE model in its current form, or to create space for cross-sectoral partnerships to develop. Cross-sectoral partnerships between institutions are essential for sustainably taking interventions like IMAGE to scale in new settings and populations. Creative institutional partnerships have the potential to take advantage of economies of scale, harness institutional synergies and deliver programmes that address a variety of community challenges. Implementing such approaches will undoubtedly require the insights, skills and expertise of a new generation of coalitions mobilized around addressing the social determinants of health.

Acknowledgements

This study builds on a huge amount of work in designing and implementing an ambitious intervention programme in rural South Africa. We thank the managing director of SEF, John de Wit, and the many staff who made this work possible. From the health training side, we thank Lulu Ndlovu and the staff who implemented the SFL programme. Thanks also to Mzamani Makhubele, who collected qualitative data during the IMAGE trial and Rico Euripidou, who extracted and ran preliminary analyses on much of the quantitative process data. We also thank John Gear for his support and guidance throughout the study.

IMAGE has over the period under study here received

financial support from the AngloAmerican Chairman's Fund Educational Trust, AngloPlatinum, Department for International Development (UK), the Ford Foundation, the Henry J. Kaiser Family Foundation, HIVOS, South African Department of Health and Welfare, and the Swedish International Development Agency. Since 2005, JH has been supported by an ESRC/MRC interdisciplinary fellowship.

Finally, we wish to thank all the people who generously gave significant amounts of time to take part in interviews and focus group discussions.

References

1. Anderson CL, Locker l, Nugent R (2002). Microcredit, social capital, and common pool resources. *World Development*, 30;95–105.

2. Anderson KG, Case A, Lam D (2001). Causes and consequences of schooling outcomes in South Africa: evidence from survey data. *Social Dynamics – a Journal of the Centre for African Studies University of Cape Town*, 27:37–59.

3. Andersson N et al. (2004). National cross sectional study of views on sexual violence and risk of HIV infection and AIDS among South African school pupils. *British Medical Journal*, 329:952.

4. Babalola S et al. (2001). The impact of a community mobilization project on health-related knowledge and practice in Cameroon. *Journal of Community Health*, 26:459–477.

5. Baumann E (2004). Imp-Act cost-effectiveness study of Small Enterprise Foundation, South Africa. *Small Enterprise Development*, 15:28–40.

6. Binswanger HP (2000). Scaling up HIV/AIDS programs to national coverage. *Science*, 288:2173–2176.

7. Blankenship KM et al. (2006) Structural interventions: concepts, challenges and opportunities for research. *Journal of Urban Health*, 83:59–72.

8. Cornwall A and Jewkes R (1995). What is participatory research? *Social Science and Medicine*, 41:1667–1676.

9. Dunford C (2002). Building better lives: sustainable integration of microfinance with education in child survival, reproductive health, and HIV/AIDS prevention for the poorest entrepreneurs. In: Daley-Harris S (ed.) *Pathways out of poverty: innovations in microfinance for the poorest families*. Bloomfield, Kumarian Press.

10. Dunkle KL et al. (2006) Perpetration of partner violence and HIV risk behaviour among young men in the rural Eastern Cape, South Africa. *AIDS*, 20:2107–2114.

11. Fenton L (2004). Preventing HIV/AIDS through poverty reduction: the only sustainable solution? *The Lancet*, 364:1186–1187.

12. Freire P (1968). *Pedagogy of the oppressed*. London, Continuum International Publishing Group.

13. Gandelman A and Rietmeijer CA (2004). Translation, adaptation, and synthesis of interventions for persons living with HIV – lessons from previous HIV prevention interventions. *Journal of Acquired Immune Deficiency Syndromes*, 37:S126–S129.

14. Garcia-Moreno C and Watts C (2000). Violence against women: its importance for HIV/AIDS. *AIDS*, 14 (Suppl 3):S253–S265.

15. Glasgow RE, Lichtenstein E, Marcus AC (2003). Why don't we see more translation of health promotion research to practice? Rethinking the efficacy-to- effectiveness transition. *American Journal of Public Health*, 93:1261–1267.

16. Hargreaves JR et al. (2010). Process evaluation of the Intervention with Microfinance for AIDS and Gender Equity (IMAGE) in rural South Africa. *Health Education Research*, 25:27–40.

17. Hargreaves JR et al (2007). "Hearing the voices of the poor": assigning poverty lines on the basis of local perceptions of poverty; a quantitative analysis of qualitative data from participatory wealth ranking in rural South Africa. *World Development*, 35:212–229.

18. IFPRI (2002). *PROGRESA: breaking the cycle of poverty*. Washington, D.C., International Food Policy Research Institute.

19. Kim JC et al. (2009). Assessing the incremental effects of combining economic and health interventions: the IMAGE study in South Africa. *Bulletin of the World Health Organization*, 87:824–832.

20. Kim JC et al. (2007). Understanding the impact of a microfinance-based intervention on women's empowerment and the reduction of intimate partner violence in the IMAGE Study, South Africa. *American Journal of Public Health*, 97:1794–1802.

21. Latkin CA et al. (2005). Neighborhood social disorder as a determinant of drug injection behaviors: a structural equation modeling approach. *Health Psychology*, 24:96–100.

22. Maluccio J, Haddad L, May J (2000). Social capital and household welfare in South Africa, 1993–98. *Journal of Development Studies*, 36:54.

23. Manandhar DS et al. (2004). Effect of a participatory intervention with women's groups on birth outcomes in Nepal: cluster-randomised controlled trial. *The Lancet*, 364:970–979.

24. Mane P, Gupta GR, Weiss E (1994). Effective communication between partners: AIDS and risk reduction for women. *AIDS*, 8 (suppl 1):s325–s331.

25. Miller RL and Shinn M (2005). Learning from communities: overcoming difficulties in dissemination of prevention and promotion efforts. *American Journal of Community Psychology*, 35(3–4):169–183.

26. Morris SS et al. (2004). Monetary incentives in primary health care and effects on use and coverage of preventive health care interventions in rural Honduras: cluster randomised trial. *The Lancet*, 364:2030–2037.

27. Oakley A et al. (2006). Process evaluation in randomised controlled trials of complex interventions. *British Medical Journal*, 332:413–416.

28. Parker RG (1996). Empowerment, community mobilization and social change in the face of HIV/AIDS. *AIDS*, 10 (suppl 3):S27–S31.

29. Parker RG, Easton D, Klein CH (2000). Structural barriers and facilitators in HIV prevention: a review of international research. *AIDS*, 14 (suppl 1):S22–S32.

30. Phetla G et al. (2008). "They have opened our mouths": increasing women's skills and motivation for sexual communication with young people in rural South Africa. *AIDS Education and Prevention*, 20:504–518.

31. Pretty JN et al. (1995). *Participatory learning and action: a trainer's guide.* London, IIED.

32. Pronyk PM et al. (2006). Effect of a structural intervention for the prevention of intimate-partner violence and HIV in rural South Africa: a cluster randomised trial. *The Lancet*, 368:1973–1983.

33. Pronyk PM et al. (2008). A combined microfinance and training intervention can reduce HIV risk behaviour among young program participants: results from the IMAGE Study. *AIDS*, 22:1659–1665.

34. Gupta GR (2002). How men's power over women fuels the HIV epidemic. *British Medical Journal*, 324:183–184.

35. Rapkin B and Trickett E (2005). Comprehensive dynamic trial designs for behavioral prevention research with communities: overcoming inadequacies of the randomized controlled trial paradigm. In: Trickett E and Pequegnat W (eds) *Community interventions and AIDS*. New York, Oxford University Press.

36. Rhodes T and Simic M (2005). Transition and the HIV risk environment. *British Medical Journal*, 331:220–223.

37. Rotheram-Borus MJ et al. (2000). Bridging research and practice: community–researcher partnerships for replicating effective interventions. *AIDS Education and Prevention*, 12:49–61.

38. Szreter S and Woolcock M (2004). Health by association? Social capital, social theory, and the political economy of public health. *International Journal of Epidemiology*, 33:650–667.

39. UNAIDS (2002). *Report on the global HIV/AIDS epidemic.* Geneva, UNAIDS.

40. UNAIDS (2006). *Report on the global HIV/AIDS epidemic.* Geneva, UNAIDS.

41. WHO (2005). *WHO multi-country study on women's health and domestic violence against women.* Geneva, World Health Organization.

42. Wong FY et al. (2008). Gender differences in intimate partner violence on substance abuse, sexual risks, and depression among a sample of South Africans in Cape Town, South Africa. *AIDS Education and Prevention*, 20:56–64.

Insecticide-treated nets in Tanzania mainland

Challenges in reaching the most vulnerable, most exposed and poorest groups

13

Jaap Koot,[1,*] Romanus Mtung'e,[2] Jane Miller[3]

[1] Jaap Koot, MD MBA, National Institute of Health Promotion, Woerden, the Netherlands

[2] Romanus Mtung'e, BSc, Population Services International, Dar es Salaam, Tanzania

[3] Jane Miller, MSc PhD, Population Services International, Dar es Salaam, Tanzania

* Corresponding author: jkoot@nigz.nl

Abstract

This case study analyses the National Programme for Insecticide-Treated Nets (ITNs) in Tanzania during the period 1995–2008, focusing on implementation issues in relation to the social determinants of health. It assesses how the poorest, most exposed and most vulnerable groups in society have benefited from the programme. Programme publications, external monitoring and evaluation reports, progress reports, as well as internal working documents of projects were analysed and, where necessary, available data were analysed. Between 1995 and 2007, Tanzania's ITN programme concentrated on social marketing; a component of vouchers (offering nets for less than US$ 1.00) for pregnant mothers was added in 2004 and for infants in 2006. Through collaboration with the commercial sector and nongovernmental organizations (NGOs), the Ministry of Health and Social Welfare created an effective and efficient system of producing and distributing mosquito nets and insecticide re-treatment kits to reach the whole country. Tanzania achieved steady growth in net ownership through this programme, and covered 65% of households with any net in 2008. However, the lowest socioeconomic groups and the rural population lagged behind in uptake and utilization of ITNs. Furthermore, the gap between net ownership and sleeping under the nets remained high. The ITN programme stepped up information campaigns and introduced rural promotion campaigns to spread malaria messages. In 2008, Tanzania changed to a "catch-up and keep-up" strategy, combining free distribution of ITNs with voucher schemes and social marketing. The combination of strategies should lead to better coverage of ITNs for the rural poor and attainment of the Abuja targets. The new approach costs 20 times more than social marketing, equal to 15% of the government's health budget; massive donor support for malaria control made this possible. The ITN programme in Tanzania was successful in expansion, but did not focus enough on the poor and rural population. Free net distribution and rural promotion campaigns can correct this, but are dependent on unprecedentedly high donor inputs.

13.1 Background

Malaria is one of the priority diseases in developing countries. It is the most serious public health problem in Tanzania, with more than 16 million cases and at least 100 000 child deaths per year (Magesa et al., 2005) caused by the malaria parasite *Plasmodium falciparum*, which is transmitted by the *Anopheles* mosquito. In most regions of Tanzania, malaria is an endemic disease (*see* Figure 1). Malaria is characterized as a disease of poverty by Gollin and Zimmerman (2007) and Barat et al. (2004). The underlying determinants of vector spread (e.g. poor housing conditions, stagnant water, bad sewerage) are predominant in poorer households (Geissbühler et al., 2007; Worrall et al., 2005; Wagstaff et al.; 2004).

Tanzania is a low-income country and poverty is highest in rural areas. Poverty in rural areas is rooted in inequitable access to productive assets, including land, financial services and livestock. Rural households have less access to safe drinking water, primary education and health services compared with urban households. According to Leonard and Masatu (2007), the quality of health services in rural areas is below par compared with urban areas. Khan et al. (2003) found pockets of poverty and ill-health in remote areas of Tanzania. Households living in high poverty concentration areas were found to have poor health outcomes and low service utilization rates.

In endemic areas, adults tend to suffer from regular attacks of malaria. In epidemic areas, where transmission is unstable, there is low immunity and all people are vulnerable to malaria (Carter and Mendis, 2002). Pregnant women and small children are more vulnerable to malaria and suffer from the more serious effects of the disease. People living with HIV or suffering from full-blown AIDS are also more vulnerable to malaria (WHO, 2004).

At the macro level, malaria has a negative impact on economic activities. Gallup and Sachs (2001) found that countries with "intensive" malaria experience a reduction in per capita income growth of 1.3% annually. Malaria costs Tanzania 3.4% of its GDP, which is more than US$ 11.00 per person. At the micro level, malaria may cause serious economic adversity due to loss of productivity and high expenditure on treatment (McIntyre and Gilson, 2005). Mortality among children below 5 years of age in rural areas of Tanzania is much higher than in urban areas: 138 vs 108 (National Bureau of Statistics, 2005). In rural Tanzania, mortality rates among children below 5 years of age following acute fever was 39% higher among the poorest compared with the least poor (Mwageni E, unpublished data, cited in Barat et al., 2004).

According to Worrall et al. (2005), the poorest suffer most from malaria because of limited access to prevention and treatment. This is called the malaria trap: poor people suffer more from malaria, and are less capable of affording treatment and prevention, further increasing the malaria burden.

Human contact with the *Anopheles* mosquito carrying the malaria parasite is the critical condition for infection. Vector control is therefore one of the ways to reduce the burden of this disease.

In the Abuja Declaration of 2000, African heads of state committed themselves to halving malaria mortality in Africa by 2010 through better prevention and adequate treatment of the disease (WHO, 2000). Tanzania has embarked on a malaria programme with a focus on prevention (insecticide-treated nets [ITNs] and indoor residual spraying), better diagnosis (clinical and laboratory) and improved treatment (artemisinin combination therapy). Expenditure on health in Tanzania is low and largely dependent on international donor support. Therefore, acquiring consistent and reliable funding for malaria interventions constitutes a problem.

Figure 1. Malaria map, Tanzania

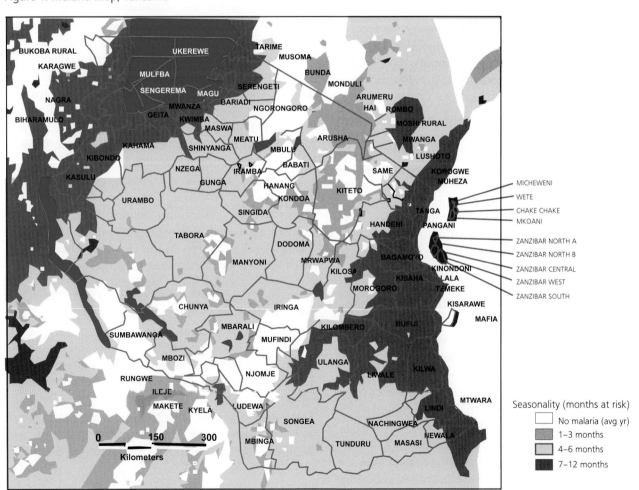

Mapping malaria risk in Africa

Tanzania: Climate model months of transmission

MOH NMCP TEHIP MARA Collaboration

May, 1999

Source: Mapping Malaria Risks in Africa (Mara) (Hay and Snow, 2006)

13.2 Methods

This chapter studies measures to prevent malaria through ITNs in Tanzania since 1995. The focus is on implementation issues in relation to the social determinants of health. What efforts were undertaken to reach the poorest, most exposed and most vulnerable groups in society? What lessons can we learn from the ITN programme in Tanzania? The study analyses the development and implementation of strategies for distribution of ITNs, based on the international and local literature, programme publications, external monitoring and evaluation reports, as well as internal working documents of projects.

The system for monitoring malaria programme activities in Tanzania is very elaborate and several research projects are implemented in the country, leading to a wealth of information. For this case study, some available data were re-analysed to answer specific questions. No new data were collected. Verification of findings took place through individual contacts with members of the National Insecticide Treated Nets programme (NATNETS) Steering Committee and through brainstorming meetings with stakeholders.

As a reference for the analysis of the ITN projects in Tanzania, the Conceptual Framework for Action on the Social Determinants of Health is used (CSDH, 2007). The five basic factors, introduced by the Commission on Social Determinants of Health (CSDH) are discussions on the socioeconomic and political **contexts**, the sociocultural and economic **position** of the people, **exposure** to diseases, **vulnerability** (or capacity to cope with diseases) and **consequences** of diseases for affected persons and their families. Interventions addressing these factors are clustered under availability, accessibility and acceptability of interventions, and assessed against context and position, exposure and vulnerability. Table 2 shows the three types of interventions and five types of factors in a matrix.

In response to the call by the WHO Priority Public Health Concerns Knowledge Network for Social Determinants of Health, this chapter describes lessons learned with regard to scaling up the programme, managing policy processes, managing intersectoral processes, adjusting design and ensuring sustainability.

13.3 Findings

Strategies

After the International ITN Conference in Dar es Salaam in 1999, the Tanzanian Ministry of Health and Social Welfare (MOHSW) formed a Task Force that formulated a national ITN policy and strategy. In 2001, a comprehensive Malaria Medium Term Strategic Plan 2002–2007 was formulated, which put ITN activities into the wider context of malaria control (MOHSW, 2002).

The NATNETS programme started in 2002 as a large integrated programme, comprising three main components: (1) a national coordination unit (ITN cell) within the national malaria control programme (NMCP); (2) strategic social marketing – SMARTNET; and (3) vouchers delivered to pregnant women and mothers of infants, the Tanzanian National Voucher Scheme (TNVS). This mechanism was designed to ensure good coordination and complementarity of all activities (MOHSW, 2002; Magesa et al., 2005; Kramer, 2005).

In 2007, a new Malaria Strategic Plan was formulated for the period 2008–2013 and a fourth component added: free distribution of ITNs to children between one and five years and possibly to other household members, if funds become available (MOHSW, 2007). This introduced in Tanzania the "catch up – keep up" policy, with mass distribution for attaining high coverage and routine distribution to ensure that vulnerable groups were sufficiently covered in between campaigns (Grabowsky et al., 2007). The reasons for this change will be discussed later in this chapter in the section on "Adjusting design".

Availability of ITNs in Tanzania

Between 1985 and 2000, a series of studies and small-scale interventions were implemented in Tanzania to study the impact of ITNs on health, and to test distribution systems, e.g. the Kilombero Net Project (KINET) (Erlanger et al., 2004). Between 1998 and 2007, Tanzania used social marketing as the main instrument for production and distribution of untreated nets, insecticide re-treatment kits (IRKs), ITNs and later long-lasting insecticidal nets (LLIN) first in the SMITN project and later in the SMARTNET project (Figure 2).[1] Bilateral donors financed the projects (Koot et al., 2006).

---

[1] In the literature it is sometimes called the total market approach, as no specific brand of net was used. Companies continue to use their own brands, while the project provides incentives for production and distribution, and implements generic marketing.

Stimulating local production had a special place in the social marketing project. The malaria programme (through SMARTNET) actively approached companies to stimulate local production. Increased local capacity reduced production costs and thus retail costs. Tanzanian factories have realized a position in the world market of nets, making Tanzania a country that now exports nets. Most nets produced in Tanzania were not treated with insecticide until 2007. IRKs were distributed separately. Since 2002, new nets were bundled with IRKs. LLINs are now produced in Tanzania, and are the main source for in-country distribution. The technology for these nets was developed by Sumitomo Chemical in Japan. Technology transfer and production was initiated through collaboration in a consortium, with financial contributions and loans from several partners (Tami et al., 2004; Carpenter et al., 2006).

The Tanzanian malaria programme made a deliberate choice of using the commercial sector for distribution in order to reduce (hidden) transaction costs in the health sector and enhance sustainability. The project built up a network of wholesalers and retailers to distribute and sell the nets. It addressed distribution bottlenecks through incentive schemes to encourage suppliers, wholesalers and distributors to achieve greater rural reach. The project also invested in creating new sales points, such as shifting markets. In all wards in Tanzania (smallest administrative unit above village level), nets are for sale in shops, kiosks or other retail units (Mponda et al., 2008). Of all the nets owned by people, 71% were purchased from a shop or pharmacy, 18% from a health facility and 11% from elsewhere (PSI, 2007). Nets have an estimated longevity of two to three years (Whiting, 2005).

Accessibility of ITNs

Initially, Tanzania concentrated on social marketing of nets, but when subsidies from the Global Fund to Fight AIDS , TB and Malaria (Global Fund) became available, the TNVS was introduced by the end of 2004, and vouchers were issued to women during their first antenatal visit to a health clinic. The TNVS aims to bring the nets within reach of the poorest and most vulnerable groups in the country. With the voucher, women can purchase standard nets at a greatly reduced price (less than US$ 1.00, instead of US$ 5.00) from accredited retailers. If women are ready to pay more, they can obtain a bigger net. In 2008, the amount of subsidy was increased, reducing the client contribution to purchase of a standard LLIN to US$ 0.40.

The redemption rate of issued vouchers (percentage of women who buy a net with the voucher) was around 80% in 2007. Having no money was the main reason for non-redemption (which amounted to 7% of all the women who received a voucher or around one third of those women who received a voucher but never went to buy a net). Other reasons for non-utilization of vouchers were losing the voucher, stock-outs in the shop, or not understanding the need for the use of a net (waiting for the wet season) (Nathan et al., 2008).

By the end of 2006, an infant voucher was launched, financed by the President's Malaria Initiative (PMI). Mothers of children who receive their measles vaccination (at 9 months of age) receive an ITN voucher. The redemption rate in 2008 was slightly lower than that for pregnancy vouchers. Not having money was mentioned as the most important cause for non-redemption, next to already having a net (Jones and Sedekia, 2008).

Through the voucher system, more than three million nets were purchased between January 2005 and December 2007. As could be expected, voucher sales have reduced unsubsidized sales; but non-subsidized sales still add up to around 50% of the total sales.

In 2005, there was free distribution of nets in Tanzania mainland for children in the regions of Lindi (162 000 nets) and Mtwara (93 000 nets) (financed by UNICEF) in a campaign, combined with vaccination, and distribution of vitamin A and mebendazole. This free distribution was not in line with the formulated ITN policy, but the result of donors offering funds for such distribution (Heierli and Lengeler, 2008). Skarbinski et al. (2007) reported that nearly 86% of eligible children below 5 years of age attended the campaign in Lindi. Of those, nearly 80% received a net. The most frequent reason for not receiving a net was that the campaign post was out of stock. Mboera et al. (2008) found an ITN coverage rate of 42.8% in Lindi Urban district, much lower than expected on the basis of the free distribution, and concluded that the nets distributed were not re-treated.

In Tanzania, NGOs and relief organizations also issue nets to specific target groups, such as refugees, orphans and vulnerable children. From the evaluations of these initiatives, it appeared that distribution problems were prominent. The logistics proved to be more demanding than envisaged. Leakages of nets to commercial markets, thefts, etc. were reported (Reed and Stephen, 2005; Koot et al., 2006).

Figure 2. Distribution trends of nets in Tanzania, 2001– 2007

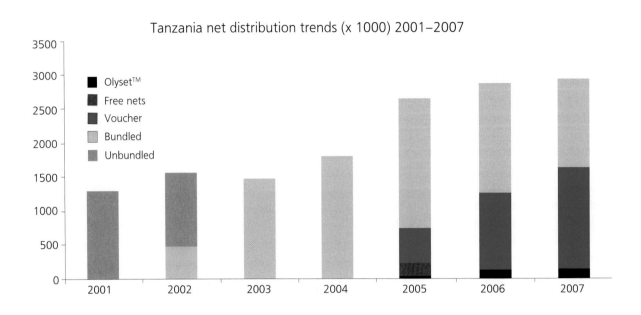

Source: Population Services International, Tanzania

Figure 3. Ownership of any net in rural, semi-urban and urban households, 2005–2007

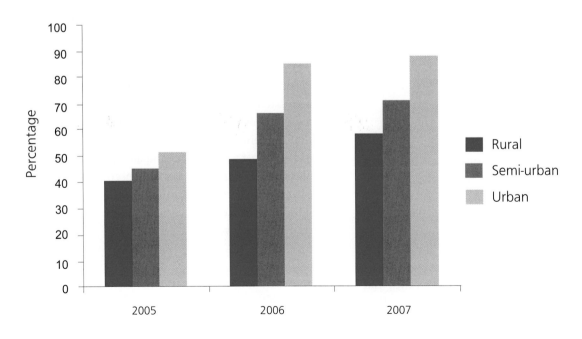

Source: Marchant TNVS survey, 2008

In 2008, Tanzania started a pilot for nationwide distribution of 5.2 million free nets to all children below the age of 5 years, with funding of US$ 53 million from the Global Fund, World Bank and PMI. The main "catch-up" campaign started in 2009. The Global Fund Round 8 has granted Tanzania US$ 113 million for 14.6 million additional nets for a universal coverage campaign, which could bring by 2010 the average number of nets to 2.5 nets per household. In the meantime, the voucher schemes continue to ensure that at all times pregnant women and infants have access to nets.

Between 2005 and 2007, the ownership of any net increased from 43.9% to 64.6% for all households in Tanzania, according to the TNVS household survey (Marchant et al., 2008) (Figure 3). The mean number of nets per household increased from 0.8 to 1.3. There were marked differences in ownership among rural and urban households. Nearly 20% of children below the age of 5 years in rural areas and 8% of children in urban areas tested positive for malaria in the Tanzania HIV–Malaria Integrated Survey, 2007–2008 (NBS, 2008).

The TNVS monitoring survey also looked at ownership per socioeconomic strata (SES) quintile (applying World Bank asset measurement). In 2007, 87.9% of the least poor households owned any net, while of the poorest households only 39.3% owned any net. The ratio of ownership among the poorest to the least poor was 0.45. (Marchant et al., 2008).

Acceptability of ITNs

Various surveys (Marchant et al., 2008; Mboera et al., 2008) have analysed factors that contribute to net ownership and net use. People in a higher SES are more likely to own and use nets than people in the lowest SES. In urban areas net ownership and use is much higher than in rural areas. In regions with a lesser mosquito nuisance, fewer people use nets. Seasonal variation is less pronounced in these areas.

There is a discrepancy between ownership of any net and sleeping under ITNs, as shown in Table 1. Apparently, many people (who still have the old nets) do not re-treat their nets with insecticide or do not sleep under an ITN even if they have one.

Understanding malaria transmission and the effects of ITNs is a precondition for increase in utilization of nets (Nganda et al., 2004). The ITN programme in Tanzania incorporates behaviour change communication (BCC) activities.

Demand creation was a crucial part of the social marketing approach. Before 2004, mainly the mass media (radio, TV, newspapers), posters and billboards were used for spreading messages related to malaria. When an evaluation in 2003 showed that the poor people in rural areas were not sufficiently reached by mass media messages, a rural promotion campaign started in 2004, mainly targeting malaria-endemic areas.

Through rural communication teams, all the high malaria-endemic districts were visited over a period of three years. The rural promotion teams travelled from ward to ward conducting meetings with local government and religious leaders to advocate for malaria prevention activities. The teams screened videos (infotainment) and performed road shows (dance, songs, music) in villages, trading centres and marketplaces. The programme distributed printed materials, e.g. child health card covers, branded soccer balls and jerseys, coffee mugs and branded T-shirts, all of them carrying malaria messages. The programme adapted the rural promotion methods of soft drink and mobile phone companies. By the end of 2006, the rural promotion campaign had covered all malaria-endemic areas in Tanzania. From January 2007 onwards, the rural promotion campaign targeted districts with a low TNVS voucher uptake to enhance voucher redemption and effective use of nets in those districts. The programme achieved higher leverage when political leaders, spearheaded by the President of the United

Table 1. Ownership of insecticide-treated net and use of nets in Tanzania

Any net in household	ITN in household	ITN used last night by all household members
64.6%	36.0%	20.5%

Source: Marchant et al., TNVS survey, 2008

Figure 4. Increase in ITN use among households, pregnant women and children below the age of 5 years between 2005 and 2007 by socioeconomic strata

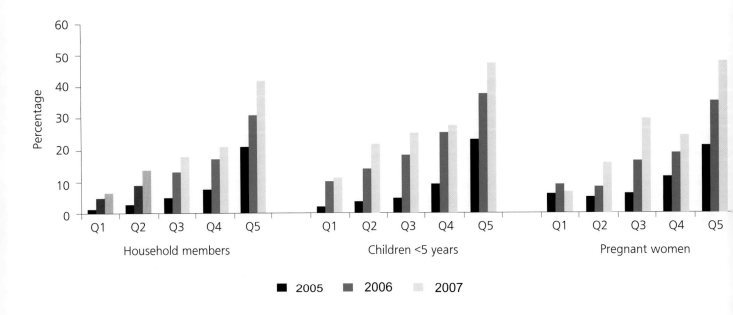

Source: Marchant et al., TNVS survey, 2008

Republic of Tanzania, joined the "Malaria… haikubaliki" (Malaria … is unacceptable) campaign, insisting that malaria is a disease to be cured and prevented. The slogan has become the national slogan for malaria campaigns.

In April 2007, the nationwide TRaC survey (monitoring tool designed by Population Services International [PSI]) reported a high level of message recall among community members as a result of the BCC activities carried out: 89% had heard of treated nets, 83% had seen or heard advertising for IRK, 26% had seen a mobile video unit (MVU) show and 35% had seen a road show. Exposure to messages is positively correlated with net ownership, net use and net treatment: 84% of those reported to own at least one net had seen an MVU show, so had 77% of caretakers of children below the age of 5 years who slept under a net the previous night, and 86% of those who had ever treated nets (PSI, 2007). Mboera et al. (2008) found that 95% of the population knew that mosquitoes are a source of malaria infection and, of these, 95% knew that nets were effective in preventing malaria.

A comparison of figures over the years shows a steady increase in the use of ITNs (Figure 4). However, the differences in usage between various SES remain significant.

13.4 Discussion

CSDH framework

Table 2 puts the findings in the analytical framework of the CSDH. Although reaching the poor was an important target from the onset of the ITN programme, in practice, it was very difficult. It is important to note the urban–rural divide, with a higher malaria burden and lower net ownership in rural areas. The poorest live in rural areas that are difficult to reach for ITN distribution activities and awareness-raising campaigns.

Sharing experiences

These are discussed under the topics of going to scale, managing policy change, managing intersectoral cooperation, adjusting design and ensuring sustainability.

Going to scale

Tanzania has one national ITN programme that combines different approaches to distribution (social marketing, voucher schemes and free distribution). Conceptualizing

Table 2. Lessons learned from the Tanzania ITN programme according to the CSDH framework

| | Level of social determinants/pathway | Availability of interventions | Accessibility of interventions | Acceptability of interventions |
	Root causes of malaria	ITNs available in the country	ITNs within reach of the poor	Make people use ITNs
Context and position	Poverty in Tanzania is widespread, but people in remote rural areas are the most disadvantaged.	The commercial sector was crucial in increasing the availability of ITNs, assisted by incentives for production and distribution.	Social marketing and TNVS are general programmes and not specifically for the poorest and most disadvantaged.	Initially, BCC was not aimed at the rural population and did not reach the poorest, who were later targeted through rural promotion teams.
Exposure	Mosquito nuisance and frequent suffering from malaria plays a role in increasing the awareness of people.	Sale of nets is dependent on the geographical area.	In the initial stages TNVS roll-out was more in the urban and rich population, and did not reach those most exposed.	There was political commitment to break through a fatalistic approach towards exposure to malaria.
Vulnerability	The poor, especially in rural areas, are more vulnerable.	Social marketing is not the most effective instrument for benefiting the most vulnerable.	Voucher scheme is a necessary complementary intervention to reach the most vulnerable groups. Free distribution will remove financial barriers.	BCC targeted at vulnerable groups would increase uptake by those groups.

the national programme was a process that took several years, starting with small research projects, expanding to districts and regions, and finally country level. Innovative approaches were used to firmly establish a competitive local industry of nets to establish a vibrant commercial distribution and retail network, and to put in place effective methods of promoting commercial rural sales. The combination of social marketing and voucher schemes resulted in nearly 65% of households owning a net by 2007.

In scaling up, pragmatic decisions prevailed: first, easy-to-reach urban areas were covered and later, remote rural areas. This increased urban–rural inequity and ignored the people most in need of malaria protection. Only at a later stage – through intensive monitoring – was this shortcoming detected and corrected.

Availability of external funding was a critical factor for scaling up and adding components. These components were gradually added when more funding became available. Over time, funding from the Global Fund and PMI replaced (and exceeded) funding from bilateral donors who stopped specific funding for malaria programmes and moved to basket funding and general budget support. Evidence from Zanzibar and other countries (and also from Lindi) shows that free mass distribution can achieve high ITN coverage in a short period of time. The poorest are more easily reached by mass distribution than by social marketing or voucher schemes. However, as in vaccination campaigns, it remains a challenge to reach the poor in very remote areas.

Managing the policy process

Developing the national ITN programme in Tanzania was a process that took years. Close consultation between policy-makers, research institutes, NGOs and donors was crucial for its success. All donors were willing to follow the national ITN policy, even if their head offices advocated other approaches, e.g. UNICEF.

The creation of an ITN cell and a NATNETS steering committee was essential for the management of the national programme. All stakeholders participated in this. NGOs working in the malaria programme were able to link to the commercial sector, which had problems in dealing directly with government organizations. Donor funding and technical assistance for the ITN cell within the NMCP made it possible to gain and maintain the momentum. This helped, for example, in mobilizing funds from the Global Fund and PMI.

The national ITN strategy and the Malaria Strategic Plans 2002–2007 and 2008–2013 guided the activities. Tanzania is now moving to the distribution of free nets, and the government works through permanent dialogues with stakeholders to keep them committed to one national programme. Partners in social marketing are also collaborating in free distribution campaigns.

Fighting malaria has become a global undertaking. The Roll Back Malaria Global Malaria Action Plan (RBM, 2008a), backed by the 2008 MDG Malaria Summit, will guide further ITN policies in Tanzania.

Adjusting design

Until 2007, Tanzania followed a strategy for ITN distribution which combined social marketing and voucher schemes. Increasingly, questions were raised as to whether the Abuja target could be achieved in this manner, and whether the poorest in society benefited sufficiently from this strategy. International pressure

was building up to incorporate free distribution into the ITN programme (Sachs, 2005; Teklehaimanot et al., 2007), fuelled by the availability of huge amounts of money through the Global Fund, PMI and World Bank. In 2007, a catch-up strategy was proposed, planning for mass distribution of 5.2 million LLINs to children below 5 years of age in Tanzania and, in 2008, the Universal Coverage Strategy, adding another 14.6 million nets for free distribution. The total budget for these distribution campaigns in 2009 and 2010 is US$ 170 million, which is equal to around 15% of the available health budget (MOHSW, 2009) and around 20 times as much as previously available for social marketing.

During the implementation of the ITN programme, it became clear that the discrepancy between net ownership and net use had to be addressed seriously to make an impact on malaria morbidity and mortality. The BCC component has evolved over the past five years. Initially, attention was given mainly to mass media campaigns, later rural outreach strategies were included, and finally distinct geographical areas were targeted where coverage of ITNs lagged behind. This fine-tuning was possible because of close monitoring of the programme, through the TNVS surveys, through PSI's TRaC surveys, and specific research activities. In the coming years, BCC will be stepped up as an important contribution to better use of ITNs.

Managing intersectoral processes

The ITN strategy document clearly indicated tasks that had to be implemented for policy development, coordination and implementation. The management mechanisms invited participation from various stakeholders, providing them guidance on the roles they had to play in the programme.

The development of the ITN programme coincided with the Tanzanian government reforms, making local government authorities responsible for service provision and planning for decentralized health services. This gave the ITN programme easy entry into the local government system, especially in the rural promotion campaign.

NGOs proved to be a suitable interface between the government and the commercial sector. SMARTNET could get confidential figures from factories, and could channel subsidies to distributors. In a direct government–private sector relation, this would have been more difficult.

In the new mass distribution campaign, one of the commercial partners that became strong during the social marketing period won the contract for production and distribution of nets, proving that capacities have been built over the years.

Sustainability

Social marketing has created a demand in Tanzania, resulting in unsubsidized annual sales of around 1.5 million nets in recent years. The mass distribution of 20 million free nets in the coming two years will reduce the commercial sales of nets by 70%, according to PSI's expectations. It may push retailers out of the market, and undermine commercial net sales. Free net distribution may also reduce the willingness of people to purchase ITNs. Whether the carefully built up infrastructure of wholesale, distribution and retail will survive in the coming years is an open question.

Promoting ITNs requires continuous sensitization, repeating the same messages over and over again. One may compare BCC for ITNs with BCC for healthy diets. The Lindi experience shows us that it cannot be a one-off campaign; it should be a continuing effort. An important lesson from the Tanzania programme is the need for specific rural promotion campaigns, which are more demanding and expensive. Probably, when the incidence of malaria in the population reduces as a result of vector control and appropriate treatment, the motivation to buy and use nets will lessen. People have to continue using nets until malaria eradication is a fact, and have to be reminded to do so time and again.

The world has adopted a high-risk approach towards malaria control. The required budget for the strategy of universal coverage of ITNs is far beyond the financial means of developing countries. During the 2008 MGD Malaria Summit, US$ 3 billion new money was committed (RBM, 2008b). The world has had bad experiences with previous commitments: during the Gleneagles meeting in 2005, G8 countries committed US$ 21.8 billion towards additional development aid, but by 2008 they had spent only 14% (DATA, 2008). With the ongoing economic crisis, western countries may have other priorities.

Not doing the job correctly has its risks: by reducing exposure and malaria transmission in developing countries, we are undermining people's natural development of immunity. The lesson from Madagascar (Carter and Mendis, 2002) and elsewhere (Rugemalila,

2006) is that failed malaria control programmes lead to higher mortality when malaria comes back, because (partial) immunity in the population has disappeared. This should not be allowed to happen again. Leaders of the western world, and especially those who claim that malaria eradication is feasible, now have the moral obligation to sustain the high level of funding.

13.5 Conclusion

Tanzania has achieved remarkable successes with its ITN programme by combining social marketing and voucher schemes. However, the focus on the poorest and on people in remote areas was not sufficient. The purchasing power of the poorest was overestimated and even the small amount of US$ 1.00 for a subsidized ITN was too high for them. Social mobilization was not appropriate for the rural population.

The new catch-up and keep-up strategy of mass distribution and new vouchers with even smaller contributions by the people, combined with intensive BCC, should achieve a break-through in net utilization and reduction of malaria.

The ambitious programme has become even more dependent on donor funding as the required budgets are far beyond the Government's possibilities.

References

1. Barat L et al. (2004). Do malaria control interventions reach the poor? A view through the equity lens *American Journal of Tropical Medicine and Hygiene*, 71(Suppl 2):174–178. Available at: http://www.ajtmh.org/cgi/reprint/71/2_suppl/174 (accessed on 20 April 2009).

2. Carpenter L et al. (2006). *Building a public–private partnership to transfer the technology of a life-saving malaria prevention tool in Africa*, World Economic Forum. Available at: http://www.weforum.org/pdf/Initiatives/GHI_Olyset.pdf (accessed on 20 April 2009).

3. Carter R and Mendis K (2002). Evolutionary and historical aspects of the burden of malaria. *Clinical Microbiology Reviews*, 15:564–594. Available at: http://cmr.asm.org/cgi/reprint/15/4/564 (accessed on 20 April 2009).

4. Commission on Social Determinants of Health (2007). *Scoping paper: priority public health conditions*. WHO, Commission on Social Determinants of Health Priority Public Health Conditions Knowledge Network version 3.1. Available at: http://www.who.int/social_determinants/resources/pphc_

scoping_paper.pdf (accessed on 20 April 2009).

5. DATA (2008). *The DATA report 2008.* Washington, DATA organisation. Available at: http://one.org/report/en/index.html (accessed on 20 April 2009).

6. Erlanger T et al. (2004). Field issues related to effectiveness of insecticide-treated nets in Tanzania. *Medical and Veterinary Entomology*, 18:153–160.

7. Gallup J and Sachs J (2001). The economic burden of malaria. *American Journal of Tropical Medicine and Hygiene*, 64(1, 2) S:85–96. Available at: http://www.ajtmh.org/cgi/reprint/64/1_suppl/85 (accessed on 20 April 2009).

8. Grabowsky M, Nobiya T, Selanikio J (2007). Sustained high coverage of insecticide-treated bednets through combined catch-up and keep-up strategies. *Tropical Medicine and International Health*, 12:815–822.

9. Geissbühler Y et al. (2007). Interdependence of domestic malaria prevention measures and mosquito–human interactions in urban Dar es Salaam, Tanzania. *Malaria Journal*, 6:126. Available at:http://www.malariajournal.com/content/pdf/1475-2875-6-126.pdf (accessed on 20 April 2009).

10. Gollin D and Zimmermann C (2007). *Malaria: disease impacts and long-run income differences.* IZA Institute of Labour, Discussion Paper No. 2997.Available at: http://ftp.iza.org/dp2997.pdf (accessed on 20 April 2009).

11. Hay SI and Snow RW (2006). The Malaria atlas project: developing global maps of malaria risk. *PLoS Medicine*, 3:e473. doi:10.1371/journal.pmed.0030473. Available at: http://www.plosmedicine.org/article/info:doi/10.1371/journal.pmed.0030473 (accessed on 20 April 2009).

12. Heiderli U and Lengeler C. *Should bednets be sold or given free? The role of the private sector in malaria control.* Berne, Switzerland, Swiss Agency of Development and Cooperation. Available at: www.swiss-cooperation.admin.ch/tanzania//ressources/resource_en_173817.pdf (accessed on 28 April 2010)

13. Jones C and Sedekia Y (2008). *Report on qualitative monitoring undertaken during October and November 2007 in six districts.* Dar es Salaam, Tanzania, Ifakara Health Institute.

14. Khan M et al. (2003). *Geographic aspects of poverty and health in Tanzania: does living in a poor area matter?* Bethesda, MD, The Partners for Health Reformplus Project, Abt Associates Inc., Technical Report No. 30. Available at: http://www.tanzaniagateway.org/docs/Geographic_aspects_of_poverty_and_health_in_Tanzania.pdf (accessed on 20 April 2009).

15. Koot J, Smithson P, Lengeler C (2006). *Output to purpose review SMARTNET programme.* Tanzania, DFID.

16. Kramer K (2005). *Netcell ITN upscaling project phase 1 final report.* Swiss Tropical Institute/National Malaria Control Programme Ministry of Health Tanzania. Available at: http://www.sdc-health.ch/priorities_in_health/communicable_diseases/malaria/netcell_final_report_phase_1

17. Leonard L and Masatu C (2007). Variations in the quality of care accessible to rural communities in Tanzania. *Health Affairs*, 26:w380–w392. Available at:http://content.healthaffairs.org/cgi/content/abstract/26/3/w380 (accessed on 20 April 2009).

18. Magesa SN et al. (2005). Creating an enabling environment for taking insecticide treated nets to scale: the Tanzanian experience. *Malaria Journal*, 4:34, Available at: http://www.malariajournal.com/content/4/1/34 (accessed on 20 April 2009).

19. Marchant T et al. (2008). *Report on 2007 TNVS household, facility services and facility users surveys (a comparison across three survey years).* Dar es Salaam, Tanzania, Ifakara Health Institute.

20. Mboera L et al. (2008). *Mosquito net coverage and utilisation for malaria control in Tanzania.* Tanzania, National Institute for Medical Research.

21. McIntyre D and Gilson L (2005). *Equitable health care financing and poverty challenges in the African context.* Paper presented to Forum 9, Global Forum for Health. Available at:, http://www.equinetafrica.org/bibl/docs/McIfin092005.pdf (accessed on 20 April 2009).

22. Mponda H, Sedekia Y, Nathan R (2008). *Report on the third round of retail census of the Tanzanian National Voucher Scheme.* Dar es Salaam, Tanzania, Ifakara Health Institute.

23. MOHSW (2002). *National Malaria Medium Term Strategic Plan 2002–2007.* Tanzania, Ministry of Health and Social Welfare.

24. MOHSW (2007). *National Malaria Medium Term Strategic Plan 2008–2013.* Tanzania, Ministry of Health and Social Welfare.

25. MOHSW (2009). *Health Sector Strategic Plan 2009–2015.* Tanzania, Ministry of Health and Social Welfare.

26. Nathan R et al. (2008). *Tanzania National Voucher Scheme, report on the 2007/8 voucher tracking study.* Dar es Salaam, Tanzania, Ifakara Health Institute.

27. NBS (2005). *Tanzania Demographic and Health Survey 2004–05.* Dar es Salaam, Tanzania, National Bureau of Statistics and ORC Macro. Available at: http://www.nbs.go.tz/DHS/

28. NBS (2008). *Tanzania HIV/AIDS and Malaria Indicator Survey 2007–08.* Prelininary report. Dar es Salaam, Tanzania.

29. Nganda R et al. (2004). Knowledge of malaria influences the use of insecticide treated nets but not intermittent presumptive treatment by pregnant women in Tanzania. *Malaria Journal*, 3:42. Available at:http://www.malariajournal.com/content/pdf/1475-2875-3-42.pdf (accessed on 20 April 2009).

30. PSI (2007). *PSI-Tanzania Project TRaC – Malaria and diarrheal disease, the PSI dashboard.* Population Services International, Tanzania.

31. RBM (2008a). *The Global Malaria Action Plan for a malaria-free world.* Roll Back Malaria Partnership. Available at: http://www.rbm.who.int/gmap/ (accessed on 20 April 2009).

32. RBM (2008b). *2008 MDG Malaria World Summit: summary report*. Roll Back Malaria Partnership, Available at: http://www.rollbackmalaria.org/docs/mdg2008SummaryReport.pdf (accessed on 20 April 2009).

33. Reed C and Stephen G (2005). *Free net distribution in Lindi Region 30.7.05–1.8.05. Monitoring and evaluation: component 2 qualitative follow-up activities*. National Malaria Control Programme, Dar es Salaam, Tanzania & Swiss Agency for Development and Cooperation, Berne, Switzerland.

34. Rugemalila J, Wanga C, Kilama W (2006). Sixth Africa Malaria Day in 2006: how far have we come after theAbuja Declaration? *Malaria Journal*, 5:102. doi:10.1186/1475-2875-5-102. Available at: http://www.malariajournal.com/content/5/1/102.

35. Sachs J, Teklehaimanot A, McCord G (2005). *The costs of making the poor pay*. Science and Development Network. Available at: http://www.scidev.net/en/sub-suharan-africa/opinions/the-cost-of-making-the-poor-pay.html (accessed on 20 April 2009).

36. Skarbinski J et al. (2007). Distribution of free untreated bednets bundled with insecticide via an integrated child health campaign in Lindi Region, Tanzania: lessons for future campaigns. *American Journal of Tropical Medicine and Hygiene*, 76:1100–1106. Available at: http://www.ajtmh.org/cgi/reprint/76/6/1100?ck=nck (accessed on 20 April 2009).

37. Tami A et al. (2004). Evaluation of Olyset™ insecticide-treated nets distributed seven years previously in Tanzania. *Malaria Journal*, 3:19. Available at: http://www.malariajournal.com/content/pdf/1475-2875-3-19.pdf (accessed on 20 April 2009).

38. Teklehaimanot A, JD Sachs, C Curtis (2007). Malaria control needs mass distribution of insecticidal bednets. *The Lancet*, 369:2143–2146. Available at: http://www.earthinstitute.columbia.edu/sitefiles/File/about/director/documents/Lancet_Malaria_control_6-21-07.pdf (accessed on 20 April 2009).

39. Wagstaff A et al. (2004). Child health: reaching the poor. *American Journal of Public Health*, 94:726–736. Available at: http://www.ajph.org/cgi/reprint/94/5/726.pdf (accessed on 20 April 2009).

40. Whiting V (2005). *PSI life of a net analysis*. Dar es Salaam Tanzania, Population Services International,

41. WHO (2000). *The Abuja Declaration and the plan of action*. Geneva, Switzerland, Roll Back Malaria Secretariat – World Health Organization (WHO/CDS/RBM/2000.17). Available at: http://www.rollbackmalaria.org/docs/abuja_declaration.pdf (accessed on 28 April 2010).

42. WHO (2004). *Malaria and HIV interactions and their implications for public health policy. Report of a technical consultation*. Geneva, World Health Organization. Available at: http://www.who.int/hiv/pub/prev_care/malariahiv.pdf (accessed on 28 April 2010).

43. Worrall E, Basu S, Hanson K (2005). Is malaria a disease of poverty? A review of the literature. *Tropical Medicine and International Health*, 10:1047–1059. Available at: http://www3.interscience.wiley.com/cgi-bin/fulltext/118667545/PDFSTART (accessed on 20 April 2009).

Addressing the social determinants of alcohol use and abuse with adolescents in a Pacific Island country (Vanuatu)

14

Patrick Harris,[1,*] Jan Ritchie,[2] Graham Tabi,[3] Tony Lower[4]

[1] Centre for Health Equity Training, Research and Evaluation, Sydney South West Area Health Service/University of New South Wales Research Centre for Primary Health care and Equity, NSW, Australia
[2] School of Public Health and Community Medicine, University of New South Wales, NSW, Australia
[3] Pacific Action for Health Project, Ministry of Health, Vanuatu
[4] Formerly with Pacific Action for Health Project, Secretariat of the Pacific Community, New Caledonia
* Corresponding author: patrick.harris@unsw.edu.au

Abstract

As with other Pacific Island countries, young people in the Republic of Vanuatu are increasingly being faced with rapid urbanization, lack of education, decreasing consumption of local foods, limited job opportunities, and the ready availability and accessibility of cheap cigarettes and alcohol. This single qualitative explanatory case study covered an integrated health promotion programme, the Pacific Action for Health Project, set up to address alcohol problems as one of the risk factors for noncommunicable diseases among urban youth in the capital of Vanuatu, Port Vila. Data were obtained from programme and policy documents, stakeholder interviews and participant observation. The findings showed achievements, supporting factors, and barriers to success emerging at both the policy and community levels that the project was designed to influence. Additional findings were managing policy change, ensuring sustainability and managing intersectoral processes. Three primary lessons can be learnt from the case. First, action on the social determinants of health is not only a health department issue but a concern of all within their respective mandates. This requires linking these interests to generate a synergistic effect over the long term, based on good understanding of the core mandates of other departments/sectors in relation to the project. Second, ultimate responsibility for mobilizing and linking these activities in a sustainable manner must come from and be formally anchored within the Ministry of Health or equivalent institution. Third, addressing the determinants in a sustained manner requires a combination of vertical short-term strategies and horizontal long-term approaches. If donors are not prepared to support this, they should stay away from engaging in such projects. Governments do not have this luxury.

14.1 Background

Since colonization by European powers formally ended in the 1970s, the small and isolated island countries of the Pacific Ocean have struggled to build their nations from subsistence existence to resource-based cash economies. Most island nations have become politically independent and overtly self-determining but, as they have little opportunity to develop this cash economy, have remained primarily economically dependent on regional donor countries and global institutions such as the World Bank. The Republic of Vanuatu is one such island country relying largely on overseas aid and funding for health, welfare and education. With urban areas attracting many families from rural locations and outer islands in the hope of material gain, a growing problem is the number of adolescents who have only a minimal education but a mind-set that attempts to adopt an affluent Western lifestyle. The majority of these young people then find themselves without employment and purpose. With the recent availability of alcohol, authorities have become concerned about its use and abuse by these urban adolescents. This case study covered an Australian-funded, integrated health promotion programme, the Pacific Action for Health Project (PAHP), set up to address alcohol problems as one of the risk factors for noncommunicable diseases (NCDs) among young people in Vanuatu.

The health problem through a literature lens

Vanuatu has recently become concerned about NCDs as these are the leading cause of death and disability worldwide. An increasing burden is being placed on low-income countries (Habib and Saha, 2008; WHO, 2005; Miranda et al., 2008; Strong et al., 2005). In both low-income and more affluent societies, it is now recognized that NCDs are more prevalent "among those who do not have the resources to pursue healthy choices easily" (Strong et al., 2005). These inequities in NCD outcomes are rooted in wider socially and structurally created conditions such as poverty and material deprivation, which form the "causes of the causes" of NCDs (WHO, 2005; Marmot, 2007; WHO, 2008). These determinants operate at the structural (e.g. political, societal and cultural), local (e.g. community) and individual levels through a web of causation and association (Miranda et al., 2008; WHO, 2008; Solar and Irwin, 2007). Across these levels, social status determines individual and population differences in exposure and vulnerability to health-compromising conditions such as NCDs (Solar and Irwin, 2007).

The evidence on alcohol use and abuse, the NCD risk factor entry point for this case study, provides a good example of the multiple factors that operate in a determinants-of-health model. Beginning with health outcomes, in terms of NCDs, the health consequences of excessive alcohol use include liver cirrhosis, pancreatitis, various cancers and injury (WHO, 2005). Individual-level or proximal risk factors that operate in the context of the drug environment include hereditary predisposition, level of strain, family dysfunction, low religiosity and failure at school (Birckmayer et al., 2004). More distal risk factors include the availability of alcohol, cultural and societal norms related to drinking, promotion of alcohol and law enforcement practices (Birckmayer et al., 2004). These are influenced by, and in turn influence, economic, social and cultural issues such as income inequality and job security, community engagement and social capital, the state of the physical environment in which people and communities live, and the policies that create or sustain these (Spooner, 2005).

To date, the majority of health promotion interventions have not aimed at the structural determinants of health that are required to fully address health inequity (WHO, 2008; Beckfield and Krieger, 2009). Instead, these have fallen within the domain of behaviour modification and health education. However, evaluations of such behaviour-based health promotion programming indicate that these approaches at best address only a small proportion of the inequitable differential distribution of health between groups; "So, if someone is not poor in relation to the society they are living in, if they are not living in absolute poverty, have a reasonably supportive social network, are reasonably free of disease, then behaviour change might make a difference to their health status. For people in whom the reverse is true, behaviour change is most unlikely to be effective" (Baum, 2002).

An alternative to behaviour-based health promotion is to take a comprehensive approach to the determinants of health by working intersectorally with those sectors that have more responsibility for the undesirable determinants of health (WHO, 2005; 2008). The purpose of intersectoral collaboration is to take action that is more effective, efficient or sustainable than that which could be achieved by the health sector working alone (WHO, 1997; in Public Health Agency of Canada, 2007). However, while intersectoral action appears simple in terms of its goals, in practice, as exemplified in this case,

it has proved more difficult, particularly at the structural levels of policy-making (Public Health Agency of Canada, 2007).

Country context

Situated in the South Western Pacific Ocean, Vanuatu's population is currently young, with 39.8% below 15 years of age (UNDP, 2008). Designated a least developed country in 2002 (UNCTAD, 2002), Vanuatu's GDP growth between 1995 and 2005 was particularly poor relative to other Pacific Island countries (IMF, 2007). Changes in government have been frequent, which has adversely affected structural reforms to the economy (IMF, 2007).

Current NCD rates are similar to those in the other Pacific Islands, all of which are currently in the grip of an epidemiological transition (Gani, 2009). As Vanuatu's young population ages and lifestyle changes such as modifications to traditional diets and lower levels of physical activity occur, the high health costs currently experienced by other Pacific Island countries have begun to appear (Coyne, 2000; WHO, 2003). As with other Pacific Island countries, young ni-Vanuatu (nationals are referred to as "ni-Vanuatu") are increasingly faced with rapid urbanization, lack of education, decreasing consumption of local foods, limited job opportunities, and the ready availability and accessibility of cheap cigarettes and alcohol (Phongsavan, 2005; UNICEF, 2001).

The Pacific Action for Health Project (PAHP)

In the late 1990s, the Pacific Island countries overtly recognized the impact that NCDs, especially diabetes, were having on their populations. The Australian Agency for International Development (AusAID) decided to support Pacific Island countries in confronting this problem by establishing a regional project in three island states: Kiribati, Tonga and Vanuatu. The project chose urban adolescents as their population of interest and each country was invited to nominate a specific risk factor as the entry point for NCD prevention. Vanuatu decided to address alcohol use and abuse among young people aged 10–19 years in the capital, Port Vila. The project was implemented between 2002 and 2005, and later extended till 2007.

Although records show that the original project was planned as a health behaviour-change intervention, a revised project design was eventually agreed upon. While PAHP was not explicitly designed to address equity through the social determinants of health, the revised design recognized that NCD risk factors are rooted in wider social conditions, and that any intervention should therefore place an explicit focus on the poverty and unemployment faced by vulnerable young ni-Vanuatu. An unusual aspect of the project plan was that the project was to be managed by the Ministry of Health with a nongovernment organization (NGO) invited to act as the implementing agency.

There were two levels of intervention for the project. The first addressed the implementation of national NCD policies. This included the establishment of multisectoral NCD Committees to oversee legislative updates covering the sale of tobacco and alcohol products, and related enforcement of this legislation, as well as the development of comprehensive chronic disease strategies for the next five-year period.

The second centred on community-based initiatives targeting young people to adopt and maintain healthy behaviours. Community-based activities including sports, drama, theatre and music were used to promote healthy lifestyle messages, with the aim of exposing whole communities to these messages. A small grants scheme to support activities developed by groups of young people was also utilized to address unemployment as the primary social determinant of the substance abuse problem.

14.2 Methods

This research project took the form of a retrospective single explanatory case study (Yin, 2003), investigating process issues raised during the implementation of the original project that addressed the social determinants of health. The case was the project itself, with embedded units of analysis being the interventions at policy and community levels, the management of the project, and the stakeholders involved.

The research question driving the case study was to investigate "How did the project attempt to address the social determinants of NCD risk factors in young people in Vanuatu?" Sub-questions included: "How did the project operate at the community and policy levels?" and "How well did this succeed?"

Due to relevant baseline and post-project health data being unavailable in this resource-poor country, the explanatory case study approach focused on operational issues of the project process occurring over time and in context (Yin, 2003), rather than seeking to measure project impact. As the theory concerning social determinants and health equity was well formulated, this single critical case was investigated to "confirm, challenge, [and] extend the theory" (Yin, 2003).

With the programme having been implemented for some years and being relatively well known by potential informants, data collection to address these two research questions occurred over one week in September 2007. Data were obtained from four primary sources: (i) electronic programme documents including formal agreements, media releases, minutes of pertinent meetings, and monitoring and evaluation records; (ii) policy documents, specifically those related to NCD and alcohol and tobacco policies; (iii) interviews with key stakeholders in their professional capacity (× 5) and with young people involved in the project (× 7); and (iv) through participant observation where the first author who collected the data recorded his personal perceptions of the project during his days on site. These data were used to develop converging lines of inquiry within the case, and to triangulate sources of evidence and findings (Yin, 2003). This researcher was known to the majority of informants and was familiar with the local culture due to previous involvement in the programme for three months in 2005.

Two frameworks were included to assist in data collection and analysis. The first was a programme logic framework which mapped PAHP's original aims and objectives against the implementation processes on the ground in Vanuatu, and their impact and outcomes (Annex 1). The second was an intervention scheme template developed for the case study investigation (CSDH, 2007) (Annex 2).

Data were analysed with NVivo computer-assisted data management and analysis software (QSR International, 2008 #44). Data were refined through iteratively developing explanations and testing these against further data sources. Triangulated data from different sources that supported the same findings were given primacy, but divergent themes that appeared to provide contrary information to other data sources were included in building explanations.

Data quality was ensured through several strategies, following Ritchie's approach (Ritchie, 2001) to matching the criteria developed for qualitative research with the equivalent concept as outlined by Yin (Yin, 2003). Trustworthiness (construct validity) was addressed through the use of multiple sources of evidence, development of a chain of evidence, and review of analyses and reports by the project team. Credibility (internal validity) was addressed through explanation building during data analysis against the two chosen frameworks. Replicability (reliability) was addressed through establishing an audit trail. Transferability (external validity) was encouraged through emphasizing the triangulation and matching of data with the wider theory.

Ethics approval for the research was granted by the Human Research Ethics Committee at the University of New South Wales, Australia, in August 2007.

14.3 Findings

The data collected from the four sources revealed strong support for the project at both the community and policy levels. As well as specific achievements at these two levels, findings began to emerge that related directly to the processes that formed the original call for case studies by the Public Health Conditions Knowledge Network: managing policy change, ensuring sustainability and managing intersectoral processes.

Community level

In the urban areas where PAHP operated, informants were adamant that the project positively influenced the lives of the young people involved and their communities. Activities included the small grants scheme, communitywide events, training and leadership building, engagement with community leaders and advocacy networks.

The small grants scheme was regarded by informants as PAHP's primary vehicle for positively influencing the lives of young ni-Vanuatu. The scheme explicitly addressed unemployment and poverty as the entry point for the social determinants influencing the health of these young people. This passage from a submission to the donor agency for an additional phase of PAHP in Vanuatu provides a relevant insight:

"This [small grants] system has allowed local groups … to choose approaches that would address the broader

socioeconomic determinants of health (education, employment, housing) and to identify how the project may be sustained … Examples have included the establishment of a lawn mowing service, a security service and motor mechanics training, all of which are now self-sustained on the revenue they raise. This system provides an opportunity for youth to become self-empowered and has proved remarkably popular and effective in reaching at-risk youth. Such an approach also integrates attention to the underlying social determinants of health into the programme."

One youth representative commented that one year on from the completion of the project, re-installation of the scheme was being requested most by young people. Others pointed out that similar schemes were being funded by other NGOs based on this model. PAHP's final completion report noted that youth activity groups in Vanuatu grew from "a handful" at the start of the programme to 89 by its completion in 2005, with actual numbers of individuals, in the estimation of the programme manager, totalling roughly "a couple of thousand adolescents".

Interestingly, informants indicated that they believed the determinant-oriented activities of the scheme acted as an entry point for youth into the project, rather than the issue of NCD prevention itself. One interviewee explained:

"I think we can say that at first when they started, probably the activities attracted them. But now we have seen that a lot of them have taken on the [noncommunicable disease] message…"

The interview data revealed that the impact of the small grants scheme was in large part due to its directly addressing the current urban situation of youth unemployment. Providing young people with constructive opportunities for group activities was seen by informants as building their self-esteem, sense of responsibility, and a sense of belonging. For example, an informant commented:

"It provided the opportunity for youth or young people to come together and to participate in these activities not only to educate themselves but also to promote a sense of being together in one community or sense of belonging together."

Interviewees also believed that it addressed community concerns regarding the large numbers of "drop-outs" hanging around with no direction or constructive opportunities to pursue. Community leaders were required to sign the application form submitted by the youth group, which provided a direct constructive and positive link between "drop-out" young people and the Chiefs – their traditional community leaders. As one informant noted *"There has been a big change. The Chiefs, for example, now trust or have confidence in their young people."*

The programme's quarterly reports revealed that much of PAHP's day-to-day focus was on a large array of communitywide events, including sports events and tournaments, theatre groups, music competitions, and the hosting of a youth forum and a youth festival by the young people themselves, all with a health theme. The reports indicated that the reach of these activities was high, often including hundreds of youth and their broader community, and involving other sectors. Moreover, events were developed with young people as decision-makers, thereby increasing their visibility in the community while building their skills and self-esteem.

Training and leadership building were through more formal educational activities attached to many of the community-level interventions, described in the final report as aiming to "develop awareness and skills in critical areas". This training included health promotion/ prevention strategies concerning alcohol consumption and smoking cessation. The notion of building leaders was an essential aspect of PAHP's design at the community level, and it became apparent that this focus on leadership fitted well with traditional Vanuatu culture – *kastom*. As one informant pointed out:

"Traditional kastom is being able to have all children, boys and girls alike, to be leaders in their own context. And I think PAHP did not disturb at all the thinking of traditional leaders. …In fact, we have encouraged it."

At the same time, according to the Director General of Health, leadership was associated with dispelling the community view that young people's behaviour was invariably negative:

"They have had a lot of leadership training … to be able to tell them what is their role in this society, and so I think they have moved out of this type of grouping together to do silly things. This is a shift, and is something that has been seen."

Advocacy networks were revealed as another important element of PAHP's community-level work. Positive relationships with established youth networks were developed, using the networks as advocacy channels

for the programme when developing alcohol harm minimization campaigns. A final list of PAHP's youth networking groups detailed more than 100 organizations, including over 1000 young people.

Equity also became an important theme at the community level. PAHP's focus on improving the status of disadvantaged youth was in and of itself an attempt to improve equity. Discussions with stakeholders and youth representatives indicated that PAHP was the first to direct support at "drop-outs". Historically, youth-focused programmes had not traditionally differentiated between groups of young people and often overlooked "drop-out" youth. In addition, PAHP emphasized gender equity, encouraging the active participation of young women at every opportunity, despite a male-oriented culture in Vanuatu.

While the overall findings were positive, particularly concerning the small grants scheme, some limitations in community-level activities were found. The Evaluation Report in 2005 questioned the reach of the health education messages promoted, with many respondents in focus groups not realizing that the community events were associated with NCD prevention. In addition, during the evaluation, a comment by a young ni-Vanuatu showed recognition that awareness-raising events may have a limited impact on structural issues facing young people:

"I think all the activities are useless – they won't help to reduce drinking and smoking and drugs. The best way is to get the Government to enforce the legal minimum age for starting these things. Sport can't help. If you consider the present situation, it is hard for young people to cope and to give up these things."

Policy level

PAHP's influence at the policy level was recognized by stakeholders. Specific achievements included the development of an NCD National Strategy document, Vanuatu's ratification of the Framework Convention on Tobacco Control, and the drafting of legislative changes for liquor licensing.

Primarily, stakeholders' impressions of PAHP's role in these successes revolved around its role as an intersectoral facilitator. For example, the multisectoral committee convened by PAHP to develop the NCD National Strategy document was chaired by the Director General of Health and included nine representatives from the Ministry of Health, two from Education, two from Youth and Sports, and one each from Trade and Industry, Customs and Quarantine, Women's Affairs, Strategic Management, Social and Economic Development, Vanuatu Broadcasting and Television Corporation, and the National Statistic Office. The evaluation in the final report noted that:

"Most of those interviewed were strongly of the opinion that the new National NCD Plan of Action could never have been developed without assistance from a project like PAHP."

During the interview with the chairman of the National NCD committee, it became apparent that the recent introduction of taxes on alcohol and tobacco by the Department of Customs was the result of discussions by the committee with one member, who subsequently become the Director of that department.

However, despite these achievements, informants generally indicated dissatisfaction that PAHP had limited reach at the policy and legislative levels. A number of reasons for this became apparent. First, the time required for policy and legislative change to occur was incongruent with the time limits of PAHP's funding, as expressed by a stakeholder in a donor agency:

"Pushing through the legislative changes in this country is enormously difficult and it's very slow…and if the pace of legislative change is really slow, actually getting things through is going to take a while. I mean, there's not a lot that a project can really do to change that."

A second reason offered by informants was the lack of government commitment to policy change, compounded by political instability and frequent changes of ministers of health throughout the project's lifetime. A good example of these difficulties was highlighted in one stakeholder interview in relation to alcohol legislation:

"The process was so lengthy, and you know the government commitments meant they have a lot of things sort of delayed, and we were all waiting for the 'yes' from the State Law. But by then remember that the timeframe for the project was coming to an end."

The final point that became apparent was poor financial management of the project by the implementing NGO, which ultimately undermined PAHP's ability to support policy and legislative change. Informants expressed regret that money which had been previously set aside for timely legislative support was mismanaged by the NGO, and lost when that organization ceased operations.

Management of the project

Project management became an important theme, particularly due to the closure of the responsible NGO during the extension phase of the project. As already mentioned, PAHP was managed through the Ministry of Health but an NGO acted as the implementing agency. This was done because the NGO had strong community links and particularly because it had the ability to enact initiatives without being limited by the Ministry's bureaucratic red tape.

During interviews, a number of stakeholders referred to the closure of the NGO as "unfortunate". However, the reports make it clear that it was the poor financial management of the NGO that undermined PAHP's ability to support policy and legislative change during its extension phase. At that point, the momentum created by earlier efforts had resulted in regular meetings of a National NCD Committee comprising multisectoral stakeholders, which could have resulted in a more immediate policy impact. Indeed, State Law had finally provided a positive response to revisions of the Liquor Licensing Act, but poor project management did not allow this to be taken forward.

A further issue concerning project management was that PAHP was driven by one dedicated individual with support from the Director General of Health. However, a consistent theme in the interviews was a concern that for PAHP to influence policy change across the board, linkages to established institutions were needed, rather than being driven by individuals.

Sustainability

Sustainability emerged as an important theme generated from all data sources. Concern over the potential lack of sustainability was expressed by many. The small grants initiatives were the only aspect of PAHP that remained functional beyond the timeframe of the project. The fact that these were "owned" by young people and their community leaders and generated income enabled a number of these initiatives to be self-sustaining. Indeed, the final report recommended that:

"An increased emphasis on addressing the underlying social and economic determinants of health is required for long-term progress to address noncommunicable diseases. As such, the interrelationships between poverty alleviation, employment and education should be promoted."

All other initiatives appeared to have ceased functioning at the end of the extension phase. The main reason for this, as suggested by informants, was the realization that the nature of short-term programme funding was incongruous with addressing long-term chronic disease issues. However, the donor representative felt that focusing solely on long-term sustainability would have been insufficient, and that vertical short-term strategies would always be appropriate for raising awareness of NCD issues that may not have previously existed, developing a required momentum for action before "the bubble burst". At the same time, all data sources recognized the need for long-term funding to address these risk factors at both the policy and community levels.

Intersectoral processes

Taking a multisectoral approach became an important theme that was touched on by all data sources. PAHP appears to have been the first programme in Vanuatu to have undertaken a multisectoral approach to NCDs. For example, in relation to the development of the National NCD Strategy, the final report across all countries commented that:

"Multisectoral collaboration…is a new approach for the Health Ministries [of the three countries] which, up to this point, have undertaken only minimal multisectoral work to address noncommunicable disease issues."

The data suggested that the social determinants of health were viewed as a conceptual driver for this intersectoral work, driven by the awareness and understanding of key individuals involved in PAHP. For example, this additional comment made by the multi-country Programme Manager stated:

"This was the first (and remains the only) project where an emphasis on the social determinants of health has been included in the Pacific. Regrettably, it is often perceived simply to be too hard to address the social determinants as it involves working across numerous sectors. In Vanuatu, we were extremely fortunate in having an exceptional local project manager with tremendous intersectoral links and a strong Director General of Health, who quickly identified the

benefits of this approach and provided unwavering support in the higher-level public service and political domains in which she functioned. Together, the personal attributes of these two individuals opened many doors to the project that would have otherwise not been accessible."

The difficulties were not underestimated, as expressed in this comment by the donor agency representative:

"It's a very siloed operation in Vanuatu, there's not a lot of cross-fertilization and engagement of ministries and that's really hard."

In addition, the donor agency representative noted the issues of core business regarding engagement with the education sector:

"I mean, it's not something's not seen as core business within the Ministry of Education and it's not seen as kind of their mandate and actually getting it on the agenda."

The siloed manner in which different government departments viewed their business in relation to acting to prevent NCDs also became important. During PAHP's extension phase, a national NCD Committee was established, chaired by the local Port Vila Municipality, and included health and other sectors involved in developing the NCD National Strategy document. A comment made by the NCD Committee chairman reflects the need to navigate the core business of other sectors:

"I think from the start we had to convince them. They thought it is an issue that's only for the Health Department. This is why they had to take this project out from the Health Department, and give it to an NGO to do. Not with a government department because the other government departments will think 'Oh, it's their responsibility, they have the budget for that and they have the officers to do that, it's theirs, and we keep to ours'."

14.4 Discussion

This explanatory case study investigated how a short-term donor-assisted project attempted to address the social determinants of NCDs in young ni-Vanuatu at multiple levels, and the extent to which it was successful. From the findings of the case study, three primary lessons can be learnt.

The **first lesson** from the case study showed that action on the social determinants of health is not only a health department issue but a concern of all within their respective mandates. Taking a social determinants' approach is about linking these interests to generate a synergistic effect. This requires understanding of the core mandates of other departments/sectors in relation to the project.

The recognition that the social determinants of health should be a concern of all sectors was present at the beginning but was strengthened as the project evolved (WHO, 2005; WHO, 2008). The initial debate around the original project was due to a concern among multisectoral stakeholders that the traditional health promotion approach in the Pacific of "telling them what they should do" was not working. As a result, the programme design was reoriented to focus at multiple levels: the structural determinants of NCDs through multisectoral policy development, and the local and individual determinants of NCDs facing young people within their community environments. It is noteworthy that the determinant-oriented activities of the small grants scheme, rather than the traditional risk factor-prevention activities, were found to be the entry point for youth into the project.

The case study also shows that creating policy change at the structural determinants level requires strategic effort to engage other sectors (WHO, 2005). For PAHP, this effort focused on mobilizing stakeholders of the appropriate health and non-health agencies to understand the relationship of their mandates to NCDs. PAHP's effort here was focused both on one-to-one policy-level meetings with agencies, establishing and resourcing the multisectoral working party, and engaging agencies (including NGOs, civil society and the wider community) in community-level events. In these, PAHP became the facilitating agent, with the goal of synergizing this multistakeholder engagement to create policy change; for example, through the drafting of the NCD Strategy and other legislative documents.

Some policy-level achievements were made, for example, in mobilizing stakeholders, drafting the strategy and legislation, and later being indirectly responsible for the introduction of taxes on alcohol and tobacco through a committee member. Indeed, these achievements are similar to the national intersectoral NCD policy achievements in neighbouring Tonga, noted by WHO as a case study in policy-level NCD prevention (WHO, 2005).

Unfortunately, however, despite the promise and initial effort, disappointment was expressed by all stakeholders that PAHP's policy-level ambitions remained unfulfilled. A number of reasons became apparent for this. PAHP may not have fully recognized the core mandate of the agencies involved, compounded by the traditionally siloed nature of the government in Vanuatu. Stakeholders apparently recognized that work on NCD risks was viewed as an additional component of the work of agencies other than the health sector, and not regarded as their core business. However, political instability led to a lack of government action and the slow progress of the government legislative machine was incongruent with the short lifetime of PAHP. Further, the initial effort at the policy level appeared to dissipate over time and more effort was given to community activities, perhaps in response to the lack of policy achievement. Finally, but perhaps most importantly, multisectoral policy coordination ceased as PAHP's funding ceased.

The **second lesson** evolving from this study was that a bounded, time-delineated project could not realistically be expected to continue its activities after the project was terminated. This indicates that the responsibility for mobilizing and linking these activities in a sustainable manner must come from and be formally anchored within the Ministry of Health or equivalent institution, as part of the shift within the health sector's core mandate toward the social determinants of health. While the impetus and support can come from outside (for example, NGOs or donors), there must be no doubt of where the ultimate responsibility and ownership lie.

During PAHP's initial design phase, it was felt that an agency operating outside the "red-tape" of the Ministry of Health would more easily facilitate and coordinate the largely intersectoral work required. However, ultimately this proved fatal. Since PAHP ceased to operate, this cooperative work stalled and all multisectoral engagement diminished.

Intersectoral action is a skilled enterprise that can take a long time to achieve results, especially in contexts such as Vanuatu where this was the first time that such an approach was taken. In the long term, the health system itself is the more sustainable mechanism for coordinating intersectoral action on the determinants of health. However, the evidence suggests there was limited activity by PAHP to build the capacity of systems. The lesson then from the case is that PAHP would have been more successful in managing intersectoral processes in the long term had it focused on establishing the structures and capacity to engage the determinants of health within the health system (Baum, 2005; Navarro, 2007), building on the support of the Director General of Health for a multisectoral approach. In this way, the health system as a whole, and not just individuals, would be in a position "to provide leadership, to provide arguments for a win–win situation, and to adapt to the agendas and priorities of other sectors" (WHO, 2005).

Finally, the **third lesson** from the case study shows that projects on social determinants to address long-term inequities associated with NCDs can benefit the community through vertical short-term strategies that show more immediate results and raise awareness, as well as horizontal long-term approaches linked with capacity building in the Ministry of Health and other systems to address the underlying determinants and support sustained impact. These findings reinforce the growing literature that ensuring sustainability is best achieved through a combination of horizontal and vertical programme planning (Ooms et al., 2008; Uplekar and Raviglione, 2007). However, this requires donor funding to appropriately target this mix of long- and short-term programming, and horizontal and vertical strategies. The lack of activity at both the community and policy levels in Vanuatu following the end of the short-term vertical funding of PAHP supports the need for long-term horizontal strategic funding. The case study shows that if donors are not prepared to support this more strategic approach they should stay away from engaging in such projects. Governments do not have this luxury.

This aspect of the case study has additional implications due to a tension between the long-term structural change required to address the social determinants and the immediacy of impact of priority public health conditions such as NCDs. Addressing structural change can be a long-term process due to its political nature. However, the priority nature of these chronic diseases themselves requires a short-term focus before the NCD "bubble" bursts. This tension underpins the need for a mix of strategies to ensure sustainability.

Given PAHP's multilevel focus, the case also provides additional lessons for developing sustainable local community activity targeted at the social determinants of NCDs. The findings suggest that ensuring sustainability extends to encouraging community ownership over all aspects of programme activities. PAHP was successful in masking "donor dependency" by encouraging youth and community ownership. The apparent sustainability of

the small grants scheme rested on community ownership and empowerment of young people within their community. In addition, PAHP's culturally appropriate focus on leadership encouraged sustainability. During the development of the case, it became apparent that the leaders PAHP had created often moved on to take paid employment positions, taking their skills and leadership with them. This creation of young leaders from the "drop-out" youth population has been recognized elsewhere as a politically astute empowerment strategy to reduce heath inequity through planting seeds for long-term future structural change (Wallerstein, 2002).

The case study also provides some pertinent lessons on project management. It was clear during the case study that while interview informants referred to the folding up of the NGO managing PAHP as "unfortunate", this was in fact a disaster. As a result, the remaining balance of PAHP's funds were lost, resulting in the cessation of all activities. One innovative strategy to address this, offered in a stakeholder interview, was for PAHP to form its own governance structure made up of cross-sectoral stakeholders including the Ministry of Health but with regular financial reporting to the donor agency, public and government.

An additional project management issue is that sound monitoring and evaluation systems are required to fully understand whether programmes influence the determinants of health and reduce health inequalities. Unfortunately, in PAHP's design, despite a focus on programme logic, there was no mechanism for monitoring and evaluating the impact of the programme on health outcomes. Incorporating the management of such data requires skills and resources. However, these are critical elements of programme design; without such information, the effect of programmes will always be doubtful.

14.5 Conclusion

This case study has explored the extent to which a health promotion intervention through a short-term donor project could influence and enable positive changes in the health of young ni-Vanuatu by focusing on the social determinants of health rather than through more conventional health educational approaches. The case provides three core lessons for other programmes attempting to address the social determinants of

NCDs. The determinants of NCDs are necessarily the responsibility of all sectors including health. However, the health sector must be the driver for action while fostering ownership of the determinants within the core mandates of collaborating sectors. At the same time, the complexity of addressing the determinants of NCDs requires programmes to take on both horizontal and vertical strategies, supported with long-term funding. Short-term funding of short-term strategies is insufficient and potentially damaging.

It is important to recognize that PAHP was operating in a context and a time where knowledge of the determinants of health was meagre in comparison with current thinking. It is a testament to the dedication of those involved in the project as they have opened themselves up to scrutiny from which others can learn.

References

1. Baum F (2002). *The new public health (2nd ed.)*. Melbourne, Oxford University Press.

2. Baum F (2005). Who cares about health for all in the 21st century? *Journal of Epidemiology and Community Health*, 59:714–715.

3. Beckfield J and Krieger N (2009). Epi + demos + cracy: linking political systems and priorities to the magnitude of health inequities—evidence, gaps, and a research agenda. *Epidemiological Review*, 31:152–177.

4. Birckmayer JD et al. (2004). A general causal model to guide alcohol, tobacco, and illicit drug prevention: assessing the research evidence. *Journal of Drug Education*, 34:121–153.

5. Commission on Social Determinants of Health (CSDH) (2007). *Scoping paper*. Geneva, WHO, Commission on Social Determinants of Health Priority Public Health Conditions Knowledge Network version 3.1. Available at: http://www.who.int/social_determinants/resources/pphc_scoping_paper.pdf (accessed on 20 April 2009).

6. Coyne T (2000). In: Langi RHAS (ed.) *Lifestyle diseases in Pacific communities*. Noumea, New Caledonia, Secretariat of the Pacific Community.

7. Gani A. 2009. Some aspects of communicable and non-communicable diseases in Pacific island countries. *Social Indicators Research*, 91:171–187.

8. Habib SH and Saha S (2008). Burden of non-communicable disease: global overview. *Diabetes and Metabolic Syndrome: Clinical Research and Reviews*, (in press).

9. International Monetary Fund (IMF) (2007). *Vanuatu: selected issues*. Washington, DC, International Monetary Fund.

10. Marmot M (2007). Achieving health equity: from root causes to fair outcomes. *The Lancet*, 370:1153–1163.

11. Miranda JJ et al. (2008). Non-communicable diseases in low- and middle-income countries: context, determinants and health policy. *Tropical Medicine and International Health*, 13:1225–1234.

12. Navarro V (2007). What is national health policy? *International Journal of Health Services*, 37:1–14.

13. Ooms G et al. (2008). The 'diagonal' approach to Global Fund financing: a cure for the broader malaise of health systems? *Globalization and Health*, 4:6 doi:10.1186/1744-8603-4-6

14. Phongsavan P et al. (2005). Health behaviour and lifestyle of Pacific youth surveys: a resource for capacity building. *Health Promotion International*, 20:238–248.

15. Public Health Agency of Canada (2007). *Crossing sectors – experiences in intersectoral action, public policy, and health*. Ottawa, Public Health Agency of Canada.

16. QSR International (2008). Available at: *http://www.qsrinternational.com*

17. Ritchie J (2001). Not everything can be reduced to numbers. In: Berglund C (ed.). *Health research*. Melbourne, Oxford University Press.

18. Solar O and Irwin A (2007). *A conceptual framework for action on the social determinants of health: discussion paper for the Commission on the Social Determinants of Health*. Geneva, World Health Organization.

19. Spooner CHK (2005). *Social determinants of drug use*. Sydney, Australia, National Drug and Alcohol Research Centre.

20. Strong K et al. (2005). Preventing chronic diseases: how many lives can we save? *The Lancet*, 366:1578–1582.

21. Thomas YF (2007). The social epidemiology of drug abuse. *American Journal of Preventive Medicine*, 32 (6 Suppl. 1):S141–S146.

22. United Nations Conference on Trade and Development (UNCTAD) (2002). *FDI in least developed countries*. New York/Geneva, United Nations.

23. UNDP (2008). *2007/2008 Human Development Report: Vanuatu 2008*. United Nations, United Nations Development Program. http://hdrstats.undp.org/en/countries/data_sheets/cty_ds_VUT.html (accessed 25 February 2010).

24. UNICEF (2001). *The state of health behaviour and lifestyle of Pacific youth. Vanuatu Report*. Suva, Fiji, UNICEF Pacific.

25. Uplekar M and Raviglione MC (2007). The "vertical–horizontal" debates: time for the pendulum to rest (in peace)? *Bulletin of the World Health Organization*, 85:413–414.

26. Wallerstein N (2002). Empowerment to reduce health disparities. *Scandinavian Journal of Public Health*, 30:72–77.

27. World Health Organization (2003). *Diet, food supply and obesity in the Pacific.* Manila, World Health Organization Regional Office for the Western Pacific.

28. World Health Organization (2005). *Preventing chronic diseases: a vital investment: WHO global report.* Geneva, World Health Organization.

29. World Health Organization (2008). *Closing the gap in a generation: health equity through action on the social determinants of health. Final report of the Commission on Social Determinants of Health.* Geneva, World Health Organization.

30. Yin RK (2003). *Case study research: design and methods* (3rd edn). Thousand Oaks, California, Sage.

From concept to practice

Synthesis of findings

15

Erik Blas[1,2]

[1] World Health Organization, Geneva
[2] The author acknowledges critical inputs to the chapter by Johannes Sommerfeld and Anand Sivasankara Kurup.

15.1 Background

The primary objective of undertaking these case studies was to review their processes of implementation and draw lessons that can be learned by others embarking on the difficult path to correct inequities in health by addressing the social determinants. It was thus not an objective to evaluate the outcomes of these programmes. In this chapter, the individual case studies are mostly referred to by the name of the country in which they are located. This is done for ease of reference as there is only one case for each country while, for example, there are nutrition programmes in three of the countries. However, the analysis and interpretations relate only to the case programmes themselves rather than the countries in general.

Equity: a perspective on social values

Equity and human rights have been discussed by social philosophers over time and with increased intensity since the 1980s. The concepts of equity and altruism are sometimes confused; however, they are distinct and have different implications for health policy. Caring and altruism are matters of preference and the level of provision is determined by the wealth of the society. Social justice or equity, on the other hand, is not a matter of preference and the source of value for making judgements is extrinsic to preferences. Social justice derives from a set of principles that define what a person ought to have as a right and requires that an equitable pattern of provision is ensured, irrespective of the sacrifice to the rest of society. As such, the concept of equity emerges from a deontological rather than a teleological perspective, i.e. *utilitarians* are primarily concerned with maximizing the sum of individuals' utilities and less with how the utilities are distributed. Within the deontological perspectives, *communitarians* focus on norms, culture and virtues of a good society primarily with respect to their own communities, while some are concerned with extending these to all societies. The primary health care (PHC) movement of the 1960s and 1970s has been viewed by some as being grounded in communitarian views (Reich, 1995). With respect to access to health care, *libertarians* view this as part of society's reward system and focus on the extent to which people are free to purchase the health care that they want. Those libertarians who are concerned about distributional issues emphasize minimum standards rather than equality. *Egalitarians*, on the other hand, view access to health care as a citizen's right and judge equity by assessing the extent to which

health care is distributed according to need and financed according to ability to pay. It is clear that, depending on which perspectives prevail in policy-making, the resulting societal organization, including health systems, will be very different.

Questions and concerns about equity are closely linked to the size, role and function of the State as the regulator, collector and distributor of resources and, as such, are deeply rooted in politics and traditions. Where different perspectives coexist, which is mostly the case, this can lead to tensions, trade-offs and outright conflicts (Blas, 2005). It can therefore be anticipated that implementation of public health programmes with a focus on equity and taking social determinants' approaches will face additional challenges compared to those faced by programmes that are more concerned about health averages than distribution.

Historical perspectives

The programmes studied in this volume have their roots in history, either because they were conceived and established long ago, such as the menstrual regulation programme in Bangladesh, or because they revived approaches developed in the past, for example, those by Indonesia and Peru. However, regardless of where and when the underlying programmatic approaches originated from, all the programmes analysed have been blended with elements from different periods and paradigms for public sector and public health development.

The twentieth century experienced three major waves of health sector reforms (WHO, 2000). These were all linked to developments in the political economy. During the 1940s and 1950s, a first generation of reforms based on the concepts of a welfare State established national health-care systems, first in the richer and later in the poorer countries. These systems came increasingly under stress during the 1960s due to escalating costs brought on by the growing volume and intensity of hospital care. In this period, disease control, such as for smallpox, malaria, sleeping sickness and tuberculosis, was mostly undertaken through dedicated programmes and campaigns. However, there was also a growing community development movement that encouraged communities to identify and find solutions for their own problems in all areas of social life (van Balen, 2004). A second generation of reforms promoted PHC as a strategy to achieve affordable universal coverage, but this did not always satisfy local demand for quality and responsiveness. The emphasis on primary care also often came into direct conflict with established medical systems that emphasized hospital care. Furthermore, as the economic situation in many developing countries worsened, it made the reforms difficult to implement.

While the first and second generations of health reforms mainly targeted the supply side, the third generation focused more on the demand side (WHO, 2000). This third generation of reforms was rooted in broader reforms aimed at reducing the role and size of the State and increasing the role of the market. Starting, again first in the richer countries, in the 1970s and 1980s, it gained momentum in poorer countries during the 1990s, attempting to shift away from central budgetary allocation of resources to providers and relying more on market or quasi-market mechanisms, and using cost-effectiveness as a key criteria for resource allocation. However, several adjustments were made to the approach, as developed countries as well as many of the poorer countries faced problems in implementation, including growing inequities resulting from these social reforms. By the beginning of the twenty-first century, the international development aid agenda largely swung back to project-driven approaches characterized under the broad terms "scaling-up" and "pro-poor" programmes, and setting specific global development and health targets.

Realizing that populations' health is not primarily a product of health care but instead a product of the social determinants, WHO established the Commission on Social Determinants of Health (CSDH) in 2005. The report of the Commission published in 2008 provided evidence of the growing inequities as well as the causal links between health outcomes and the social determinants of health (CSDH, 2008). The *World health report* released in the same year advocated for revival of PHC (WHO, 2008). In 2010, the report of the Priority Public Health Conditions (PPHC) Knowledge Network of the Commission provided analysis and proposals on how public health programmes could incorporate equity and social determinants approaches into their work (Blas and Sivasankara Kurup, 2010).

15.2 The case studies within the PPHC framework

Several very different interventions can be considered to address inequities. These can be specifically targeted to particular situations such as lack of access to services, lack of financial means, and so on. Taking a social determinants approach to reducing inequities, however, means targeting the root causes on the pathways that result in inequitable health outcomes and grounding interventions in the three principles for action of the Commission on Social Determinants of Health (CSDH, 2008):

- Improve conditions of daily life – the circumstances in which people are born, grow, live, work and age.

- Tackle the inequitable distribution of power, money and resources – the structural drivers of those conditions of daily life – globally, nationally and locally.

- Measure the problem, evaluate action, expand the knowledge base, develop a workforce that is trained in the social determinants of health, and raise public awareness about the social determinants of health.

The report from the Commission's PPHC Knowledge Network points to what public health programmes can do individually and collectively to address the social determinants that drive health conditions and the outcomes of each major public health programme. The report identifies promising entry points, possible interventions and key movers in a five-level framework (Blas and Sivasankara Kurup, 2010).

The upstream levels of the PPHC framework (*see* chapter 1 of this volume), namely, *context* and *position*, *differential exposure* and *differential vulnerability*, can be usefully considered in relation to a classification of structured interventions that:

- acknowledge health as a function of social, economic and political power and resources, and thus seek to manipulate power and resources to promote public health;

- are based on the assumption that health problems result from the lack of or, conversely, the excessive availability of products, tools, behaviours or settings, and thus seek to influence their availability;

- recognize that the health of a society and its members is partially determined by its values, cultures and beliefs, and thus seek to alter the social norms (Blankenship, 2000).

At the two individual levels of the framework – *differential health-care outcomes* and *differential consequences* –

the design characteristics of services may contribute to increasing inequity. There are four steps in coverage that have all to be negotiated before service use can start: availability, accessibility, acceptability and contact (Tanahashi, 1978). Once an effective contact with the health services has been established, there are still three steps to complete before a successful outcome is achieved: diagnostic accuracy, provider compliance and consumer adherence (Tugwell et al., 2006). The obstacles to successfully completing each of these seven steps depend on a combination of service provision factors and social determinants related to the user.

The report of the PPHC Knowledge Network proposes concrete actions that public health programmes could take to effect change at each level of the framework (Blas and Sivasankara Kurup, 2010). These are in summary:

Context and position: provide setting-specific, timely and relevant evidence; provide examples of good practices; review and propose policy options; and engage in public debate to incorporate health equity issues into economic and social strategies and plans.

Differential exposure: generate evidence and advocate for appropriate interventions to address social norms; influence the health ministry to shift attention upstream to policies that produce good population health; and actively participate in public education, regulation, infrastructure planning and design, and taxation work, for example, regulating the price of certain goods and services.

Differential vulnerability: identify vulnerable population groups and the causes of differential vulnerability; ensure that health delivery systems are culturally and socially appropriate; sensitize vulnerable populations to the health benefits of programmes; and extend service coverage and reduce barriers to access.

Differential health-care outcomes: identify the sources and causes of inequity within health-care services; influence priority setting and service provision, financing and organization; and create awareness of and demand for equity in health-care outcomes.

Differential consequences: analyse and identify the causes of differential consequences and the resulting needs; strengthen standard referral and follow-up procedures in health and across social systems; and facilitate appropriate responses from all actors.

The 13 case studies presented in the chapters of this book have analysed real-life situations where people, nongovernmental organizations (NGOs) and government programmes have worked to reduce inequities through influencing the social determinants of health at different levels of the PPHC framework.

Collectively, the 13 case studies address four of the five levels of the PPHC framework, all the five themes, and cover a variety of public health challenges through a range of different interventions (Table 1).

Policy/legislation: intervening to regulate the availability and control of services, resources and commodities such as alcohol and tobacco with the aim of modifying the *context and position* determinants of health (**Nigeria, Peru, Vanuatu**)

Norm change: Addressing *differential exposure* by modifying what the society formally or informally encourages or discourages, for example, in terms of what to eat, what women can or cannot do, and what young people value and do (**Canada, Chile, Pakistan and Vanuatu**)

Community empowerment: handing over control of institutions and/or public funds in full or in part, for example, from civil service structures to communities, thus involving some transfer of power and control with the potential to reduce *differential exposure* (**Pakistan, Indonesia and Peru**)

Community development: releasing the potential within communities to make them take things in their own hands and thereby reducing group or individual *differential vulnerability*. It involved provision of information and training and, in some cases, loan opportunities and direct injection of resources (**Canada, Indonesia, Iran, Kenya, Pakistan, South Africa, Vanuatu**).

Commodity access: reducing barriers to access of commodities such as healthy food and insecticide-treated nets (ITNs) and thus aiming to modify the *differential vulnerability*. This included making these available at subsidized prices or for free (**Chile, Iran, Pakistan and Tanzania**).

Service access: reducing barriers to access of selected health-care services for certain population groups in order to reduce their *differential vulnerability*, including making services available, removing or reducing fees, etc. (**Bangladesh, China, Kenya, Nigeria, Peru**)

Table 1: Summary description of the 13 case studies according to public health challenges, nature of interventions, entry points and main themes covered

Country of case study programme	Main public health challenge	Generic nature of core interventions	Main entry point in PPHC Framework	Main themes covered				
				Going to scale	Managing policy change	Managing intersectoral processes	Adjusting design	Ensuring sustainability
Bangladesh	Reproductive health	Service access / Service responsiveness	Vulnerability / Health-care outcome	✓✓	✓✓✓	✓✓	✓✓	✓✓
Canada	Mental health (suicide)	Norm change / Community development	Exposure / Vulnerability	✓	✓	✓	✓✓ ✓	✓✓✓
Chile	Noncommunicable diseases	Norm change / Commodity access	Exposure / Vulnerability	✓	✓	✓✓✓		
China	Maternal and child health	Service access and responsiveness	Vulnerability / Health-care outcome	✓✓	✓✓✓	✓		✓✓
Indonesia (Gerbangmas)	Primary health care	Community empowerment / Community development	Exposure / Vulnerability	✓	✓✓	✓✓✓		✓✓
Iran	Child nutrition	Community development / Commodity access	Vulnerability	✓✓		✓✓✓		✓✓
Kenya (MVP)	Primary health care	Community development / Service access	Vulnerability	✓✓✓	✓	✓✓✓		✓✓
Nigeria (REW)	Immunization	Policy/legislation / Service access	Context and position / Vulnerability	✓	✓✓✓	✓		✓✓✓
Pakistan (Tawana)	Girls' nutrition	Norm change / Community empowerment / Commodity access	Exposure / Vulnerability	✓✓		✓✓✓		✓✓
Peru (CLAS)	Primary health care	Policy/legislation / Community empowerment / Service access / Service responsiveness	Context and position / Exposure / Vulnerability / Health-care outcome	✓✓	✓✓✓	✓		✓
South Africa (IMAGE)	HIV/domestic violence	Community development	Vulnerability	✓✓	✓	✓✓✓		✓
Tanzania (ITN)	Malaria	Commodity access	Vulnerability	✓✓✓	✓✓	✓✓	✓✓	✓✓✓
Vanuatu	Noncommunicable diseases	Policy/legislation / Norm change / Community development	Context and position / Exposure / Vulnerability	✓	✓	✓✓✓		✓✓

Service responsiveness: modifying the way that pregnancy, delivery and general PHC services are provided in order to make these better correspond to the needs of and usability for certain population groups with the aim of reducing the differential in health-care outcomes experienced by these groups (**Bangladesh, China, Peru**)

15.3 Lessons learned

Going to scale

A small-scale operation means a situation where all internal and most external elements of a programme can be relatively easily controlled by a single or a few individuals. These persons will often be those who conceived of and initiated the operation, thus understanding the concepts and strategies and having a strong sense of ownership – wanting to see it succeed, even if the price is high. When new challenges occur, such as those due to unforeseen combinations of internal weaknesses or external threats, they will view the challenges in light of the original concept, values and strategies, and put their full innovative power and energy to ensure that problems are resolved without compromising the core ideas. A large-scale project means that many more factors interact and combine in new ways. It also means that many more people are delegated managerial responsibilities. Such people might not always understand the ideas and concepts as well as the "original few" and, for them, working on the programme might be a job just like any other. Managing implementation involves repeated cycles of monitoring, interpreting, taking decisions, and acting in real-world, often complex situations. It is therefore not surprising that almost all of the case programmes faced challenges during the scale-up process.

Two main generic types of scale-up can be identified in the 13 cases studied – expansion and replication. In the **expansion or organic growth type**, there is a defined line of command structures. As the operation expands, the organization grows and the lines of command get longer and new branches might be added. However, at least in principle, problem resolution can be referred back to one point. Examples of this type of scale-up are represented by the menstrual regulation programme in Bangladesh, programme for prevention of noncommunicable diseases in Chile, community development programme in Indonesia, Millennium Villages Project (MVP) in Kenya, Tawana programme in Pakistan, IMAGE

project in South Africa, ITN programme in Tanzania, and adolescents' interventions in Vanuatu. In the other type of scale-up, **replication or cloning**, there is no univocal overall line–command structure linking the management of implementation with the keeper of the core idea. One subgroup of this type is covered by the case studies on independent First Nations communities in Canada and the autonomous community associations in Peru. The other subgroup involved implementation across government administrative structures, such as the migrant maternal health programme in China, where the centre of innovation lay in one of the districts; immunization coverage in the federal states and local government areas of Nigeria; and the provinces in Iran. Some of the organic growth cases, such as those in Kenya and South Africa, eventually expected to be replicated. However, during the period covered in this book, these had not yet reached that stage.

Diverting from established interventions is a risk when scaling up and involving more actors. However, addressing equity is not just about procedures; **fidelity to the values** enshrined in the equity and social determinants approach is just as important as **fidelity to the set strategies and operational procedures**. Transferring the values from the original dedicated migrant delivery centre in Minhang district in China to other centres was identified in the case study as one of the most important obstacles to successful replication, and the authors suggest establishing professional teams, skilled in values transfer, to support the process. The two cases that most directly addressed the values dimension in their scale-up were Canada and Indonesia. In both cases, the programmes worked with the local custodians of values to enhance and integrate with those aspects of the local values that supported the equity and social determinants approach.

A special challenge to fidelity occurred when the CLAS programme in Peru, grounded in communitarian values, for a time joined forces with the International Bank for Reconstruction and Development (IBRD) Programmatic Social Reform Loan, based on liberal market-oriented values with a shared goal of scaling up the coverage of CLAS. The result was a dramatic increase in the number of health facilities operated by each CLAS, thus turning these into businesses. Some ran up to 40 facilities and distanced themselves from the communities. A similar alliance occurred in South Africa between the HIV/violence prevention and the micro-finance projects. While the cooperation facilitated a controlled scale-up, the **difference in values** was a constant challenge to the day-to-day management of the common programme.

Some of the case programmes studied grew to a considerable size during the period of study, in particular, Bangladesh, Pakistan, Peru and Tanzania, while others remained relatively small. Of course, there are many factors that limit the size of a programme, such as available resources, as was the case for Vanuatu; or the need for change in national or global contexts, as was the case with the MVP in Kenya. Common to the four large programmes was that they embraced some form of **pull mechanism** to draw resources and services. In Peru, particularly during the early phases, there was a strong demand from communities, possibly resulting from a strained relationship with the government and its institutions. At one point, there was a waiting list of more than 200 communities awaiting approval. In Bangladesh and Pakistan, NGOs acted as proxies to articulate and legitimize the needs of individuals and population groups within communities, and translate these into demands and actions to draw services in the case of Bangladesh, and resources in the case of Pakistan. Social marketing methods and a voucher system were used in Tanzania to pull ITNs through the private for-profit sector.

Pilot or demonstration projects were used in several of the cases. These projects can be categorized into four broad groups:

Proof of principle – this was most clearly used by the programmes in Kenya, South Africa, Pakistan, China and Iran. In these cases, the pilot projects covered limited geographical areas. They were relatively well-resourced, with managerial attention and pre-defined success criteria, baselines and targets.

Demonstration projects to support the "pull effect" – this kind of demonstration projects were used in Indonesia and Peru. Several small projects were launched at the same time, not so much to demonstrate that the approach could work but to generate a demand from other communities.

Demonstration projects to support the "push effect" – here, the objectives were to gain support from policy-makers and potential funders. This type of project model was used in Peru and Kenya. Particularly in the case of Kenya, the core of the project's strategy was to draw the attention of the international society to increase development assistance and allocate resources in support of rural development.

Projects to test scale-up – despite the widespread challenges in scaling up programmes, it was only the Kenya and South Africa cases that invested in a phase after the initial pilot to try and test what happens when a project moves out of a closely controlled environment. For both of these programmes, the driving actors were university-based researchers.

Before embarking on scaling up from a controlled setting, it is important to identify what will be the main driver of the scale-up, then test and monitor its feasibility and fidelity to values, strategies and procedures in order to make the necessary corrections to implementation.

Managing policy change

Achieving improved health equity through addressing the social determinants of health is a value-based and often political process involving changes to policies at the institutional, national or international level. All changes trigger resistance, in particular, change that relates to redistribution of power and resources. Sometimes, the **right moment and circumstances** are present to kick-start programmes. This was the case in post-war Bangladesh, where there was an international concern about population growth, a burning social need to support the "heroines of war" as well as a new technology for uterine evacuation. In Peru, economic and political problems combined with the international trend of decentralization, including splitting purchaser and provider functions, and the availability of new community development tools provided a launch that was conducive for the CLAS programme. However, these as well as the other case study programmes described in this volume faced challenges in triggering changes to policies, and had to use a variety of tools and approaches.

Three different strategies were used to generate support for or address potential public resistance to social policy change. The migrant delivery programme in China was the only case where the values debate took place in the **public forum**, initially raised by the media with reference to individual events, hospital statistics and research reports. However, throughout the process, the programme ensured a continued media coverage via advertising and organizing celebrity events, creating wide public support. Converse strategies were used in Bangladesh and Peru. In particular, in Bangladesh, resistance was deemed too strong to face head-on and a number of **work-around approaches** were pursued. This had the advantage of letting the programme function successfully for decades. However, it had the disadvantage of locking the programme into one way of operating, making it difficult to introduce new technologies. While the CLAS programme in Peru initially also took the strategy of **not publicizing** for fear of adverse reactions from the medical profession, it eventually took the legal political route to consolidate policy change. In this latter process, compromises were made, giving in to the unions and thus reducing community control over the CLAS health facilities. The Vanuatu programme included from the beginning **political and legislative work** as one of the prongs of its strategy; however, it faced challenges due to incompatibility of the donor's funding time frame with the length of the political processes as well as political instability.

Two of the case programmes, the MVP in Kenya and IMAGE in South Africa, used research as their main strategy to back and encourage policy change. The idea was to show that investing in changing the social determinants of health would have lasting positive effects on health and other social outcomes. For the CLAS programme in Peru, research and evaluations were important strategy elements to instigate change. However, while the evaluations convinced donors and other funding agencies, they did not convince the politicians. It seems a much more forceful approach to combine **research and the media** as was done in China. Here, research fed into the debate through the media, creating a public demand for change that prompted politicians to support the Dedicated Migrant Delivery centre initiative when this was proposed.

The cases describe a number of **operational or strategic alliances** by which the programmes enhanced their power to change policy. However, the alliances of the Five-a-Day programme in Chile with commercial fruit exporters as well as other commercial partners were not without problems, as the interests of the various parties coincided only partially. In Peru, alliances with an international NGO devoted to PHC and community development and a local health advocacy group greatly facilitated the final push during the legislative process in the Congress. A more strategic or legitimizing role of alliance partners was found in Bangladesh, where a group of intellectual and social elite young doctors provided important policy support during the first years of the menstrual regulation programme. The First Nations suicide prevention programme in Canada gained more clout and legitimacy vis-à-vis government agencies through forming an alliance with the University of Victoria.

In the Reach Every Ward (REW) programme in

Nigeria, the policy had been to support the worst-off local government areas to reach at least the same immunization coverage levels as the average. However, during implementation, this policy was twisted because the strongest diverted resources for their own benefit. The programme ended up increasing instead of decreasing inequities. The two programmes that most directly addressed the operationalization of policy change were the Chinese and Indonesian *Gerbangmas* programmes that designed comprehensive incentive schemes for staff in China, and multiple sectors within communities in Indonesia. Both incentive schemes focused on achievement of outcome rather than process and output measures, thus reducing the risks of the schemes becoming perverted. Further, to reinforce the incentive scheme, the *Gerbangmas* programme also used disincentives in the form of official warnings in case of non-compliance.

In five of the cases, Bangladesh, Nigeria, Peru, Tanzania and Vanuatu, donor money played a critical role in the implementation, and **donor values and interests** became important for how policies were formulated, amended and implemented. The lead donor, who at the beginning was instrumental in formulating the policy as well as in training paramedics in uterine evacuation care in Bangladesh, later pulled out completely due to domestic antiabortion pressure and the programme was left to find an alternative donor or to close down. In Tanzania, the original national ITN policy had been distribution through social marketing and voucher schemes. However, international pressure backed by the availability of huge amounts of money through the Global Fund to fight AIDS, Tuberculosis and Malaria (Global Fund), the President's Malaria Initiative (PMI) and the World Bank changed the policy to include free distribution, possibly challenging the investments in social marketing channels and outlets, and making the programme even more donor dependent. During the short period of expansion of the CLAS programme in Peru, donor and funding agencies played a key role in steering policy through providing funds and setting conditions. However, the policy got diverted from the original concept of community empowerment towards cost-effectiveness, and subsequently the CLAS policy was not supported by the new government, which stopped further expansion.

The role of **leadership**, which constitutes formulating the policy vision and getting people on board, was visibly carried out in China and Indonesia by omnipresent individuals who interacted up and down through political and institutional hierarchies as well as in the public forum. In both cases, the reach was limited to one administrative jurisdiction. However, within these boundaries, they were able to get comprehensive and cohesive policies formulated and implemented. The drifting policy in Nigeria and the diluted policy in the case of Peru could possibly be attributed to the absence of a consistent leadership to carry the vision through to expansion in the case of Nigeria, and over time in Peru.

Introducing as well as implementing policies for reducing inequities through addressing the social determinants rely on a combination of choosing the right moment of opportunity, providing the evidence, and taking control of public perception through leadership and skilful media work. These call for values and politics more than management, administration and procedures.

Managing intersectoral processes

In all the case studies, addressing the social determinants of health meant more than providing health-care services. In most cases, it meant expanding the traditional scope of the health sector and dealing with new partners. The programmes often found that these partners had different value bases, success criteria, constraints and management cultures, which frequently made coordination and joint action challenging; at times creating conflicts. Difficulties were documented across government sectors, as in Iran, Kenya, Nigeria and Vanuatu; across the government–private sector divide in Chile, Pakistan, Peru and Tanzania; and within the private sector in Chile.

In Kenya and Vanuatu, the compartmentalized structure in which the government and donors work was found to create barriers to effective coordination and integration. In the South Africa case study, it was noted that dealing with different sectors meant dealing with staff from different backgrounds, technical skills and different views of the world. In both Kenya and South Africa, significant differences between approaches to risk-taking were found between micro-finance and public health partners. In Pakistan, giving money to village women did not fit in with any format that the civil servants could handle. Finally, lack of adequate human and financial resources prevented the district education sector in Kenya from participating actively, despite appreciation of both the goals and the means. The issues emerging from the case studies with respect to managing intersectoral processes

can be grouped into *coordination, incentives, role of NGOs*, and *leadership*.

The Chile case study suggests a common conceptual framework as the indispensable starting point for effective **coordination**, something which is echoed by several of the other programmes. The most comprehensive of such common frameworks was probably the one provided by the case from Indonesia. Here, everything was predefined in policies and guidelines, providing the foundation for the "common vehicle". Such a framework would not only involve improved understanding of the structural interventions, as proposed by the Kenya study, but also an understanding of one's own and others' roles, interests, constraints and need to change. Only then can the necessary mutually supportive learning and action commence, as suggested by the Pakistan and Iran studies.

While communities can understand and appreciate the linkages between interventions, decision-making processes at the community level rarely follow the compartmentalized structure of government and donor programming, as noted in the Kenya case study. Different approaches were tried by the programmes. Over time, the IMAGE project in South Africa shifted from what they call a "linked" model, i.e. integration at the point of delivery to the clients, towards a partial "parallel" model during scale-up, where attempts were made to harmonize approaches and interventions at a senior management level. Eventually, the project returned to the "linked" model. In Canada and Vanuatu, traditional chiefs played controlling roles in anchoring multisectoral action within their communities. In Indonesia and Peru, the anchoring and controlling points for the purpose were created and officials elected. Reportedly, these approaches worked well. There were more mixed experiences with top-level coordination mechanisms. In Pakistan, clear choices had been made in the original programme design. However, when it came to implementation, there was no functioning forum to articulate and explain these choices, and to integrate the interest of the different sectors at district, provincial or federal level. Similarly, the oversight and coordinating committees in Bangladesh and Iran rarely met and had little impact on programme coordination.

It might be tempting to suggest that interventions dealing with a relevant set of social determinants be grouped within a single organizational entity to overcome the difficulties of coordination. For example, the three interlinked determinants – nutrition, education and gender – were all seen as falling within the mandate of the Ministry of Women and Development (MoWD) in Pakistan when this ministry initiated the Tawana project. However, as large-scale operations began, more sectors and line ministries soon became involved and the MoWD was ill-equipped to undertake the required coordination. The experiences at the operational level from the IMAGE project in South Africa indicate that, despite the difficulties in coordination, it is probably more effective to develop institutional partnerships than to attempt integrating the interventions into a single institution.

Effective collaboration requires that all involved sectors have a sense of ownership. It is questionable if health indicators are sufficient to maintain engagement of other sectors when external resources are no longer available, as was found when rolling out the nutrition programme in Iran. In general, the case studies found that, for meaningful participation, at the core of the collaboration there must be some **incentives** for each collaborator to engage whole-heartedly. These incentives took many forms and shapes in the programmes studied, ranging from perceptions by the private fruit exporters in Chile of positive and negative externalities to fear of being reprimanded for failure to achieve targets in Indonesia.

A key condition for successful collaboration was the realization by the partners that complementarity and dependency of action were required to achieve their sector-specific outcomes. This was the case in the MVP in Kenya, the community project in Vanuatu and the IMAGE project in South Africa. The collaborators found that simultaneous coordinated action in multiple sectors had a synergistic effect, and the returns were greater than if they had gone alone, whether this was measured in terms of poverty reduction, health, alcohol use or loan repayment.

The most elaborate example of an incentive scheme to drive multisectoral collaboration is described in the study of the *Gerbangmas* programme in Indonesia. Here, based on the concept that health is the outcome of all sectors, the health goals were transformed into the interest of multiple sectors through 21 indicators (14 for human development, one for economy and six for household environment). After assessments in the individual communities, targets were set for each of these indicators, and sectors were held accountable for delivering their part. Further, the local government provided a flexible economic stimulant through the common community vehicle to be matched by the community towards achieving the 21 targets. One indication that the sectors saw benefits of the participation was that they also

channelled their own funds through the common vehicle rather than maintaining vertical mechanisms.

In several of the government programmes described by the case studies, **nongovernmental organizations** (NGOs) played key roles as intermediaries between different actors, as in Vanuatu, Tanzania and Pakistan, or as proxy government agents, as in Indonesia and Bangladesh. This was found to provide several advantages, including bypassing red tape, forming a bridge between government sectors and bureaucracy and the community, providing linkages between the government and the private commercial sector, and providing controversial services.

The case studies showed that the advantages of using NGOs for multisectoral collaboration were grounded in key characteristics of NGOs. They were not bound by formal government hierarchies and explicit policies and rules; had independent sources of funding; were trusted by the community or the private sector where the government was not, and were accountable to their constituencies for making a change and showing tangible results. However, while the studies showed several benefits, they also indicated some potential pitfalls. Despite being fully funded by the government, the Tawana project's operational dependency on its NGO partners prevented uptake, integration and ownership by government sectors. The civil services did not understand what it required to work with the community and the NGOs did not understand how the government worked and what it required, for example, in terms of audit trails. This was the Achilles heel that eventually brought the project down. In Vanuatu, when independent funding ceased for the intermediary role, so did multisectoral engagement and collaboration. The arm's length distance between the policy-level structures of the government and service provision through the NGO sector in Bangladesh proved an obstacle to updating policies to reflect new technologies, after decades of effective collaboration.

About half of the case studies addressed the **role of leadership** to formulate and carry the vision. Leadership was required to get sectors and organizations on board to integrate and internalize the goals and objectives within the respective structures and action plans of these sectors. The role of leadership played out differently in the different cases. The cases in China, Indonesia and Vanuatu experienced support and commitment generated by an individual with exceptional charisma, through personal insight, abilities and skills. The vision for multisectoral action during the pilot projects in Kenya, South Africa and Pakistan were provided by university-based research groups and, in the case of Iran, by an international organization. However, when it came to scaling up the projects, those who were expected to provide the multisectoral leadership did not do so, e.g. the MoWD and local governments in Pakistan and Governors-general in Iran. The torch of vision had not been effectively passed on to them. The torch was successfully passed on in Indonesia from the head of the District Health Office to the *Bupati* (the political head of the District), who made it his own vision and had the power to orchestrate multisectoral action.

The vision for multisectoral action on the social determinants of health needs to germinate within the health sector, including identification of required actions by and potential benefits to other sectoral actors. Only then is the vision ripe for convincing and passing on to someone who can navigate the core agendas of other sectors.

Adjusting design

The case programmes studied have, over the years, undergone several changes. However, many of these changes have been in the form of "cutting a heel and clipping a toe", and meant compromising and giving in to various external pressures or specific interests of stakeholders. As a result, objectives, targets and approaches drifted. Only a few of the changes were made to align features of the programme with the response, as in cases where the desired results were not achieved, or because of wrong or changing assumptions. This is remarkable, as all the programmes faced challenges to implementation; significant resources and efforts went into all of them, and several of them used logical framework approaches for their planning. The programmes in Chile, China, Iran, Nigeria, Pakistan, Peru and Vanuatu, in one way or the other, fell short of meeting the expectations, which became obvious during their implementation. Yet, as documented in the case studies, the appropriate adjustments to the design were not made.

Of the programmes that developed beyond the pilot phase, corrective adjustments to the design were made during implementation only in Bangladesh, Canada and Tanzania. In Bangladesh, the weight of programme leadership moved from the government to the NGO sector in order to counter anti-abortion pressures on the government from donors and religious conservatives. In Tanzania, an elaborate monitoring and research system detected that the ITNs were not reaching the populations

as intended, and inequities in access to and use of ITNs for malaria prevention increased rather than decreased. As a result of these findings, the design of the programme was adjusted to include new strategies for ITN distribution, improved voucher systems and new approaches to health promotion and communication. The suicide prevention programme in Canada faced multiple challenges in relation to its heterogeneous and geographically dispersed target populations, lack of official recognition and difficulties in funding. The programme remained focused on youth suicide prevention through addressing the social determinants but developed into an open design with emphasis on leadership and community development, while increasingly spending managerial resources on pursuing opportunities for partnerships and funding.

Programmes that did not adjust their designs despite not evolving as anticipated had the following common denominators: ill-defined measures and/or unrealistic targets for what was to be achieved; lack of timely monitoring and appropriate research systems; and absence of appropriate mechanisms or functioning forums for making decisions to adjust the design. For several of these programmes, the data providing evidence of the need for design adjustments were collected and analysed only as part of the work done for the case studies. This meant that even in cases where decision-making bodies existed, these did not have the information to realize the need for adjusting programme design. The absence of appropriately defined measures and targets, timely information and effective decision-making bodies is particularly critical in large programmes because the intended and unintended effects will show up in different sectors, often only after a long time. Further, the vastness and multifaceted nature of these programmes often cause long lead times in reacting to design changes.

Ensuring sustainability

The question of sustainability is particularly important for programmes that seek to influence the social determinants of health, as the results will materialize only after continued efforts over a long time, and after new ways of thinking, planning and allocating resources have been fully embedded in all the relevant areas, bodies and policies. However, sustainability has many faces, including: the observation made in the MVP case study from Kenya that external government and donor support to sustain the various achievements attained in the health, education and other social sectors would need to continue; the finding by the Tanzania programme that the world has adopted a high-risk approach towards malaria control, requiring sustained resources far beyond the financial means of developing countries for the strategy of universal coverage of ITNs; and, as suggested in the Vanuatu study, that the time horizons for dealing with the social determinants of health are much longer than the planning time frames of both donors and governments. The findings of the case studies under the theme "sustainability" can be grouped under five broad headings: *financial, political, institutional* and *impact sustainability*; and the *use of short-cuts*.

The concept of **financial sustainability** differs, depending on the perspective applied. In the South Africa case, for the microfinance partner, it meant a drive to reduce reliance on donor funds. Conversely, in the public health sector part of the programmes, as in South Africa, Kenya and Nigeria, virtually all interventions required some form of subsidy or external support. The question of financial sustainability, therefore, meant securing a continuous flow of resources, regardless of whether the source was national or international. Two of the cases studied experienced impacts due to shifts in direction of donor resource flows from factors unrelated to the programmes but these had a significant impact on their financing and, to some extent, design. In Tanzania, the bilateral donors who originally provided the majority of the funding for the ITN activities shifted their contributions to basket funding and general budget support. When the Global Fund and the PMI stepped in on a large scale, they had a different philosophy requiring a change of strategy. Thus, while the overall resources increased, so did the cost of sustaining the programme. The study suggests that the costs are now far beyond the government's capabilities. The menstrual regulation programme in Bangladesh experienced challenges twice due to donors redirecting their resource flows. First, when the original donor decided to stop funding due to domestic pressures and policies; second, when the new donor decided to provide funding through a sectorwide approach and, due to the official government "arms-length policy", funds could not be allocated from within government mechanisms.

Expanding the scope of interventions and improving equity is easiest to do when more resources become available. The CLAS model in Peru provides an example where the combination of community-controlled health-care provision and social insurance financing through the demand side formed an efficient mechanism to increase the equity, quality and quantity of services

in a sustainable manner. However, more resources are not always required to pursue social determinants approaches. For the dedicated migrant delivery services in China, reprioritization within the health services was done to finance the reduction in fees and improve service quality. However, internally as well, there were examples of dependency on resource flows that did not follow the usual government channels. For example, removal of the non-sectoral stimulant resources that provided the mortar between the sectoral bricks in the community programme in Indonesia would be detrimental to the programme. The risk of such removal is tightly linked to the **political sustainability** of the programme.

The end of office and subsequent change of the *Bupati*, the seniormost politician in the district, would possibly mean potential loss of political support, policy change and erosion of the financial foundation of the community programme in Indonesia. Several strategies were pursued in order to increase the chances of sustaining the programme through the political transition, including making an official book, incorporating the programme in the accountability (hand-over) report and formulating a district regulation to be ratified by the district legislature. While the analysis of the Indonesian programme only covered the terms of office of a single political head, the CLAS case study in Peru covered several government periods, some with supportive political leadership and some with governments directly opposing the programme. While it survived long enough to be become covered by a Congressional law, political pressure from medical associations and health workers' unions removed the core tenet of community ownership and control over staff. In Nigeria and Vanuatu as well, the programmes experienced the effect of political instability resulting in a lack of action, prolongation of processes and unwillingness or inability to take on critical processes of reallocation of resources to address inequities, such as in access to appropriate immunization services.

The menstrual regulation programme in Bangladesh provided politically and religiously controversial pregnancy termination services to disadvantaged women. It remained in a constant state of unstable balance over its forty years of existence, from being fully integrated into the government services in the 1970s through a period of distancing of activities from the State during the 1980s and 1990s, with direct marginalization from 1998. The programme survived through this flux by resting on three pillars: government–NGO–donor; when support from one lessened, the support of another was strengthened.

The fact that, almost since its inception, the programme has remained at odds with the key political establishment hindered its **institutionalization**.

The conclusion from the Tawana case study in Pakistan was that sustaining a large-scale and nationwide programme that addressed social norms hinges on government buy-in and complementary action by the government and nongovernment actors. Further, as suggested by the Vanuatu case study, the responsibility must be formally anchored within the Ministry of Health or equivalent institution as part of the shift within the health sector's core mandate toward the social determinants of health. The impetus and support for a shift can come from outside, such as from donors. But unless there is an effective handing over of ownership and responsibility to the government, programmes and achievements are unlikely to be sustained or scaled up, as was seen in the cases of Iran, Nigeria and Vanuatu. In all three cases, the programmes were seen as largely donor owned.

The Canada case study proposes that institutional sustainability of public health programmes that address the social determinants of health needs a functioning interface between an informal and flexible community-based approach and the officialdom. Steering from the top must be combined with a demand from below. At the same time, programmes should be solidly linked to the local administration rather than to political agendas in order to ensure policy coherence and sustainability as found in the REW programme in Nigeria. The lessons from the Tawana case study imply that NGOs could have a critical role to play at the interface between the administration and the community in challenging and educating both. This role could be more important for sustainability than participating directly in the implementation.

Elaborate examples of institutionalization at the district level were provided in the case studies from Indonesia and China. In the latter case, this was achieved through a values-based complete overhaul of staff profiles, training procedures, incentives, monitoring systems and performance criteria. However, both cases also illustrate the potential challenges in replicating this for wider geographical application.

One of the most important threats to the sustainability of Tawana was probably that the programme never came to grips with whether it was an NGO project implemented with government money or a government programme implemented by NGOs. Instead of addressing the challenges to institutionalization, **instant short-cuts** were sought, creating friction and distrust between the civil servants and the NGO implementers. As a result, the focus shifted from outcome to process, and the rural village women consequently lost out.

Two examples of short-cuts were found in relation to the MVP in Kenya. The first was the instant short-cut to attract qualified staff by offering a higher-than-standard government pay. This resolved an acute capacity problem, but created a sustainability problem with respect to integrating staff into the health-care system as government employees. The second short-cut was related to the question of whether even the seemingly broad and comprehensive investment in agriculture was unsustainable. The case study suggests that for agriculture to become a sustainable vehicle for rural economic and social growth, investments in physical and logistical infrastructure need to be made together with ensuring economically viable sizes of land plots. Thus, sustainability would require structural interventions at the level of socioeconomic context and position, and in differential exposure in the form of basic infrastructure. This finding was echoed by that of the REW in Nigeria; while it is possible to drive specific average and equity targets, short-cut driven approaches increase the risk of collapse, and could even make the situation worse than before.

The mass distribution of 20 million free nets in Tanzania would, according to estimates referred to in the case study, reduce the commercial sector by 70%, push retailers out of the market, and undermine the infrastructure of wholesale distribution and retail commercial net sales that had been carefully set up over several years. Further, free net distribution would also reduce the willingness of people to purchase ITNs. This brings up the issue of **impact sustainability** or, as stated in the Canadian case study, "*The proof of sustainability is in the interventions and impact.*" Failed malaria control programmes lead to higher mortality when malaria resurfaces, because (partial) immunity in the population has disappeared. This brings in a moral obligation to sustain the high level of funding to continue not only the short-cut measure, i.e. provision of free nets, but also to support a continuous sensitization, repeating the same messages over and over again. ITN promotion cannot be a one-off campaign undertaken only during the distribution of nets; it should be a continuing effort.

Public health approaches to addressing equity and the social determinants of health require a continuous flow of new or redirected resources and they cannot, in a narrow sense, become financially self-sustaining. Interventions are required in the socioeconomic context and at the position level to institutionalize them legally and managerially in the general public policy and administration. Finally, the findings from Canada, Pakistan and Vanuatu suggest that investing in and empowering the people might have a high pay-back in terms of sustainability. "*Had the programme continued, it could have built a self-sustaining social base for greater participation of women for bettering the conditions of the poor and the disadvantaged*" (Tawana case study).

15.4 Conclusion

The case studies presented in this book represent a wealth of experiences from very different settings. The case programmes were concerned with different public health problems and took different approaches. Some of the programmes were small and in a pilot stage, others were large and complex, and some were more comprehensive in their approaches than others. However, common to all of them was that they addressed the social determinants of health and tried to redress the inequities in health outcomes rather than simply providing health-care services in the usual way.

There are many lessons to be learned from each of these case studies, and the major common lessons have been synthesized in this chapter. Three key messages might emerge if one were to step back and reflect on what, in hindsight, could have been done better were the case programmes to be started today with the combined lessons learned from the other case studies.

Even before thinking about interventions, gather the evidence and establish the baseline. These are needed to guide programme development and, equally important, to support the public and institutional information-sharing and popularization that will be paramount for any progress in addressing the social determinants of health. Once the programme gets started, systematic monitoring and repeated evaluations are indispensable for continuously adjusting and refining the programme design, as well as for keeping politicians and the public abreast with the progress and challenges.

Reducing inequities through influencing the social determinants is a values-based endeavour that needs careful mapping of perspectives and vested interests of key actors. It also calls for a change in the incentives and the attitudes of staff across multiple sectors and organizations at the local and facility levels. However, it is important to realize that, in the long haul, the final battle for equity takes place in the public space. Through the media and intelligent use of the evidence and partners, influencing the public debate is within the reach of the health sector.

Piloting and full-scale programming are two very different stages and at least three phases should be considered in scaling up. *Phase one* is proof of principle, where the interventions are tested and refined in a controlled environment. *Phase two* is testing the scalability of the programme with particular focus on the drivers of expansion and how to transfer the values torch. *Phase three* is roll-out with strong monitoring of the processes, managerial behaviours and practices, as well as outputs. All three phases must be accompanied by public information and a research component to measure and debate intended and unintended impacts, as well as causality between intervention and effect.

While all of the cases studied faced significant challenges in their implementation, and several of them today are very different from what was aimed for when they were initiated, the lessons learned point to the ways forward and provide hope for a future with a more equitable distribution of health in the population.

References

1. Blas E (2005). 1990–2000: *A decade of health sector reform in developing countries*. Göteborg, Nordic School of Public Health.

2. Blas E and Sivasankara Kurup A (2010). *Equity, social determinants and public health programmes*. Geneva, World Health Organization.

3. Blankenship KM, Bray SJ, Merson MH (2000). Structural interventions in public health. *AIDS*, 14 (Suppl 1):S11–S21.

4. Commission on Social Determinants of Health (2008). *Closing the gap in a generation: health equity through action on the social determinants of health. Final report of the Commission on Social Determinants of Health*. Geneva, World Health Organization.

5. Reich MR (1995). The politics of health sector reform in developing countries – 3 cases of pharmaceutical policy. *Health Policy*, 32 (1–)3:47–77.

6. Tanahashi T (1978). Health service coverage and its evaluation. *Bulletin of the World Health Organization*, 56:295–303.

7. Tugwell P, De SD, Hawker G, Robinson V (2006). Applying clinical epidemiological methods to health equity: the equity effectiveness loop. *British Medical Journal*, 332(7537):358–361.

8. van Balen H (2004). Disease control in primary health care: a historical perspective. *Tropical Medicine and International Health*, 9.6:A22–A26.

9. WHO (2000). *The world health report – health systems: improving performance.* Geneva, World Health Organization.

10. WHO (2008). *The world health report – primary health care.* Geneva, World Health Organization.

Annexes to Chapter 14

Annex 1
Programme logic framework mapping PAHP's original aims and objectives against the implementation processes on the ground in Vanuatu, and their impact and outcomes

Annex 2
Intervention scheme template, Vanuatu

Annex 1

204

Programme logic framework mapping PAHP's original aims and objectives against the implementation processes on the ground in Vanuatu, and their impact and outcomes

Objective	Process 1 – multicountry design	Process 2 – contextual adjustment in Vanuat
Objective 1. National NCD policy implementation – healthy public policies are implemented to address priority NCD risk factors in young people.	• Planning processes strengthened at the national level to develop multisectoral support for healthy public policies for the selected NCD risk factors of tobacco and alcohol use • NCD policy response plans for priority risk factors affecting young people implemented • Revised national policy, action plan or draft legislation documented • Mobilization of community and NGO support and advocacy for required reforms	• Response plans to address prioritized gaps in improving public policy agreed upon an documented • Current NCD public policy framework reviewed • Initial meetings held with government departments outside of health
Objective 2. Community-based interventions – young people between 10 and 19 years of age adopt and maintain healthy behaviours to reduce the risk of developing NCDs.	• Urban community-based capacity to coordinate and implement selected interventions established • Programme of modelling of positive behaviours for young people within the family and in the community • Healthy alternative activities for young people available within the urban community • Advocacy networks for young people established and functioning effectively • Influential young people within communities provide leadership and promote healthy behaviour • Small grant funds rationally and effectively applied, grant fund application and award system documented and operational	• NGOs contracted and project coordinators appointed • Cross-sectoral consultations held • Programmes developed with regard to fac such as young peoples' level of risk factor knowledge, decision-making skills, and pe pressure and self-esteem issues • Youth and community involved in designir and implementing initiatives • MOH certifies that programmes implemer align with guidelines developed • Emphasis on youth leadership • Build relationships with community leaders • Build relationships with existing youth gro

Programme impacts	Programme outcomes	Health outcomes
National NCD committee established, with subgroups, comprising good multisectoral representation Impact on tobacco and customs and excise legislation Draft legislation developed "Walk for life" Wednesday afternoon activity	• NCD strategy developed and supported by Cabinet/Government • Legislative change concerning tobacco, customs and excise	
Young people effectively engaged at the community level to plan, coordinate and implement appropriately designed and effective programmes Communitywide events developed by the youth themselves to promote their status in the community and raise awareness of NCD issues Large numbers of youth involved in events Raise profile of sport as an activity for young people Cross-sectoral engagement in community-level initiatives Community leaders engage with youth initiatives Conforming grant fund applications received, and amounts and purposes approved Advocacy networks commenced and ongoing Development of youth leadership Increase in visibility of influential young people providing leadership Training events offered and attended by both genders Engagement with large numbers of existing youth groups	• Builds self-esteem, sense of responsibility, and sense of belonging • Small grants increase access to programme • Provides a positive contribution to community life • Raises the profile of drop-out youth • Provides a direct link to community leaders • Lack of structural change in the community • Youth forum (one-off) provides a voice for drop-out youth • Change in perception of community leaders concerning abilities of young people	• Changes in knowledge, attitudes and behaviours arising from urban-based community interventions targeting young people individually, young people in the family and young people in the community compared with baseline assessments • Number and type of advocacy networks for young people operating effectively

Public health condition(s) addressed: Noncommunicable diseases
Population size covered by the programme: N/A – Under 19 population in Vanuatu is around 108 000, or 52% of the populatio
Programme started (year): 1999 (2002)
Programme ongoing (Y/N): Y in principle, N in practice
Is documentation of effect on health outcome available (Y/N): N
Has programme been externally evaluated (Y/N): Y
Programme implemented by: Foundation of the Peoples of the South Pacific, Vanuatu
Programme funded by: AusAID

LEVEL	SOCIAL DETERMINANTS/PATHWAY	AVAILABILITY INTERVENTIONS Are based on the assumption that health problems result from the lack of or, conversely, the excessive availability of products, tools, behaviours, or settings and, as such, seek to influence their availability
Context and position	• Lack of awareness of, capacity to address, and action to be taken to address NCD risk factors at senior levels • Lack of policy activity and legislation regarding NCD risk factors • No "whole Government" approach to NCDs • Limited capacity at MoH level to address NCD risk factors through the social determinants of health (some health education activity) • Limited capacity within MoH to develop intersectoral "healthy public policy" approach to NCD risk factors • Structural obstacles to "drop-out" youth in Vanuatu society leading to a lack of opportunity (e.g. education and employment) • Lack of action on structural obstacles facing "drop-out" youth • "Drop-out" youth not empowered to make changes at senior levels in Vanuatu society	• Development of National NCD Strategy (but limited implementation, and no reference to disadvantaged youth) • National NCD Committee established to enhance healthy public policy and enact supporting legislation • Inclusion in NCD Committee of stakeholders invited from a range of relevant sectors and backgrounds • Act as facilitator for intersectoral engagement on NCD issues • Limited mobilization of policy support for required policy reform • Updated legislation covering sale of tobacco products to young people • Submission of updated legislation on liquor licensing • Increased taxes on alcohol and tobacco • Engagement at policy level with NCD risk factors, but limited action beyond "Wednesday afternoon off" for civil servants • Limited actions resulting from engagement of government departments regarding NCDs

ACCEPTABILITY INTERVENTIONS
Recognize that the health of a society and of its members is partially determined by its values, cultures and beliefs, or of sugroups within it and, as such, seek to alter the social norms

ACCESSIBILITY INTERVENTIONS
Acknowledge that health is a function of social, economic and political power and resources and, as such, manipulate power and resources to promote public health

- Mobilization of community and NGO support for required policy reform

- Limited mobilization of policy support for required policy reform

- Development of National NCD Strategy (but limited implementation, and no reference to disadvantaged youth)

- Behaviour change evident at government level through Wednesday afternoon physical activity for civil servants

- Inclusion in NCD committee of stakeholders invited from a range of relevant sectors and backgrounds

- Limited increase in MOH's capacity for healthy public policy development

- National NCD Committee established

- Raised profile of "drop-out" youth at senior levels of Vanuatu society

- No focus on structural obstacles facing youth or "drop-out" youth in legislative reform

- Raised awareness of health and NCD risk factors, and impacts at senior levels of government and across sectors and communities, resulting in limited engagement

- National NCD Committee established to enhance healthy public policy and enact supporting legislation

- Good cross-sectoral representation on National NCD Committee

- Development of National NCD Strategy (but limited implementation, and no reference to disadvantaged youth)

- Provided "voice" for young people at government level through Youth Forum

- Raised profile of "drop-out" youth at community leader level

- No focus on structural obstacles facing youth or "drop-out" youth in legislative reform

- Limited actions resulting from engagement of government departments regarding NCDs

- Limited approach to build capacity of entire government

- Initial approaches made to MoH to engage system in NCD prevention

continued...

LEVEL	SOCIAL DETERMINANTS/PATHWAY	AVAILABILITY INTERVENTIONS Are based on the assumption that health problems result from the lack of or, conversely, the excessive availability of products, tools, behaviours, or setting and, as such, seek to influence their availability
Exposure	• Social environments of ni-Vanuatu youth contribute to overuse and abuse of alcohol and tobacco • Lack of opportunity for secondary or vocational education • Lack of employment • Limited links between young people and community leaders • Lack of awareness of NCD risk factors in community and other intersectoral partners (NGO donors, NGOs and government representatives and departments) at community level • Lack of appreciation for positive potential of young "drop-outs" • Lack of opportunity for constructive activities at community level	• Programmes available to young people to provide acceptable and positive opportunities for support socially and financially • Updated legislation covering sale of tobacco products to young people • Submission of updated legislation on liquor licensing • Increased taxes on alcohol and tobacco • Small grants scheme provided constructive opportunities and income for young people within their community • Social marketing and awareness-raising at community level through the use of media • Engagement with community leaders and intersectoral partners (donors, NGOs and government representatives and departments) at community level on NCD risk factors and the youth • Raised the profile of gender equity
Vulnerability	• Low status of "drop-out" youth in community and society • Poverty among and exclusion of "drop-out" youth • Illiteracy, lack of education and associated lack of knowledge and skills • Lack of opportunity for constructive activities • Lack of self-esteem • Limited sense of responsibility • Low frequency of contact with between "drop-out" youth and community leaders, health and other professionals	• Mobilization of advocacy networks set up and available for young people • Training offered by health and other professionals to develop skills • Limited enforcement of legislative changes • Engagement with other sectors to raise profile of the youth • Unclear whether "within" group disadvantage existed or if it was addressed • Raised profile of gender equity • Built self-esteem, sense of responsibility and sense of belonging

ACCEPTABILITY INTERVENTIONS
Recognize that the health of a society and of its members is partially determined by its values, cultures and beliefs, or of sugroups within it and, as such, seek to alter the social norms

ACCESSIBILITY INTERVENTIONS
Acknowledge that health is a function of social, economic and political power and resources and, as such, manipulate power and resources to promote public health

- Raised profile of "drop-out" youth at community level
- Communitywide events developed by the youth themselves to promote their status in the community and raise awareness of NCD risk factors
- Limited capacity building of MoH to engage with young people on NCD risk factors
- Links made between "drop-out" youth and community leaders
- Small grants scheme provided constructive opportunities and income for young people within their community
- Community leaders mobilized to support young people's involvement in programme activities
- Raised the profile of healthy choices among young people and their communities
- Links to existing youth groups established
- Encouraged "responsible" behaviour change in groups of young people
- Good "fit" of programme to cultural context, but limited actions to address the structural obstacles facing young people

- Engagement with community leaders and intersectoral partners (donors, NGOs and government representatives and departments, and private sector) at community level on NCD risk factors and youth
- Links made between "drop-out" youth and community leaders
- Community leaders mobilized to support young people's involvement in programme activities
- Provided a "voice" for young people at government level through Youth Forum
- Limited structural changes at community level
- Small grants scheme provided income
- Development of youth leaders
- Limited capacity of MoH or NGO sector to move beyond health education approaches, although some evidence that NGOs are addressing the structural determinants of health
- Initial approaches made to incorporate NCD prevention in MoH staff workplans

- Young champions as role models for healthy lifestyle behaviour
- Development of youth leaders provided opportunities for the leaders and role models for others
- Communitywide events developed by the youth themselves to promote their status in the community
- Limited capacity built of MoH or NGO sector to engage with youth beyond health education approaches, although some evidence that NGOs are addressing the structural determinants of health
- Provided opportunities for constructive group behaviour
- Built self-esteem, sense of responsibility and belonging
- Links to existing youth groups established
- Encouraged "responsible" behaviour change in groups of young people

- Small grants scheme provided opportunities for youth to undertake acceptable income-generating activities, designed by the youth themselves, supported by communities
- Unclear whether "within" group disadvantage or vulnerability existed or if it was addressed
- Youth involved in the planning and design of communitywide events
- Youth forum concept developed and run once, as opportunity for "drop-out" youth to voice their concerns